Math Calculations

for Pharmacy Technicians, a Worktext

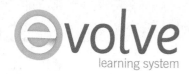
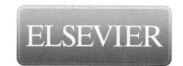
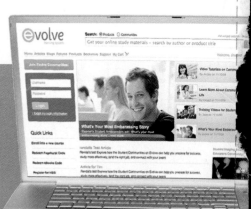
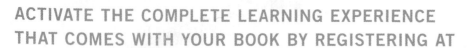

Math
Calculations

for Pharmacy Technicians

A Worktext

Robert M. Fulcher
BS Chem, BSPh, RPh

Pharmacist
CVS Pharmacy
Waynesboro, Georgia

Eugenia M. Fulcher
BSN, MEd, EdD, RN,
CMA (AAMA)

Allied Health Instructor

SECOND EDITION

ELSEVIER

3251 Riverport Lane
St. Louis, Missouri 63043

MATH CALCULATIONS FOR PHARMACY TECHNICIANS: ISBN: 978-1-4377-2366-3
A WORKTEXT, SECOND EDITION

Notices

Knowledge and best practice in this field are constantly changing. As new research and experience broaden our understanding, changes in research methods, professional practices, or medical treatment may become necessary.

Practitioners and researchers must always rely on their own experience and knowledge in evaluating and using any information, methods, compounds, or experiments described herein. In using such information or methods they should be mindful of their own safety and the safety of others, including parties for whom they have a professional responsibility.

With respect to any drug or pharmaceutical products identified, readers are advised to check the most current information provided (i) on procedures featured or (ii) by the manufacturer of each product to be administered, to verify the recommended dose or formula, the method and duration of administration, and contraindications. It is the responsibility of practitioners, relying on their own experience and knowledge of their patients, to make diagnoses, to determine dosages and the best treatment for each individual patient, and to take all appropriate safety precautions.

To the fullest extent of the law, neither the Publisher nor the authors, contributors, or editors, assume any liability for any injury and/or damage to persons or property as a matter of products liability, negligence or otherwise, or from any use or operation of any methods, products, instructions, or ideas contained in the material herein.

Library of Congress Cataloging-in-Publication Data

Fulcher, Robert M.
  Math calculations for pharmacy technicians: a worktext / Robert M. Fulcher,
Eugenia M. Fulcher.—2nd ed.
    p. ; cm.
  Includes bibliographical references and index.
  ISBN 978-1-4377-2366-3 (pbk. : alk. paper)
  I. Fulcher, Eugenia M. II. Title.
  [DNLM: 1. Pharmaceutical Preparations—administration & dosage—Problems and Exercises. 2. Mathematics—Problems and Exercises. QV 18.2]
  LC classification not assigned
  615.1′401513—dc23

                          2011053249

Publishing Director: Andrew Allen
Content Manager: Ellen Wurm-Cutter
Content Developmental Specialist: Kelly Brinkman
Publishing Services Manager: Catherine Jackson
Senior Project Manager: Mary Pohlman
Design Direction: Karen Pauls

Printed in Canada

Last digit is the print number: 9 8 7 6 5 4 3

To our parents, Robert M. and Lucy F. Fulcher and Harold L. and Rosabel L. Mills, we give thanks for our genetic and educational backgrounds in all areas but especially in the math field. Their diligence to lovingly provide for us and give us roots and wings, love, and allow personal growth, ensured that we are who we are today with the abilities that we have. We only wish that they could enjoy this publication with us. We know they would be proud as both of our mothers were educators.

To our sons, Lee and Gene Fulcher, we wish for you the very best in the remainder of your lives. You are wonderful children and we are proud of your accomplishments. Lee, your inclusion of your business background in this text only strengthens the educational materials. Thanks.

To our grandchildren, Mac and Allie Fulcher, may your lives always be as fun and fruitful as ours have been and are. You are the apples of our eyes and we love both of you dearly. We wish you the best throughout your lives. May you grow into wonderful adults who know the firm foundation provided by our families.

All of you are so special in making us who we are, and we love you and are proud of your accomplishments.

To the students who will use this text, we wish you the best in your chosen careers. May you have a long professional life in the field of pharmacy or other health care fields. We have enjoyed our many years in the medical field and we wish you the best in the future.

Contributors and Reviewers

CONTRIBUTOR

John L. Fulcher, BBA, CPA
John L. Fulcher, CPA, LLC
Waynesboro, Georgia

TECHNICAL EDITOR

MaryAnne Hochadel, PharmD, BCPS
Saint Petersburg, Florida

TECHNICAL REVIEWER

Dianna M. Black, RPh, FSVHP
Veterinary Clinical Pharmacist
University of Illinois Veterinary Teaching
    Hospital;
Instructor of Pharmacy Technology
Parkland College
Champaign, Illinois

REVIEWERS

Alaric Barber, CPhT, MBA
Santa Ana, California

Karen Davis, AAHCA, CPhT
Allied Health Program Specialist
Virginia Colleges
Birmingham, Alabama

**James J. Mizner Jr., BS Pharmacy,
    MBA, RPh**
Pharmacy Technician and AHT Program
    Director
ACT College
Arlington, Virginia

**Joshua Neumiller, PharmD, CDE,
    CGP, FASCP**
Assistant Professor
Department of Pharmacotherapy
College of Pharmacy
Washington State University
Pullman, Washington

Bobbi Steelman, BS, MA, CPhT
Pharmacy Technician Program Director
Daymar Colleges Group
Bowling Green, Kentucky

Preface

In our 50-plus years in the fields of pharmacy and nursing respectively, we have realized that patient safety depends on the ability of health care professionals, especially those responsible for the distribution of medication, to calculate medication dosages and doses. Pharmacy technicians must learn this skill early in their studies and use it continuously throughout their careers. This text, that meets the guidelines prepared by the American Society of Health-System Pharmacists (ASHP) for accredited pharmacy technician programs, is intended to provide the basic—and not so basic—mathematical concepts that are applied to pharmacy.

Our goal with *Math Calculations for Pharmacy Technicians: A Worktext* is to assist pharmacy technician students and other appropriate allied health students who need this background with mastering the mathematical calculations necessary when delivering medications safely. This text provides students with the knowledge to perform calculations for dispensing or administering medications in both ambulatory care and inpatient arenas as well as basic accounting procedures used in retail and some hospital pharmacy. Although some sections of the text are more related to ambulatory care and others are more relevant to hospital settings, both are necessary for the professional pharmacy technician.

As with most mathematical texts, this book includes the traditional methods of calculating medicinal dosages and doses: ratio/proportion, dimensional analysis, and formula method. Even though we show each method, we don't expect you to use all the methods with each problem. You should complete these exercises using the method that works best for you. We have also included other unique ways of obtaining correct calculations. Ultimately, we want to help you find the method that works best for you.

The book is organized from basic mathematical calculations (fractions, percentages) to basic medication calculations to more complicated dose and dosage calculations related to prescriptions and hospital orders. Each chapter builds on the previous knowledge base to ensure that information has been gleaned and processed for use in more exacting situations. For example, reading prescriptions is presented before using the prescription to count medications for dispensing to a patient.

A new chapter on business math presents the routine accounting procedures completed in retail pharmacy on a daily, monthly, or yearly basis with some concepts such as inventory also being used in inpatient pharmacy practice. Business calculations for reimbursement of prescriptions are included for practice prior to the actual need for these concepts. The new chapter provides a brief introduction to the calculations needed for business practices in the pharmacy field, especially in a retail setting, and provides a quick look into these practices for the student who decides to go into the nonhospital pharmacy option. It provides the basic skills for use in a community pharmacy. Inventory control and calculations for reimbursement for medications may be found in all areas of pharmacy and the basic business math concepts are needed to keep the pharmacy efficient.

Because adequate practice is so important, the text includes over 1300 practice problems that cover a wide range of concepts. The concepts of pharmaceutical mathematics build with each chapter, with reinforcement of previous materials throughout the text. The worktext format allows students to work at a pace that is right for them and meet the needs of the instructor and course objectives. The time devoted to each chapter may vary depending on the student's mathematical level. For this reason, the student's prior mathematical competence is tested with each chapter. Be sure that the math calculations are shown with each problem; this allows the person to find where errors occurred so these errors are not carried forward without accomplishing the needed understanding of the math principle.

ORGANIZATION OF MATERIAL

The text is divided into five sections: Section I, Introduction and Basic Math Skills, which includes an assessment of math skills needed in this field, as well as a review of basic math skills; Section II, Measurements Used in Health Care and Conversions between Measurement Systems, which explores all aspects of the different measurement systems used in the pharmacy; Section III, Medication and Prescription Orders and Their Calculations, which focuses on the calculations needed to fill common prescriptions; Section IV, Special Medication Calculations, which covers special medications, diverse populations, and less commonly used pharmaceutical calculations; and Section V for Basic Business Mathematical Calculations.

CHAPTER FEATURES

Each chapter begins with a set of learning objectives and a list of key words.

OBJECTIVES

- Read labels of powders or crystals (lyophilized) medications to determine correct diluent and correct volume necessary to reconstitute powders
- Check labels for expiration dates and storage conditions before and after reconstitution of solid medication to a liquid form
- Understand the importance of labeling reconstituted medications with date, time, and initials of person performing the medication reconstitution
- Determine the appropriate amount of diluent necessary when using a single-dose container of a powder or crystals
- Determine the appropriate amount of diluent necessary when preparing a multidose container of a powder or crystals
- Determine the appropriate dilution concentration when more than one dosage strength in the multidose container is possible, and then determine amount of diluent necessary to meet the desired concentration
- Calculate the amount of medication of a reconstituted medication to be dispensed to meet the physician's order

KEY WORDS

Diluent Agent that dilutes a substance; in pharmacology, the liquid added to a powder to change the powder to a liquid or the liquid used to dilute another liquid

Graduates Containers marked with progressive series of lines or markers, usually in the metric system, for measuring liquids or solids

Lyophilized Freeze dried

Powder displacement Amount of solute that causes displacement in the total volume of medication

Powder volume Space occupied by dry powder or freeze-dried (lyophilized or crystalline)

active ingredient related to total volume of medication following reconstitution with indicated diluent volume

Reconstitution Process of adding fluid, such as distilled water, sterile water for injection, or sterile saline, to a powdered or crystalline form of medication, making a specific liquid dosage strength

Vehicle Inert substance in which a medication is mixed for administration

---

Included in each chapter is a pretest that indicates the level of student understanding of the calculation principles to be presented.

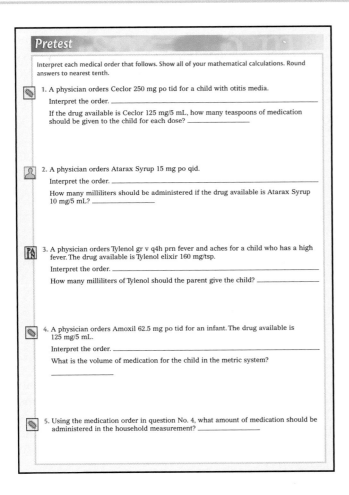

Pretest

Interpret each medical order that follows. Show all of your mathematical calculations. Round answers to nearest tenth.

1. A physician orders Ceclor 250 mg po tid for a child with otitis media.

   Interpret the order. _____

   If the drug available is Ceclor 125 mg/5 mL, how many teaspoons of medication should be given to the child for each dose? _____

2. A physician orders Atarax Syrup 15 mg po qid.

   Interpret the order. _____

   How many milliliters should be administered if the drug available is Atarax Syrup 10 mg/5 mL? _____

3. A physician orders Tylenol gr v q4h prn fever and aches for a child who has a high fever. The drug available is Tylenol elixir 160 mg/tsp.

   Interpret the order. _____

   How many milliliters of Tylenol should the parent give the child? _____

4. A physician orders Amoxil 62.5 mg po tid for an infant. The drug available is 125 mg/5 mL.

   Interpret the order. _____

   What is the volume of medication for the child in the metric system?

   _____

5. Using the medication order in question No. 4, what amount of medication should be administered in the household measurement? _____

If the materials presented are understood at a level on which to build a good comprehension of the materials, the student may find that only a review in that area is essential. Students should move onto the next chapter only if they feel comfortable with the material presented, and have demonstrated that they understand the subject matter.

Students who complete the exercises in each chapter should retake the pretest before taking the posttest at the end of the chapter to ensure that they have learned the material. A student who continues to have problems with the posttest should study the chapter again. The importance of proper calculations cannot be overemphasized, and a working knowledge of accurate calculations is essential. Just as in the pharmacy, this material may not be used every day, but students must have this knowledge base for patient safety.

The practice problems presented are designed to be used for practice in class as well as for homework. Be sure the knowledge base for each exercise is understood so any previous mistakes are not made in subsequent calculations. Understanding the bases for pharmaceutical calculations is essential in preventing errors in actual practice. If an answer looks wrong, always look at the calculation and refigure for accuracy. Ask for assistance by the professional as appropriate to ensure patients safety.

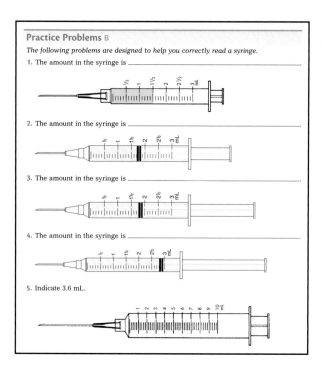

The answers to every third problem are presented in the Answer Key so students can check their individual work and also determine if they have completed the calculations correctly. If the answer is incorrect, the student has immediate feedback. Instructors should require students to show all mathematical calculations, so instructors can see the point at which mistakes occurred and can correct the concept before students advance to more difficult calculations.

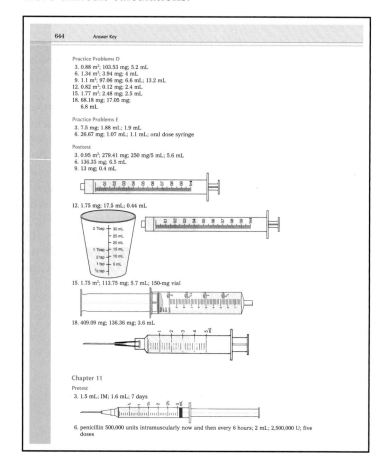

Throughout the text, when medications are used in practice problems, icons indicate the main body system affected by certain drugs. In this way, students learn the mathematical calculations and are also exposed to the medications and their uses. The following icons are included in the text:

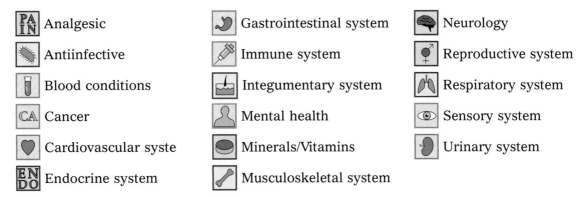

PAIN Analgesic	Gastrointestinal system	Neurology
Antiinfective	Immune system	Reproductive system
Blood conditions	Integumentary system	Respiratory system
CA Cancer	Mental health	Sensory system
Cardiovascular syste	Minerals/Vitamins	Urinary system
ENDO Endocrine system	Musculoskeletal system	

We have included **Tech Notes** boxes to highlight important concepts. Another set of boxes called **Tech Alerts** have been added to assist students in perceiving areas where comprehension is important to reduce patient care errors and to enhance patient safety.

> **TECH NOTE**
> Whole numbers are used in strengths of medications, doses of medications, inventory, and costs of medications, to give just a few examples of the need to understand this concept.

> **! TECH ALERT**
> The use of household measurement utensils provide only an approximation of a needed dose and may result in either an overdose or too little of the medication. When an approximate dose is given, therapy may be varied and may not provide the therapeutic results desired.

Key mathematical concepts and formulas used in each chapter are repeated at the end of the chapter for students who need a quick review. This feature also provides a quick reference for those working in both retail and hospital pharmacy professions.

At the end of the book, there are answers to every third question and a glossary.

ANCILLARIES

Instructor Ancillaries Available on Evolve

New and Improved TEACH Instructor's Resource: The TEACH Instructor's Resource provides instructors with customizable lesson plans and PowerPoint slides based on learning objectives. With these valuable resources, instructors will save valuable preparation time and create a learning environment that fully engages students in classroom preparation. The lesson plans are keyed to each chapter and are divided into 50-minute units. The PowerPoint slides are unique to each chapter in the text.

ExamView Test Bank: Contains over 500 questions. It also includes additional practice problems divided by chapter and answers to all of the problems in the book.

Special Chapters on TPN and Chemotherapy Calculations: New content focusing specifically on calculations needed to prepare TPN and Chemotherapy solutions.

Additional Practice Problems: Provide even more practice for students using these additional problems.

Full Answer Key: Allows instructors to easily check answers to every problem in the book.

Image Collection: Contains all the images in the text so they can be used as teaching aids.

Student Ancillaries Available on Evolve

Student Practice Problems: Enhance calculation skills with additional practice problems that correspond to every chapter in the text.

Comprehensive Posttest: This interactive posttest tests students' knowledge and mastery of all content.

SPECIAL NOTE

To comply with current The Joint Commission (TJC) and Institute for Safe Medication Practices (ISMP) recommendations, we have not included abbreviations found on the official "Do Not Use" lists in the text. However, because pharmacy technicians may still see the older abbreviations in many settings, we have included the table here to show the old abbreviations along with the new terminology for reference.

Official "Do Not Use" List[1]

DO NOT USE	POTENTIAL PROBLEM	USE INSTEAD
U, u (unit)	Mistaken for "0", the number "4" or "cc"	Write "unit"
IU (international unit)	Mistaken for IV (intravenous) or the number 10 (ten)	Write "International Unit"
QD, Q.D., qd, q.d. (daily)	Mistaken for each other	Write "daily"
Q.O.D., QOD, q.o.d, qod (every other day)	Period after the Q mistaken for "I" and the "O" mistaken for "I"	Write "every other day"
Trailing zero (X.0 mg)*	Decimal point is missed	Write X mg
Lack of leading zero (.X mg)		Write 0.X mg
MS	Can mean morphine sulfate or magnesium sulfate	Write "morphine sulfate"
MSO_4 and $MgSO_4$	Confused for one another	Write "magnesium sulfate"

[1]Applies to all orders and all medication-related documentation that is handwritten (including free-text computer entry) or on pre-printed forms.

*Exception: A "trailing zero" may be used only where required to demonstrate the level of precision of the value being reported, such as for laboratory results, imaging studies that report size of lesions, or catheter/tube sizes. It may not be used in medication orders or other medication-related documentation.

Copyright The Joint Commission, 2012. Reprinted with permission.

In addition, please see the ISMP List of Error-Prone Abbreviations, Symbols, and Dose Designations at www.ismp.org/tools/errorproneabbreviations.pdf. In order to test pharmacy technician students from a realistic perspective, not all medication orders/prescriptions in the text contain the route of administration when it is by mouth (PO). This is to ensure students learn that capsules and tablets should be taken by mouth even if not specifically identified. All other routes of administration are included.

Robert M. Fulcher
Eugenia M. Fulcher

Acknowledgements

Several people have worked diligently to make this text the best possible. Many hours of persistent calculations of the materials in the text have been spent—but the time spent has been necessary to be sure the text is as accurate as possible.

First we want to thank Andrew Allen, Vice President and Publisher, for listening to our desire to be sure a calculations text that covered both retail and hospital pharmacy materials was available for the pharmacy technician students. He heard the need and acted on this step several years ago. Again, Andrew, you are wonderful to work with and we appreciate you.

To Sue Hontscharik, Andrew's former Administrative Assistant, thanks for lending your ear as we worked our way through both editions of the text. You are a friend in need and a friend indeed.

Ellen Wurm-Cutter, Content Manager, has been a major player in both editions of the text. Thanks for being so patient even when we persevered in our thoughts and desires for the text. We are glad that we had your guidance with both editions. You and your team showed creativity and a commitment to excellence that ensured a high-quality text that will be helpful to both faculty and students alike.

Kelly Brinkman, Content Development Specialist, has been our go-between for day-to-day decisions. You have also been patient and have assisted in so many ways. We hope that we did not cause too much confusion for you and we thank you for your support and guidance with a good humor when needed.

We feel so lucky to have worked with Mary Pohlman, Senior Production Manager, in production on both this text and the *Pharmacology: Principles and Applications, 3rd Edition.* You are so efficient and your desire to work with authors for the best ever textbook is apparent in finding the needed materials, being sure the text is correct, and finding little errors that would make a difference. You are the greatest when working on this project. We cannot thank you sufficiently for a job well done.

To our son, Lee, we are proud of your contribution to this edition of the text. Your accounting expertise provides the professional level needed in the business math section. To the reviewers who painstakingly calculated the many problems in the text and provided feedback, you have assisted in the completion of this project while being sure that the accuracy is at the highest level possible. Your comments and suggestions were analyzed carefully and most were used to raise the text to a new standard. Thanks so much for time and expertise.

To create a textbook is no small feat. We hope that the faculties that adopt the text and students who use this book will find it a basis for pharmaceutical calculations for years to come. A good learning experience that can be used in the "real world" of pharmacy is our desire for it use. To our family we are grateful for the patience and support you have provided during this endeavor. You have been the reason for the time and diligence we have placed in this edition. We want you to be proud of your parents and grandparents so that you will provide the best you can in your futures. Finally thanks to our friends and colleagues who have assisted us on both editions of this text. Your friendships are a blessing and the sharing of your knowledge base has helped us meet the standard of excellence that we so desire and what we know our users expect. All of you are special to us.

Bobby and Genie Fulcher

Contents

SECTION V   Business Math, 603

APPENDICES

CHAPTER 1

Assessment of Mathematical Calculation Skills Needed for Pharmacy Technicians

OBJECTIVES

- Explain why proficiency in basic mathematical skills is essential for pharmacy technicians and other health occupations
- Use medical and pharmaceutical abbreviations
- Assess basic mathematical skills needed to proficiently perform calculations in a pharmaceutical setting

KEY WORDS

Active ingredients Chemicals in pure, undiluted forms that affect body function

Ambulatory care Patient care in an outpatient setting; health care provided on an outpatient basis so that those who are treated in a health care facility depart on the same day as treatment

Anatomy Study of the body structure and body organs

Apothecary system One of the oldest measurement systems used to calculate drug orders using such measurements as grains and minims

Chemistry Study of elements, their compounds, and the molecular structure and interactions of matter

Inpatient Patient who has been admitted to a health care facility such as a hospital for at least a 24-hour or overnight stay

Metric system Decimal measurement system considered to be the international standard for scientific and industrial measurements, using grams, liters, and meters

Microbiology Study of microscopic organisms

Pharmacology Study of drugs, their uses, and their interactions with living systems

Physiology Study of the processes and functions of the human body

Psychology Study of behavior and the functions and processes of the mind, as related to the social and physical environment

Round To express a number to its nearest place value such as tenths, hundredths, thousandths

1

Pretest

Interpret the following abbreviations.

1. #, lb _____

2. ↓_____

3. npo _____

4. ↑_____

5. gtt _____

6. qid _____

7. q4h _____

8. mL _____

9. hs _____

10. fl _____

11. tbsp, T _____

12. mcg _____

*13. U _____

14. cap(s) _____

15. gr _____

16. noc _____

17. OTC _____

18. non rep _____

19. bid _____

20. qh _____

21. q2h _____

22. kg _____

23. IM _____

24. IV _____

Pretest, cont.

25. ad lib _____

26. R _____

27. tid _____

*28. qod _____

29. rep _____

30. qs _____

31. prn _____

32. tab _____

33. ung _____

34. syr _____

35. inj _____

36. supp _____

37. elix _____

38. $\overline{\overline{aa}}$ _____

39. $\overline{3}$ _____

40. 3 _____

41. qam _____

42. tsp, t _____

43. po _____

44. $\overline{P}$ _____

45. $\overline{a}$ _____

46. qpm _____

47. stat _____

48. q12h _____

Continued

Pretest, cont.

49. qd _____   50. $\overline{ss}$ _____

51. TO _____   52. q _____

53. $\overline{s}$ _____   54. $\overline{c}$ _____

After completing this exercise, note the abbreviations that you missed and start learning them. You will use these daily in your duties as a pharmacy technician and you must be proficient using these abbreviations.

*These abbreviations are found on the TJC Do Not Use List and ISMP's List of Error-Prone Abbreviations, Symbols, and Dose Designations due to medication safety issues. They should not be used. You are being tested on them here because these abbreviations may still appear in the pharmacy setting.

THE NEED FOR A PHARMACY TECHNICIAN TO HAVE MATHEMATICAL SKILLS

Pharmacology is the study of medications and their uses. It is a science that draws from many disciplines such as **anatomy, physiology, chemistry, microbiology**, and **psychology**. Medications are powerful in treating conditions and diseases when prepared and used appropriately. When a drug is not prepared accurately, it may become a potentially deadly chemical. With many conditions and prescriptions, the difference between toxic and curative may only be the careful calculation of the correct dose or dosage of the drug.

All chemicals used as medications, or drugs, are the basis of pharmacology. Different chemical preparation does not contain the same concentration of **active ingredients** in solid or liquid form. Rather, each drug has its own distinct concentration of active ingredient in a dose. This safe amount of medication has been tested and given acceptable limits by the U.S. Department of Health and Human Services' Food and Drug Administration (FDA). The FDA is also responsible for the *U.S. Pharmacopeia* and the *National Formulary*—manuals that provide the exact ingredients found in medications and the strengths of medications that may be prescribed in the United States. Therefore each prescription has its own dose, and each time a prescription is written the dose must be calculated for that prescription on the basis of the patient's age, medical condition, weight, and gender.

Pharmacy technicians must calculate the amount of medication necessary to provide each dose. Pharmacy technicians must also ensure that there are sufficient numbers of doses for the desired length of time as prescribed by the physician. Although math is not a basic pharmacology science, it is used daily in preparation of medications whether in an **inpatient** setting or an **ambulatory care** setting, such as a pharmacy where the prescription is prepared for the person to take at home. Math is used on a daily basis in all calculations of doses, dosages, and the administration of medications.

This mathematical responsibility that accompanies the preparation of medications is one that must be taken seriously so that dangerous drug levels are not reached. Ethically, you, as a pharmacy technician, must know your level of mathematical skills and must understand the language of the profession by using abbreviations that accompany prescriptions. You must be familiar with acceptable limits—both minimum and maximum—of medications that you are preparing to dispense. Legally, you are responsible for the medications you prepare, although a pharmacist double-checks the medications. Therefore legally, ethically, and morally, you are responsible for your actions, which are heavily dependent on mathematical skills. The course of pharmacology covers the skills required to master acceptable dosages and the expected results of the medication. This text deals with the mathematical skills necessary for the safe administration of the amount of medication prescribed for the patient. The effects of medications on the body are found in another course.

Then why is calculation so important? It does not matter if the correct medication is prescribed or ordered if calculations of medicine to be given for the weight, age, and route of administration are not correct. Calculations are the important steps that you as a pharmacy technician check and recheck for the correct dosage so that patient safety is maintained. To perform pharmaceutical calculations, you must have the math skills covered in this text.

Basic fundamental math skills are necessary in dosage calculation. Fractions, decimals, and whole numbers are used to obtain the correct amount of medication to be given. These skills are used for dosage calculation in the three measurement systems—household measures such as drops, teaspoons, and tablespoons, which are used almost daily because these measurements are easily understood in the United States; **metric system** measures such as grams, liters, and meters, which are used throughout the world for common measures; and the **apothecary system** such as grains, drams, and ounces, which has been the basis of pharmacology since Greek and Roman times but is now used less often. You must understand all systems of measurement and be able to convert among these systems to prepare prescriptions for administration.

Special mathematical conversions that are not directly related to medication dosage are also necessary. The conversion between 24-hour time and military time is a necessary skill, because military time is often used in an inpatient setting for medication administration. The standard 24-hour time is used in most ambulatory care situations, so the ability to give the correct time in either place is necessary. Conversions between Fahrenheit and Celsius temperatures and the use of Arabic versus Roman numerals are also important in prescription reading. Clearly, many factors are necessary to be sure the math for pharmacology is accurate and used correctly.

INTERPRETING THE ABBREVIATIONS USED IN MEDICAL LANGUAGE

Pharmacology also has a language of its own, including shorthand, that allows physicians and other health professionals to avoid writing an entire order. Interpretation of this shorthand is a necessary component for properly dispensing prescriptions and educating patients as they take medications at home. Abbreviations are used to refer to the route or method of administration, the frequency with which a drug is to be given, and to general terms such as those found in measurement systems or those related to food and sleep. These abbreviations as well as their interpretation need to be memorized. Chapter 6 discusses using abbreviations to interpret drug orders, but learning abbreviations should start now to ensure success in interpreting orders and prescriptions later.

Routes of Administration

PARENTERAL
IM—intramuscularly
SC, SQ, Subq—subcutaneously
IV—intravenously
ID—intradermally

BY MOUTH
PO, po—by mouth (per os in Latin)
SL, subling—sublingually

FOR EASE OF LEARNING
"q" means every
"id" means the number of times in a day (in die)
"c" means cibus, or food, in Latin

Frequency of Administration

RELATED TO DAYS/WEEKS/MONTHS
qweek—every week
qmonth—every month

RELATED TO HOURS
qh—every hour
q2h—every 2 hours
q4h—every 4 hours
q6h—every 6 hours

RELATED TO MORE THAN ONCE DAILY
bid—twice a day
tid—three times a day
qd—everyday
qid—four times a day
*qod—every other day

RELATED TO SPECIFIC TIMES
ac—before meals
pc—after meals
hs—hour of sleep/bedtime
stat—at once, immediately

Forms of Administration

SOLIDS
tab—tablet
cap—capsule

LIQUIDS
gtt(s)—drop(s)
fl, f—fluid
Liq, liq—liquid
Syr—syrup
elix—elixir

MISCELLANEOUS
ung—ointment
supp—suppository
inj—injectable

Measurements of Medication

METRIC SYSTEM
mg, mG—milligram
ml, mL—milliliter

G, g, gm—gram
L, l—liter
K, kg—kilogram
mcg—microgram

HOUSEHOLD SYSTEM
tsp, Tsp, t—teaspoon
tbsp, Tbsp, T—tablespoon
c, C—cup
#, lb—pound
″, in—inch
′, ft—foot
oz—ounce
pt—pint
qt—quart

APOTHECARY SYSTEM
gr—grain
dr, ℥—dram
oz, ℥—ounce
m, ℳ—minim
s̅s̅—one half

MISCELLANEOUS MEDICATION MEASUREMENTS
mEq—milliequivalent
*U—unit

General Abbreviations

c̄—with
s̄—without
=—equal to
≠—not equal to
<—less than
>—greater than, more than
℞—prescription, treatment, take this drug
OTC—over the counter
VO—verbal order
TO—telephone order
NKA—no known allergies
NKDA—no known drug allergies
ā—before
p̄—after
ad lib—as desired
prn—as needed
a̅a̅—of each
↑—higher than, increase
↓—lower than, decrease
non rep—do not repeat
NPO, npo—nothing by mouth (nil per os in Latin)
noc—night

*These abbreviations are found on the TJC Do Not Use List and ISMP's List of Error-Prone Abbreviations, Symbols, and Dose Designations due to medication safety issues. They should not be used but may still appear in the pharmacy setting.

WHAT ARE YOUR BASIC MATH SKILLS?

You use basic math skills daily to perform calculations in the pharmaceutical world. Many of the skills required for calculating doses and dosages are simply the basic arithmetic of daily living taught in elementary school. However, they may become the source of frustration when described as "math" or when these skills have not been used for an extended time.

Understanding whole numbers, fractions, decimals, percentages, Roman numerals, ratio and proportion, and basic problem solving is essential to perform calculations. Basic insertion of numbers into formulas and then solving for an unknown are other skills that you will use daily. These skills are necessary for safe and accurate calculation of medication doses and dosages for the patients.

During practice exercises throughout the text, you may use a calculator if your instructor permits, but remember that a calculator may not always be available in pharmacy situations. Practicing the math skills that you may not have used for years will sharpen your thinking skills to perform calculations with confidence. Using math skills without a calculator is a way to increase your analytical skills—skills that enable you to solve equations and take components of a whole to form relationships among its parts. Analysis of pharmacological problems is an important step in ensuring accurate calculations with each medication order. If your answers seem incorrect, always check your answers. Calculations are analytical skills that will increase with use.

Prerequisite skills of adding, subtracting, multiplying, and dividing whole numbers are essential before you can begin drug calculations. You must also be able to work with decimals, fractions, ratios/proportions, and percentages. Following is a self-test to be used as a tool to help you determine your math skill strengths and weaknesses. It is also an indicator of your readiness to proceed through the text. Proficiency in these basic math concepts is gauged by attaining a grade of 90% or better. In Chapter 2 you may skip basic skills in which you are proficient, but do not skip any part that gives you difficulty on this test. Having proficiency in basic math skills is of utmost importance.

General rules for taking the self-test are as follows:

- Allow yourself at least 1 hour to take the test. Each question is worth 2 points. Thus you may miss 5 questions and achieve 90%. If all the questions you miss are similar, please take time to use the materials in Chapter 2 for review of this material. In this scenario, you may pass the test yet not understand a basic math principle.

SELF-TEST OF PROFICIENCY IN BASIC MATH SKILLS

Directions

1. Figure all decimals to three places but **round** answers to two places, so 1.454 would become 1.45 and 7.5685 would become 7.57.

2. Always express fractions in their lowest possible terms; for example, 4/8 should be expressed as 1/2.

3. Complete ratio and proportion problems to the lowest terms (e.g., 5:10 should be reduced to 1:2).

4. Do your work on paper, without a calculator, and keep your paperwork attached so that, if you made an error you can return to the paper and find the mistake.

Basic Math Skills Proficiency Self-Test

1. Express the following sum in Arabic numerals: XXV + LX = _____

2. 156.90 + 368 = _____

3. 4.65 − 3.056 =   _____

4. 3.50 × 43.5 =   _____

5. $12.56 + $152.47 + $4.98 + $68.08 =   _____

6. $52.43 × 0.25 =   _____

7. 0.7 ÷ 0.0035 =   _____

8. 78 + 0.186 =   _____

9. $\dfrac{3}{4} + 7\dfrac{7}{8} =$ _____

10. 25 − 13 = (express in Roman numerals)   _____

11. $15.43 × 25 =   _____

12. 5025 − 4995 = (express in Roman numerals)   _____

13. 1932 ÷ 102 =   _____

14. $\dfrac{1}{5} + \dfrac{4}{10} + \dfrac{3}{15} + \dfrac{5}{6} =$ _____

15. $\dfrac{5}{6} \div \dfrac{3}{8} =$ _____

16. $\dfrac{1}{200} \times 150 =$ _____

17. 0.6% of 36 =   _____

18. Express 0.4 as a fraction.   _____

19. Express 0.006 as a %.   _____

20. $\dfrac{1}{4}$% of 20 =   _____

21. $1\dfrac{1}{3} + 3\dfrac{3}{4} =$ _____

22. $9\dfrac{1}{4} - 6\dfrac{3}{8} =$ _____

23. $1\dfrac{3}{8} \div \dfrac{1}{4} =$ _____

24. Which fraction has the greatest value? 1/150, 1/200, 1/500   _____

25. Which decimal has the least value? 0.012, 0.12, 0.0125   _____

26. Change 3/4 to a percentage.   _____

27. Change 3½ to a decimal.   _____

28. $\dfrac{2.2}{4.4} \times 60 =$ _____

29. $\dfrac{12.75}{2.25} =$ _____

30. Which has the greatest value? 3.75, 3¾, 3⅞   _____

31. If a medication container holds 20 tablets, how many containers would you need for 120 tablets?   _____

32. A prescription is written for 150 tablets. How many containers containing 50 tablets will it take to fill the prescription?   _____

33. A prescription is written for a solution to contain 10% of an active ingredient. How many milliliters of active ingredient would be necessary in a 100-mL solution?   _____

34. If 1 inch contains 2.54 cm, how many centimeters are in 10 inches?   _____

35. Express 70:350 in its lowest terms.   _____

36. Solve for x. $\dfrac{50}{25} x = 120$ _____

37. Solve for x. $\dfrac{1}{100} \times 350 = x$ _____

38. $7 \times -5 =$ _____

39. 1 g = 1000 mg. How many milligrams are in 5.5 g?   _____

40. If one kg equals 2.2 lb, how many kg are in 88#?   _____

41. $906.2 \times 1.34 =$ _____

42. If one kg equals 2.2 lb, how many pounds are in 11 kg?   _____

43. Express 4% as a ratio in its lowest term.   _____

44. $3\dfrac{2}{3} - 1\dfrac{5}{6} =$ _____

45. A stock bottle of medicine contains 500 tablets. How many prescriptions of 25 tablets can be filled with that bottle of medication?   _____

46. Subtract the following and express in Roman numerals. XIX – XIV =   _____

47. $3.6 \div 0.0005 =$ _____

48. $\$4.28 + \$5.65 + \$0.78 + \$15.39 =$ _____

49. $195.46 - 35.86 =$ _____

50. $5\dfrac{5}{6} - 3\dfrac{7}{30} =$ _____

After grading this test, look at the problems you missed. If you did not score 90% or higher, continue working on basic skills in Chapter 2. If you missed a group of problems that are related and you scored 90% or higher, review your areas of weakness. Be sure your basic mathematical skills are adequate for learning the more advanced skills that are used in pharmaceutical calculation. Self-confidence in your math skills will make learning less frustrating and calculating math fun. Be fair with yourself and spend the time necessary for basic mathematical skills.

CHAPTER 2

Review of Basic Mathematical Skills

OBJECTIVES

- Add, subtract, multiply, and divide whole numbers
- Add, subtract, multiply, and divide fractions and reduce fractions to the lowest terms
- Add, subtract, multiply, and divide mixed numbers and reduce to the lowest terms
- Add, subtract, multiply, and divide decimals and round them to a specific number place value
- Convert fractions to decimal fractions
- Convert among fractions, decimals, and percentages
- Express numbers in ratio and proportion and solve for unknowns

KEY WORDS

Complex fraction Fractions in which the numerator, denominator, or both are fractional units

Decimal Number system based on the number 10 and progressions of 10s

Decimal place Place values found to the right of the decimal point

Denominator Bottom number of a fraction

Dividend Number being divided in division

Divisor Number by which another number is divided

Extremes First and last number found in a proportion (or) $\dfrac{B \qquad B}{1:2:3:4}$

Fraction Part of a whole number with a numerator and denominator

Improper fraction Fraction in which the numerator is equal to or greater than the denominator; a fraction that is equal to or greater than 1

Inversion To turn upside down, as with a fraction, or to interchange the terms of a ratio

Lowest term Form of a fraction in which no common number will divide into both the numerator and denominator evenly

Means Second and third numbers found in a proportion (or) $\dfrac{A \ A}{1:2::3:4}$

Mixed number Number containing a whole number and a fraction

Multiplicand Number to be multiplied by another

Multiplier Number used to multiply another number

Numerator Top number found in a fraction

Percentage A means of expressing a portion of 100 parts

Product Number obtained by multiplying two numbers together

Proper fraction Fraction in which the numerator is less than the denominator

Proportion Comparative relationship among the parts; one or more ratios that are compared

Quotient Number obtained when one number is divided by another

Ratio A means of describing the relationship between two numbers

Remainder Number left after completing subtraction; in division the number left after division (number left after steps of division have been completed)

Rounding To calculate a number to a desired place value when the exact number is not desired

Scored tablet Tablet containing an indention for ease of breaking into equal parts

Whole number Numeral consisting of one or more digits; number that is not followed by a fraction or decimal

Pretest

Complete the following answers, and show all of your work. **Round all decimals to the closest thousandth unless otherwise stated.**

1. $\dfrac{4}{5} + \dfrac{5}{6} + \dfrac{7}{30} =$ _____

2. $154 + 1063 + 25 + 2376 =$ _____

3. $163 - 69 =$ _____

4. $256 \times 42 =$ _____

5. $256 \div 16 =$ _____

6. $3655 - 29 =$ _____

7. $25.6 + 1456 + 35.67 =$ _____

8. $354.29 - 45.390 =$ _____

9. $12.56 \times 65.031 =$ _____

10. $655.08 \div 1.2 =$ _____

11. $\dfrac{1}{2} + \dfrac{3}{4} + \dfrac{7}{8} =$ _____

12. $\dfrac{5}{8} - \dfrac{1}{6} =$ _____

13. $\dfrac{1}{8} + \dfrac{5}{12} + \dfrac{5}{6} =$ _____

14. $\dfrac{3}{5} \times \dfrac{7}{8} =$ _____

15. $\dfrac{5}{8} \div \dfrac{1}{4} =$ _____

16. $\dfrac{2}{3} \times \dfrac{14}{15} =$ _____

17. $16 \times \dfrac{5}{8} =$ _____

18. $36 \div \dfrac{4}{9} =$ _____

19. $45\dfrac{1}{4} + 12\dfrac{1}{3} + 10\dfrac{5}{6} =$ _____

20. $12\dfrac{1}{2} - 11\dfrac{5}{6} =$ _____

21. $5\dfrac{3}{8} + 2\dfrac{1}{12} + 4\dfrac{1}{3} =$ _____

22. $2\dfrac{3}{5} - 1\dfrac{1}{3} =$ _____

23. $4\dfrac{1}{10} \times 2 =$ _____

24. $\dfrac{2}{9} \times 3\dfrac{3}{5} \times \dfrac{5}{6} =$ _____

Pretest, cont.

25. $3 \div \dfrac{1}{4} =$ _____

26. $\dfrac{9}{10} \div \dfrac{3}{5} =$ _____

27. $12 + \dfrac{7}{8} + \dfrac{3}{4} + 2\dfrac{1}{2} =$ _____

28. $100.2 \times 100.03 =$ _____

29. $721 - 0.01 =$ _____

30. $12.02 \div 6.01 =$ _____

31. A roll of adhesive is 10½ inches long. The physician asks you to be sure the person has sufficient amount to apply bandages daily for 2 weeks using approximately 1½ yards per bandage. How many rolls of adhesive should you be sure the patient buys?

32. A solution contains 4½ cups of water. How many milliliters would be in ⅔ of the solution?

Round the following to the nearest one hundredth.

33. 75.0023 _____

34. 12.015 _____

35. 6.12453 _____

36. 126.444 _____

Change the following to decimal fractions.

37. $\dfrac{3}{5}$ _____

38. $1\dfrac{3}{25}$ _____

39. $1\dfrac{3}{4}$ _____

40. $\dfrac{7}{20}$ _____

Continued

Pretest, cont.

Change the following to ratios and reduce to the lowest terms possible.

41. $\dfrac{23}{95}$ _____

42. $\dfrac{34}{68}$ _____

43. $\dfrac{25}{75}$ _____

44. $\dfrac{12}{96}$ _____

Solve the following proportions.

45. $x:3::15:30 =$ _____

46. $5:15::8:x =$ _____

47. $3:x::11:33 =$ _____

48. $1:50::x:40 =$ _____

49. A pharmacist is able to fill six prescriptions in 10 minutes with the assistance of a pharmacy tech. How many prescriptions can be completed in 1 hour?

50. A prescription calls for 15 mL of water to reconstitute a medication in a 20-mL vial. How many milliliters of water would be needed proportionally to reconstitute 50-mL vial of the same medication?

Interpret the following abbreviations.

51. mL _____

52. tsp _____

53. mg _____

54. g _____

55. gr _____

56. mcg _____

57. tbsp _____

58. ℥ _____

59. ℈ _____

60. pt _____

INTRODUCTION

In calculation of medications, accuracy is extremely important for patient safety. Remember, the patient depends on your calculations and the pharmacist expects you to correctly make these calculations. Answers must be precise—partially correct answers are unacceptable and may endanger patient safety. Basic math skills are an important component in finding the correct answers. You learned many of these skills in early grade school, but you may not use them on a regular basis, so they may be forgotten.

WHOLE NUMBERS

What Is a Whole Number?

A **whole number** is the basic mathematical symbol that we use on a daily basis. In the math world, whole numbers represent numerals consisting of one or more digits. The digits used in math are 0, 1, 2, 3, 4, 5, 6, 7, 8, and 9. Numbers may also be written in words, such as one, two, ten, one thousand, ten million one hundred three, and the like. The word "and" should not be used between digits in a whole number. In the medical field, commas are not placed in numbers with more than four digits or seven digits, such as 1275 or 2356302. A comma might be misinterpreted as a **decimal** when used in whole numbers, causing a medication error.

A whole number does not have a decimal, **fraction**, or **percentage**. When you add, subtract, or multiply whole numbers, the answer will always remain a whole number such as 10, 25, or 100. For example, $45 + 12 = 57$ or $5 \times 45 = 225$ because all of the numbers are whole numbers. In some cases if dividing whole numbers, the answer may be found as a whole number, a decimal number, or a whole number with a decimal number. For example, 10 divided by 2 is 5 or 11 divided by 3 would be $3.66\overline{6}$; all the numbers in this example contain whole numbers, but they are not evenly divisible and may have decimal **remainders**.

EXAMPLE 2-1

$$
\begin{array}{cccccc}
3 & 8 & 10 & 12 & 24 & 12 \\
+5 & -5 & -8 & -12 & \div12 & \times2 \\
\hline
8 & 3 & 2 & 0 & 2 & 24
\end{array}
$$

> **INTERESTING FACT**
> The word digit used in numbers actually came from the Latin word digitus, meaning finger. Just as with our hands, each digit has its own value depending on where it is found in the number or numeral.

A whole number is always to the left of a decimal point. The numeral 0 is a whole number with the decimal understood to be at the right side of the zero. In pharmaceutical mathematics, if no number is to the left of a decimal, a zero (0) is placed in the whole number place.

> **TECH NOTE**
> Whole numbers are numbers found to the left of the decimal point and may have one digit or more. Fractions and decimals may be added to a whole number, but the whole number is to the left in each of these cases. Examples: 25, 25.1, $25\frac{1}{2}$.

Whole numbers are used in strengths of medications, doses of medications, inventory, and costs of medications, to give just a few examples of the need to understand this concept.

Adding and Subtracting Whole Numbers

When adding or subtracting whole numbers, align the digits from the right and then add or subtract one set of digits at a time starting from the right (from ones to tens to hundreds, etc.). Addition is finding a sum or total of two numbers. Subtraction is finding the difference between two numbers.

EXAMPLE 2-2

$$
\begin{array}{r} 25 \\ +\ 5 \\ \hline 30 \end{array}
\qquad
\begin{array}{r} 236 \\ -\ 24 \\ \hline 212 \end{array}
\qquad
\begin{array}{r} 1302 \\ +\ 205 \\ \hline 1507 \end{array}
\qquad
\begin{array}{r} 10584 \\ -10263 \\ \hline 321 \end{array}
$$

Practice Problems A

Calculate the following problems, being sure to show your work and stating measurement designations as appropriate.

1. 25 + 56 = _____

2. 105 + 235 = _____

3. 1243 + 356 = _____

4. 50 g + 100 g = _____

5. 25 mg + 90 mg = _____

6. 240# + 133# = _____

7. 125,000 units + 250,000 units = _____

8. 7500 mL + 1000 mL = _____

9. 78 − 56 = _____

10. 285 − 168 = _____

11. 1549 − 1374 = _____

12. 725 mL − 650 mL = _____

13. 525 g − 175 g = _____

14. 156# − 48# = _____

15. 65 mL – 30 mL = _____

16. 350 mg – 125 mg = _____

17. 1250 mg – 615 mg = _____

18. 266 kg – 15 kg = _____

19. A bottle of antibiotic needs to be reconstituted with 100 mL of distilled water. You have a calibrated graduate that holds 50 mL. How many times will you have to fill the container with water to reconstitute the medication? _____

20. A vial of anesthetic contains 10 mL. The pharmacist asks that you add 30 mL of distilled water to prepare an anesthetic compound for mouth ulcers. How many milliliters will be in the bottle of prepared medication? _____

Multiplying Whole Numbers

Multiplication of whole numbers is actually a shortcut to repeated addition of numbers. When multiplying whole numbers, align the numbers or factors as you would for addition or subtraction. The use of "×" denotes that the numbers should be multiplied to find a **product.** Either number may be the **multiplier** or **multiplicand** and the product will not be affected. However, it requires less calculating if the multiplier has the fewer digits. You should also remember that if a number is multiplied by zero, the product is zero. First multiply the number in the multiplicand (number that is to be multiplied or is multiplied by another or the number on top of the problem) by the number at the far right of the multiplier (number that is used to multiply another number or that on the bottom of the equation).

EXAMPLE 2-3

3 (multiplicand) × 4 (multiplier) = 12 (product)

Multiply the remaining numbers in the subsequent digits, moving from right to left. Be sure to keep the numbers to the far right in alignment with the numbers in the multiplier. Finally, add the numbers that have been multiplied to obtain the product.

EXAMPLE 2-4

```
    125 Multiplicand
×    15 Multiplier
    625
+125
   1875 Product
```

EXAMPLE 2-5

$$
\begin{array}{r}
225 \text{ Multiplicand} \\
\times \quad 10 \text{ Multiplier} \\
\hline
000 \\
+225 \quad\; \\
\hline
2250 \text{ Product}
\end{array}
$$

Please notice the zero or "0"s are now in the first product line and then multiply the numbers following the zero or "0" in the multiplicand in the usual manner. Be sure to keep the alignment correct.

 TECH ALERT

If the multiplier is divisible by ten (or ends in "0") align the multiplier so the "0" is to the right of the multiplicand to shorten the computation of the problem. The number of "0s" to right of first number above zero in the multiplier will then be found to the right of the first line of numbers multiplied.

Dividing Whole Numbers

Division is a way of determining how many times one number can be found in another. It is actually repeated subtraction steps. Division is represented by either "÷" or ")‾‾‾‾." The number being divided is called the **dividend**, and the number used to divide is the **divisor**. The result of the division is the **quotient**.

EXAMPLE 2-6

35 (Dividend) ÷ 5 (Divisor) = 7 (Quotient)

OR

5 (Divisor))$\overline{35 \text{ (Dividend)}}$ = 7 (Quotient)

Any number that is remaining when numbers are not exactly divisible is called a **remainder**. In math, when rounding numbers, any amount in the remainder (the number that remains after subtraction) that is less than half of the divisor is usually discarded and the number in the quotient remains the same. Conversely, when rounding, if the remainder is more than one half of the divisor, the number in the quotient is increased by one number. For example, 30 divided by 9 is 3, with 3 as a remainder. In this instance, the quotient would remain at 3. But if 33 is divided by 9, the quotient is 3 with a remainder of 6. Six is more than half of 9, so the quotient will become 4.

LEARNING TIP

Remember that any number divided by itself equals 1 and any number divided by 1 equals that same number. Zero divided by any number remains 0. (Zero can never be the divisor; i.e., 9 ÷ 0 has no meaning, and the answer remains 9.)

When dividing whole numbers, the number in the divisor must be smaller than the number in the dividend to be able to do the calculation. When the divisor is a single digit, the first number of the dividend must be divisible by the divisor or the second digit in the dividend is also used.

EXAMPLE 2-7

$360 \div 9$

In this example, 3 cannot be divided by 9, so you must move to 36 to be able to use the divisor 9. Nine will divide into 36 four times, and 9 will divide into 0 zero times, so $360 \div 9 = 40$.

When there are multiple digits in the divisor, the divisor is rounded to the nearest 10 to estimate the quotient digit. The entire divisor is then used to complete the calculation.

EXAMPLE 2-8

$275 \div 25$

Estimate to the nearest 10 digit or go from 25 to 30. If you divide 275 by 30, the answer is 9 (3 into 27), but when you multiply 25 by 9, the answer is 225 with 50 as a remainder. If you divide by 10, the answer still has a remainder of 25. So then try 11, and the answer is correct. $11 \times 25 = 275$ or $275 \div 25 = 11$.

LEARNING TIP

When dividing by two, three, or more digit numbers, estimate the numbers before doing the calculation. This will cut down on the errors by helping to discover whether the calculated answers are near to the exact number needed after calculation. Round to the nearest multiple ending in zero. For example, in Example 2-8, the estimation of the divisor would become 25 to show that the quotient should first be close to 10. Thus, your answer of 11 is basically correct.

Practice Problems B

Calculate the following problems, being sure to show all your work. Estimate your work first. Round to the nearest hundreth as appropriate.

1. $56 \times 10 = $ _____

2. $76 \times 11 = $ _____

3. $100 \times 87 = $ _____

4. $768 \times 2 = $ _____

5. $3500 \times 265 = $ _____

6. $345 \times 70 = $ _____

7. $\begin{array}{r} 653 \\ \times \quad 30 \end{array} = $ _____

8. $\begin{array}{r} 275 \\ \times \quad 310 \end{array} = $ _____

9. $\begin{array}{r} 362 \\ \times \quad 65 \end{array} = $ _____

10. $\begin{array}{r} 563 \\ \times \quad 715 \end{array} = $ _____

11. $105 \div 5 =$ _____

12. $840 \div 40 =$ _____

13. $296 \div 4 =$ _____

14. $1125 \div 15 =$ _____

15. $150 \div 15 =$ _____

16. $162 \div 18 =$ _____

17. $15 \overline{)600} =$ _____

18. $12 \overline{)276} =$ _____

19. $152 \overline{)2432} =$ _____

20. $25 \text{ mg} \times 40 \text{ mg} =$ _____

21. $275 \text{ mL} \times 4 \text{ mL} =$ _____

22. $24\# \times 16\# =$ _____

23. $150 \text{ mg} \times 15 \text{ mg} =$ _____

24. $30 \text{ kg} \times 400 \text{ kg} =$ _____

25. $21 \text{ qt} \times 28 \text{ qt} =$ _____

26. $1250 \text{ mg} \div 125 \text{ mg} =$ _____

27. $250{,}000 \text{ units} \div 150 \text{ units} =$ _____

28. $2400 \text{ kg} \div 48 \text{ kg} =$ _____

29. $300 \text{ mg} \div 15 \text{ mg} =$ _____

30. You are asked to fill a prescription that has 10 tablets containing 250 mg each. What is the total actual ingredient of the medication? _____

31. The physician orders 100 tablets of a medication that is to be taken as 1 tablet four times a day until all the medication has been taken. The physician asks that these medications be placed in separate bottles for each week. How many tablets would you put in each bottle? How many bottles of medication should you have available for the pharmacist to check? _____

32. A prescription costs $15, and the customer gives you $50. How much money should you refund to the person? How many $5 bills would you refund to the patient? _____

33. The manufacturer's label tells you to add 375 mL of water to a medication for reconstitution. You have a container that will hold 125 mL of water. How many times will you need to fill the container to reconstitute the medication correctly? _____

34. Mrs. Jones comes to the pharmacy and tells you that her child has lost her allergy medication. You look at the prescription and read that the original prescription is for 30 tablets to be taken once daily. Fourteen days have passed since Mrs. Jones filled this medication. After consulting with the pharmacist, you are told to replace the lost medication. How many tablets do you need to give Mrs. Jones so that her child can complete her treatment? _____ How many weeks of medication did the child take? _____

35. You are asked to provide the pharmacist with vials of medication to total 1000 mg. Each vial of medication holds 250 mg. How many vials of medication does the pharmacist need? _____

FRACTIONS

What Is a Fraction?

When a whole number or unit is divided into parts, the parts are called fractions. Fractions are designated as proper and improper. A **proper fraction** is one in which the **numerator** is less than the **denominator** or is part of a whole. An **improper fraction** is defined as a fraction in which the numerator is equal to or greater than the denominator, a fraction that is equal to or greater than one, or a fraction that can be changed to a whole number or a whole number plus a proper fraction. **Complex fractions,** found later in the text, are fractional expressions in which the numerator, denominator, or both are expressed as fractions such as $\dfrac{1/4}{1/8}$ or $\dfrac{1/4}{2}$.

Fractions may be expressed in the form a/b such as $3/4$ or $\dfrac{a}{b}$ such as $\dfrac{3}{4}$.

The "a" is called the *numerator* (top number found in a fraction). The "b" is the *denominator* (bottom number of a fraction). Both numbers must be whole numbers, and the denominator cannot be 0 or the resultant answer becomes 0. The denominator also tells how many times the whole unit has been divided.

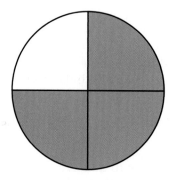

The circle pictured shows a proper fraction. The shaded area shows the part of a whole. Can you tell the number in the numerator and denominator? If you said ¾ you are correct. Try with this example:

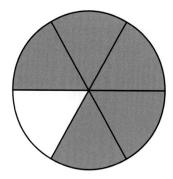

If you said the numerator is 5 and the denominator is 6, you are correct.

TECH NOTE

Fractions are used in pharmacy in both household and apothecary quantities as well as in business math calculations.

Practice Problems C

In the following examples, please indicate the numerator and the denominator.

1. $\dfrac{5}{7}$ Numerator _____   Denominator _____

2. $\dfrac{8}{11}$ Numerator _____   Denominator _____

3. $\dfrac{7}{15}$ Numerator _____   Denominator _____

4. $\dfrac{135}{356}$ Numerator _____   Denominator _____

5. $\dfrac{5}{6}$ Numerator _____   Denominator _____

A fraction can also be thought of as indicating division—the numerator may be divided by the denominator. So when $\frac{2}{3}$ is written, the fraction actually means $2 \div 3$. The following illustrates this in pharmaceutical terms:

If a patient has 25 tablets in a prescription and takes 13 tablets, what is the fractional use?

Answer: $\frac{13}{25}$

A pharmacist has a bottle of medication that contains 90 tablets. He uses 50 tablets. What is the fractional use?

Answer: $\frac{50}{90}$ or $\frac{5}{9}$. (When $\frac{50}{90}$ is divided by 10 in both the numerator and the denominator, the result is $\frac{5}{9}$.)

TECH NOTE

Whole numbers are actually fractions in which the numerator is an exact multiple of the denominator. When whole numbers are shown in a graph, the entire area of the graph is shaded versus the shading of parts of the entire area in fractions.

This figure represents the whole number 1.

This figure represents the fraction $\frac{1}{4}$.

A proper or simple fraction is a fraction in which the numerator is less than the denominator, such as $\frac{2}{3}$ and $\frac{5}{8}$. An improper fraction is one in which the numerator is equal to or greater than the denominator, making the fraction a number of one or more such as $\frac{9}{8}$ or $1\frac{1}{8}$ and $\frac{14}{7}$ or 2. If the numerator and denominator are the same, the number becomes 1, such as $\frac{9}{9}$ or $\frac{10}{10}$. An improper fraction may be written as a **mixed number** (a whole number and a fraction) or as an improper fraction (a fraction that has a numerator equal to or greater than the denominator). To change an improper fraction to a mixed number, the numerator is divided by the denominator and any remainder is written over the denominator, such as $\frac{43}{8}$ (an improper fraction) = $5\frac{3}{8}$ (a mixed number). (When 43 is divided by 8, the answer is 5 with a remainder of 3, so $\frac{43}{8}$ as a mixed number is $5\frac{3}{8}$.) The remainder is the amount that is left over after the whole number has been divided into the numerator the maximum number of times (in this problem, 3 is the remainder that now is seen as $\frac{3}{8}$). An improper fraction should always be reduced to a mixed number after calculations have been completed.

A mixed number is a whole number with a proper fraction, such as $3\frac{3}{4}$ and $6\frac{5}{9}$. To change a mixed number to an improper fraction, multiply the whole number by the denominator and add the amount found in the numerator (e.g., $4\frac{1}{8}$ actually means that 4 is multiplied by 8 to provide the whole number of 32 and the 1 found in the numerator of the fraction is added to the total, or $32 + 1 = 33$). The denominator remains the number found as the denominator of the mixed number, or $4\frac{1}{8} = \frac{33}{8}$. Another example of changing a mixed number to an improper fraction is $2\frac{2}{3}$: $2 \times 3 + 2$ with the same denominator of 3 or $\frac{8}{3}$.

Practice Problems D

Change the following improper fractions to mixed numbers or whole numbers. Show all of your work. Be sure to indicate measurement as appropriate.

1. $\dfrac{16}{3}$ = _____

2. $\dfrac{24}{7}$ = _____

3. $\dfrac{35}{4}$ = _____

4. $\dfrac{223}{110}$ = _____

5. $\dfrac{16}{15}$ = _____

6. $\dfrac{21}{7}$ = _____

7. gr $\dfrac{5}{4}$ = _____

8. $\dfrac{9}{8}$ c = _____

9. $\dfrac{3}{2}$ L = _____

10. $\dfrac{3}{2}$ tab = _____

11. $\dfrac{6}{6}$ tab = _____

12. $\dfrac{5}{4}$ c = _____

Change the following mixed numbers to improper fractions. Be sure to indicate measurement as appropriate.

13. $3\dfrac{1}{2}$ = _____

14. $9\dfrac{7}{9}$ = _____

15. $2\dfrac{7}{8}$ = _____

16. $3\dfrac{1}{4}$ = _____

17. $10\dfrac{9}{10}$ = _____

18. $4\dfrac{5}{7}$ = _____

19. $2\frac{1}{2}$ c = _____

20. $6\frac{3}{4}$ qt = _____

21. $4\frac{1}{2}$ tab = _____

22. $3\frac{1}{3}$ c = _____

23. $5\frac{1}{4}$ c = _____

24. gr $1\frac{3}{8}$ = _____

Indicate the fraction or mixed number for each of the following shaded areas.

25. 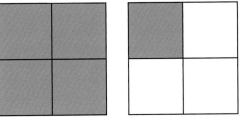 = _____

26.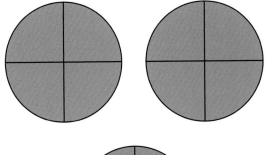

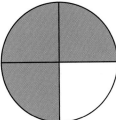 = _____

27.

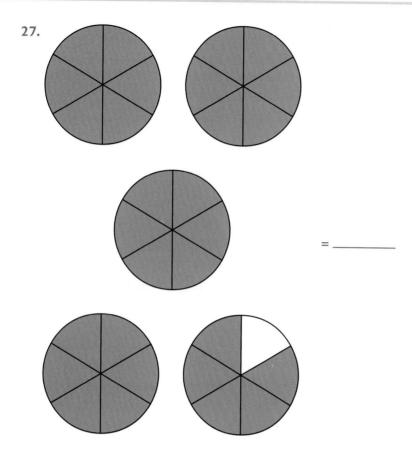

= _____

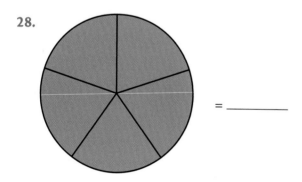

28.

= _____

29.

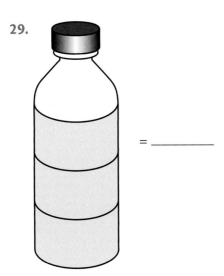

= _____

30.

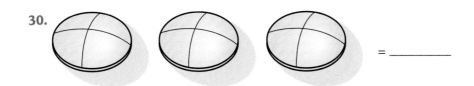

= _____

31. A pharmacist has a medicine cup that is divided into eight equal sections. She fills to the line to indicate five parts. What is the fractional amount that the pharmacist has filled? _____

32. A customer asks you to show him how to divide a tablet (i.e., a **scored tablet** that is divided into four equal parts) into ½ of a tablet. Fill in the following tablet to show this fraction.

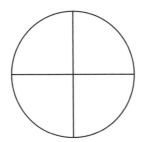

33. A medication requires that the customer mix granules in ⅓ of a glass of water. On the glass, show ⅓ of the glass of water.

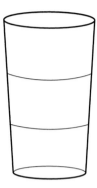

34. A customer is supposed to take a dose of 1½ tablets four times a day. The prescription drug is in whole tablets. Show what the customer should do.

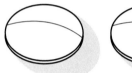

35. A customer is supposed to give her child ¾ of a medicine dropper of medication. Indicate on the medicine dropper what you would show the customer as a dose.

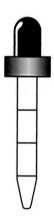

Reducing Fractions to the Lowest Term

Some fractions, called equivalent fractions, have the same equivalency without having the same portions of a whole. The fraction ½ could be ²⁄₄, ³⁄₆, or even ⁵⁰⁄₁₀₀. For example, with ²⁄₄, the numerator and denominator can both be divided by 2 to give ½; or with ³⁄₆, both parts of the fraction can be divided by 3 for ½; finally, with ⁵⁰⁄₁₀₀, both components of the fraction can be divided by 50 for $\frac{1}{2}$. Each of these fractions is actually one half of the total number of equivalent parts of a whole.

TECH NOTE
Any fraction that has a denominator of 1 is equal to the number in the numerator, such as $\frac{6}{1} = 6$.

Reducing or simplifying fractions to the **lowest term** is actually the process of finding the lowest equivalent fraction through division of the numerator and denominator by the same number (e.g., the fraction $\frac{2}{4}$ can be reduced by dividing by 2 [$2 \div 2 = 1$ and $4 \div 2 = 2$] = $\frac{1}{2}$, or $\frac{3}{6}$ can be reduced by 3 [$3 \div 3 = 1$ and $6 \div 3 = 2$] to = $\frac{1}{2}$). In each case the reduced fraction contains the same amount of space in each whole. The difference is that the number of divided pieces of the whole has changed. The fractions are comparable, although the actual numerators and denominators have been altered by division with a number that is common to both parts of the fraction. This is dividing by a common factor of the numerator and denominator (e.g., with the fraction $\frac{15}{50}$, both the numerator and denominator can be divided by 5, so the fraction can be reduced to $\frac{3}{10}$).

LEARNING TIP
Failure to reduce fractions to lowest terms can be cause for the answer to be incorrect because the higher the numbers used, the more difficult the calculations.

TECH NOTE
If the lowest common denominator is not readily apparent, finding this number may require other steps. One way is to multiply the two denominators together and use that number as the common denominator, or the denominators may be multiplied by 2, 3, or 4 to find a common denominator (e.g., if the denominators are 3 and 4, a common denominator could be 12 because $3 \times 4 = 12$). If the denominators were 6 and 9, multiplying the 6 by 3 would provide denominator of 18 and multiplying 9×2 would also provide the denominator of 18. So in this case the common denominator would be 18, and the math could be calculated using the common denominator.

Practice Problems E

Reduce the following fractions to the lowest term. As always, show your calculations.

1. $\dfrac{3}{6}$ = _____

2. $\dfrac{6}{9}$ = _____

3. $\dfrac{8}{12}$ = _____

4. $\dfrac{25}{125}$ = _____

5. $\dfrac{7}{35}$ = _____

6. $\dfrac{27}{108}$ = _____

7. $\dfrac{6}{48}$ = _____

8. $\dfrac{125}{750}$ = _____

Solve the following problems and reduce to the lowest term. Be sure to indicate measurement as appropriate.

	Answer	Lowest term

9. $\dfrac{1}{2} + \dfrac{3}{4} =$ _____   _____

10. $\dfrac{25}{75} + \dfrac{25}{125} =$ _____   _____

11. $\dfrac{4}{10} + \dfrac{6}{8} =$ _____   _____

12. $\dfrac{5}{4} + \dfrac{6}{8} =$ _____   _____

13. $20\dfrac{1}{3} + 10\dfrac{5}{6} =$ _____   _____

14. $\dfrac{7}{9} - \dfrac{2}{3} =$ _____   _____

15. $2\dfrac{4}{5} - 1\dfrac{2}{10} =$ _____   _____

16. $\dfrac{18}{81} - \dfrac{1}{9} =$ _____   _____

17. $gr\, \dfrac{2}{3} + gr\, \dfrac{1}{6} =$ _____   _____

18. $1\dfrac{1}{2}\, c + \dfrac{5}{6}\, c =$ _____   _____

19. $2\dfrac{1}{2}\, tab + \dfrac{3}{4}\, tab =$ _____   _____

20. $gr\, 7\dfrac{1}{2} - gr\, 5\dfrac{1}{5} =$ _____   _____

Adding and Subtracting Fractions

When adding or subtracting fractions, the denominators must be the same numeral. If the denominators are the same number, the numerators may either be added or subtracted (e.g., $\frac{3}{5}$ + $\frac{1}{5}$ can be added by adding the numerators, or 3 and 1 [3 + 1] and placing the answer over the denominator of 5. This provides an answer of $\frac{4}{5}$. To subtract $\frac{3}{5}$ − $\frac{1}{5}$, subtract 1 from 3 [3 − 1]/5 for an answer of $\frac{2}{5}$).

Finding Common Denominators

For denominators to be the same for adding or subtracting fractions, the lowest common denominator, must be found. The smallest whole number that can be divided evenly by the denominators within the problem is the common denominator. Sometimes the lowest common denominator is easily found because one denominator is readily divided by the other denominator. For example, a common denominator for $\frac{3}{5}$ + $\frac{2}{15}$ could easily be found because 15 is divisible by 5. To change $\frac{3}{5}$ to the common denominator, divide the denominator 5 into the denominator 15 (3); then multiply the 3 (numerator) times 3 to calculate $\frac{9}{15}$. Therefore $\frac{9}{15}$ + $\frac{2}{15}$ would provide an answer of $\frac{11}{15}$.

TECH NOTE

When estimating fractions, use 0, $\frac{1}{4}$, $\frac{1}{2}$, $\frac{3}{4}$, 1, and so on to estimate the answer with any calculations with fractions. Estimate either slightly larger or slightly smaller numbers. Remember that this is an estimate not a specific answer. It is for comparison for your exact answer.

LEARNING TIP

Estimation, even if mentally calculated, is important in accuracy with calculation of doses and dosages later. Please practice this as you go through this section as means to be sure your answer is reasonable. First estimate, then compute, and then check your answer to the estimation.

To change fractions to their equivalent fractions for adding or subtracting of fractions, first find the lowest common denominator and divide the denominator of the fraction to be changed into the lowest common denominator. Then multiply the numerator of the fraction being changed by the quotient found in the first step. Finally, place the product or answer found in this step over the lowest common denominator. In the previous example, in $\frac{3}{5}$ + $\frac{2}{15}$, the lowest common denominator is 15. The problem with the common denominator is $\frac{9}{15}$ (15 ÷ 5 = 3; 3 × 3 = 9; so $\frac{3}{5}$ = $\frac{9}{15}$) + $\frac{2}{15}$ = $\frac{11}{15}$.

EXAMPLE 2-9

$$\frac{3}{10} + \frac{3}{5} = ?$$

The fraction $\frac{3}{10}$ is okay. The common denominator for both fractions will be 10.

10 is divisible by 5; 2 × 5 = 10

So, the fraction $\frac{3}{5} = \frac{6}{10}$

$$\frac{3}{10} + \frac{6}{10} = \frac{9}{10}$$

LEARNING TIP

Numbers ending in even numbers are divisible by 2; numbers ending in 5 or 0 are divisible by 5; and numbers ending in 0 are divisible by 10.

If a mixed number is in the expression, the mixed number should be changed to an improper fraction before finding the common numerical denominator. Then change both fractions to the lowest common denominator and add or subtract as indicated. For example, $\frac{3}{4} + 3\frac{5}{8} = $ _____ ($3\frac{5}{8} = \frac{29}{8}$), so now the problem is simply $\frac{3}{4} + \frac{29}{8}$. The next step is to find the lowest common denominator; in this problem it is 8; $8 \div 4 = 2$; $2 \times 3 = 6$; leading to the fraction $\frac{6}{8}$. The problem is now $\frac{6}{8} + \frac{29}{8} = \frac{35}{8}$. This improper fraction can then be converted back to the mixed number of $4\frac{3}{8}$ ($35 \div 8 = 4$ with a remainder of 3 or $4\frac{3}{8}$). Here is one more example: $\frac{5}{6} + 2\frac{11}{12}$. First, change the mixed number to an improper fraction ($12 \times 2 + 11 = \frac{35}{12}$). The problem now becomes $\frac{5}{6} + \frac{35}{12}$. The lowest common denominator is 12. To convert $\frac{5}{6}$ using the lowest common denominator would be $\frac{10}{12}$ ($12 \div 6 = 2$; $2 \times 5 = 10$; so $\frac{5}{6} = \frac{10}{12}$). Next, $\frac{10}{12} + \frac{35}{12} = \frac{45}{12}$, or $3\frac{9}{12}$ ($45 \div 12 = 3$ with a remainder of 9, or $3\frac{9}{12}$ or $3\frac{3}{4}$). In this problem the fraction may be reduced.

TECH NOTE

When reducing fractions or when finding a common denominator, the numerator and the denominator must be divided by the same nonzero number. For example, $\frac{3}{12}$ can be reduced to $\frac{1}{4}$ by dividing the numerator and denominator by 3.

Practice Problems F

Solve the following problems and reduce fractions to the lowest term as appropriate. Show all of your calculations. Be sure to indicate measurement as appropriate.

1. $\dfrac{1}{3} + \dfrac{1}{3} = $ _____

2. $\dfrac{3}{8} + \dfrac{4}{8} = $ _____

3. $\dfrac{2}{7} + \dfrac{3}{7} = $ _____

4. $\dfrac{3}{10} + \dfrac{4}{10} = $ _____

5. $\dfrac{1}{6} + \dfrac{4}{6} = $ _____

6. $\dfrac{5}{8} - \dfrac{1}{8} = $ _____

7. $\dfrac{8}{9} - \dfrac{5}{9} = $ _____

8. $\dfrac{13}{15} - \dfrac{10}{15} = $ _____

9. $\dfrac{6}{7} - \dfrac{5}{7} = $ _____

10. $\text{gr } \dfrac{1}{4} + \text{gr } \dfrac{1}{4} = $ _____

11. $\text{gr } \dfrac{1}{3} + \text{gr } \dfrac{1}{3} =$ _____

12. $\dfrac{3}{8}\,c + \dfrac{2}{8}\,c =$ _____

13. $\text{gr } \dfrac{5}{8} - \text{gr } \dfrac{1}{8} =$ _____

14. $\dfrac{5}{6}\,c - \dfrac{1}{6}\,c =$ _____

15. $\dfrac{7}{8}\,\text{oz} - \dfrac{1}{8}\,\text{oz} =$ _____

16. $1\dfrac{1}{3} + \dfrac{4}{9} =$ _____

17. $3\dfrac{2}{3} + 1\dfrac{3}{5} =$ _____

18. $1\dfrac{3}{16} + 2\dfrac{3}{8} =$ _____

19. $\dfrac{4}{7} + \dfrac{3}{11} =$ _____

20. $\dfrac{5}{12} + \dfrac{3}{4} =$ _____

21. $3\dfrac{1}{8} + \dfrac{2}{3} =$ _____

22. $\dfrac{2}{3}\,c + \dfrac{1}{6}\,c =$ _____

23. $\dfrac{1}{3}\,\text{tsp} + \dfrac{1}{6}\,\text{tsp} =$ _____

24. $2\dfrac{1}{2}\,\text{qt} + \dfrac{1}{4}\,\text{qt} =$ _____

25. $\text{gr } \dfrac{1}{100} + \text{gr } \dfrac{1}{150} =$ _____

26. $\dfrac{1}{8}\,\text{qt} + \dfrac{3}{4}\,\text{qt} =$ _____

27. $3\dfrac{1}{2}\,c + 5\dfrac{1}{8}\,c =$ _____

28. $3\dfrac{1}{4} - 2\dfrac{1}{4} =$ _____

29. $4\dfrac{1}{5} - 2\dfrac{9}{10} =$ _____

30. $5\dfrac{5}{16} - 2\dfrac{3}{16} =$ _____

31. $5\dfrac{2}{3} - 3\dfrac{3}{8} =$ _____

32. $3\dfrac{3}{8} - 1\dfrac{1}{2} =$ _____

33. $3\dfrac{1}{4} - 1\dfrac{3}{16} =$ _____

34. $1\dfrac{7}{8}$ c $- 1\dfrac{3}{16}$ c $=$ _____

35. $2\dfrac{3}{8}$ tsp $- 1\dfrac{1}{6}$ tsp $=$ _____

36. $4\dfrac{3}{4}$ qt $- \dfrac{1}{16}$ qt $=$ _____

37. gr $1\dfrac{1}{2} -$ gr $\dfrac{3}{4} =$ _____

38. gr $2\dfrac{1}{2} -$ gr $1\dfrac{1}{16} =$ _____

39. $3\dfrac{5}{16}$ # $- 1\dfrac{3}{8}$ # $=$ _____

40. $12\dfrac{1}{2}$ oz $- 6\dfrac{3}{4}$ oz $=$ _____

41. A bottle of medication granules contains $12\frac{1}{2}$ oz of the desired medication. A newer medication container holds $11^{15}\!/_{16}$ oz of the medication. A customer asks you to calculate the difference in the amount of medication in the two bottles. What is your answer? _____

42. You are using a gallon bottle of distilled water to reconstitute dry antibiotics. The first medication requires $\frac{1}{8}$ gallon. The second medication uses $\frac{1}{24}$ gallon. The third medication needs $\frac{1}{12}$ of a gallon. What is the total amount of distilled water used? _____

43. How much distilled water is left in the container? *Hint: Remember that a fraction for a whole number has the same numerator and denominator.* _____

44. The pharmacist asks you to find the common denominator for medications expressed in grains. You have prescriptions for gr $\frac{1}{4}$, gr $\frac{1}{6}$, and gr $\frac{3}{4}$. Express the medication doses in a common denominator. _____ What is the total amount that has been used? _____ If the total medication is gr v, how many grains are left following the completion of the prescription preparations? _____

45. You have $3\frac{3}{4}$ oz of a specific medication. In a day, you have used $2\frac{3}{16}$ oz of that medication. How much medication will you have left for use to fill prescriptions the next day? _____

Multiplying Fractions

Multiplication of fractions is straightforward. To find the product of fractions, multiply the numerators and then the denominators. The product should then be reduced to the lowest term. The calculations are easier than with addition or subtraction, which require a common denominator. For example, $\frac{5}{6} \times \frac{3}{5}$ ($5 \times 3 = 15; 6 \times 5 = 30$) $= \frac{15}{30}$. In this example, 15 is a number that can be used to reduce to lowest terms ($15 \div 15 = 1; 30 \div 15 = 2$), giving the final answer of $\frac{1}{2}$.

When multiplying or dividing fractions, you may shorten the steps by simplifying the numbers before finding the final product. If the numbers in the numerator and denominator can be divided by a common number, this step should be accomplished before multiplying the fractions. When completing this step, the numerator and denominator are on opposite sides of the "×". An example follows:

$$\frac{1}{4} \times \frac{4}{5} \qquad \frac{1}{\cancel{4}_1} \times \frac{\cancel{4}^1}{5} = \frac{1}{5}$$

> **TECH NOTE**
>
> Remember that to multiply (or divide) mixed numbers, you must change the mixed number to an improper fraction (e.g., $3\frac{1}{6}$ would be changed to $\frac{19}{6}$ by multiplying 3×6 and adding the 1 in the numerator of the fraction, with the denominator remaining the same).

Dividing Fractions

To divide fractions or mixed numbers, you must change the mixed numbers to improper fractions. The next step in the multiple-step process is **inversion** (turn the fraction upside down) of the divisor (or the second number in the expression, which is the number to the right of the division sign) so that the numerator now becomes the denominator. For example, if $\frac{4}{5}$ is inverted, the fraction would become $\frac{5}{4}$. In the problem $\frac{1}{2} \div \frac{2}{3}$ ($\frac{2}{3}$ is the number to be inverted), the problem becomes $\frac{1}{2} \times \frac{3}{2}$ after the inversion of the numbers. After the inversion is complete, the remainder of the problem is actually multiplication of fractions. Remember to cancel any numbers that can be simplified to make the problem easier to solve. (Canceling numbers was shown earlier with the multiplication example.) To cancel a number, divide both the numerator and the denominator by a common number that will divide into both numbers evenly, or without a remainder. This is a shortcut used to reduce the value of the numerals in the fractions for ease of calculation. (Cancellation is used when fractions are being multiplied. Canceling cannot be accomplished if sums or differences are in numerators or denominators. If you question whether you can cancel, do not do it.) Then reduce the fraction further if this is possible. In the previous example, solving the problem gives an answer of $\frac{3}{4}$. Another example is $\frac{4}{5} \div \frac{5}{10} = ?$ In this example, the problem is now $\frac{4}{5} \times \frac{10}{5}$ or simplified to 4×2 ($10 \div 5$) $= 8$, and 1 ($5 \div 5$) $\times 5 = 5$, so the fraction is $\frac{8}{5}$. This can be changed to a mixed number of $1\frac{3}{5}$.

> **TECH NOTE**
>
> In division of fractions, after inverting the numerator and denominator of the fraction to the right of the division sign, continue with the steps as for multiplication—multiply the numerators and multiply the denominators, placing the products with the numerators over the denominators. Finally, reduce the resultant fraction to the lowest possible terms.

Practice Problems G

In the following problems, perform the multiplication or division and then reduce the fractions to the lowest terms. Show all of your calculations. Indicate measurement as appropriate.

1. $\dfrac{2}{3} \times \dfrac{3}{5} =$ _____

2. $\dfrac{1}{8} \times \dfrac{6}{9} =$ _____

3. $\dfrac{3}{5} \times \dfrac{5}{8} =$ _____

4. $\dfrac{3}{25} \times \dfrac{15}{21} =$ _____

5. $\dfrac{1}{3} \times \dfrac{3}{4} =$ _____

6. $\dfrac{1}{3} \times \dfrac{4}{5} =$ _____

7. $\dfrac{7}{12} \times \dfrac{5}{9} =$ _____

8. $\dfrac{3}{8} \times \dfrac{1}{3} =$ _____

9. $\text{gr } \dfrac{1}{4} \times \text{gr } \dfrac{1}{2} =$ _____

10. $\dfrac{2}{3} \text{ c} \times \dfrac{1}{8} \text{ c} =$ _____

11. $\dfrac{7}{8} \text{ c} \times \dfrac{5}{6} \text{ c} =$ _____

12. $1\dfrac{1}{2} \text{ qt} \times \dfrac{5}{6} \text{ qt} =$ _____

13. $\dfrac{9}{10} \text{ L} \times \dfrac{7}{8} \text{ L} =$ _____

14. $\dfrac{5}{12} \text{ oz} \times \dfrac{6}{7} \text{ oz} =$ _____

15. $2\dfrac{1}{3} \times 3\dfrac{4}{5} =$ _____

16. $5\dfrac{6}{7} \times \dfrac{7}{8} =$ _____

17. $4\dfrac{3}{4} \times 3\dfrac{5}{9} =$ _____

18. $1\dfrac{3}{8} \times 7\dfrac{8}{9} =$ _____

19. $8\dfrac{1}{9} \times 2\dfrac{3}{4} =$ _____

20. $5\dfrac{1}{4} \times 6\dfrac{4}{5} =$ _____

21. $2\dfrac{3}{4}$ c $\times 5\dfrac{1}{2}$ c = _____

22. $1\dfrac{2}{5}$ tsp $\times 2\dfrac{3}{4}$ tsp = _____

23. $66\dfrac{1}{2}$ # $\times 4\dfrac{1}{2}$ # = _____

24. $1\dfrac{7}{8}$ oz $\times 3\dfrac{5}{6}$ oz = _____

25. gr $3\dfrac{1}{2}$ $\times$ gr $7\dfrac{1}{2}$ = _____

26. $2\dfrac{1}{3}$ c $\times 5\dfrac{3}{4}$ c = _____

27. $\dfrac{9}{10} \div \dfrac{2}{5}$ = _____

28. $\dfrac{2}{5} \div \dfrac{3}{4}$ = _____

29. $3 \div \dfrac{1}{3}$ = _____

30. $\dfrac{1}{4} \div 3$ = _____

31. $\dfrac{3}{4} \div \dfrac{4}{7}$ = _____

32. $\dfrac{3}{4} \div \dfrac{8}{9}$ = _____

33. gr $\dfrac{1}{4} \div$ gr $\dfrac{1}{2}$ = _____

34. gr $\dfrac{1}{3} \div$ gr $\dfrac{1}{4}$ = _____

35. $\dfrac{1}{8}$ c $\div \dfrac{1}{6}$ c = _____

36. $4 \div \dfrac{3}{4}$ = _____

37. $5\dfrac{1}{3} \div \dfrac{2}{6}$ = _____

38. $4\dfrac{1}{3} \div 2\dfrac{2}{25}$ = _____

39. $4\dfrac{4}{5} \div 6\dfrac{1}{10}$ = _____

40. $7\dfrac{2}{3} \div 2\dfrac{2}{5}$ = _____

41. $4\dfrac{3}{4} \div 3\dfrac{1}{6}$ = _____

42. gr $\dfrac{1}{6} \div$ gr $\dfrac{1}{3}$ = _____

43. $\text{gr } 1\dfrac{1}{2} \div \text{gr } \dfrac{1}{4} = $ _____

44. $\text{gr } 5 \div \text{gr } 1\dfrac{1}{2} = $ _____

45. $1\dfrac{1}{2} \text{ c} \div \dfrac{1}{6} \text{ c} = $ _____

46. $1\dfrac{3}{4} \text{ qt} \div \dfrac{1}{4} \text{ qt} = $ _____

47. $7\dfrac{1}{2} \text{ tsp} \div 1\dfrac{1}{2} \text{ tsp} = $ _____

48. A medication order is for gr 2¼ of a drug to be given tid. You have gr ¾ tabs in stock. How many tablets would you give with each dose? _____ How many tablets would you give in a day? _____ How many tablets would you need to fill this prescription for a 30-day supply? _____

49. Your stock bottle of medication contains 500 tablets. You have used ¾ of the bottle. How many tablets do you have left in stock for filling future prescriptions? _____

50. A bottle of liquid antibiotic contains 150 mL of medication or 30 teaspoons. If each dose is 1½ tsp, how many doses are in the bottle? _____. If the medication is given four times a day, how many days will this medication last? _____

DECIMALS

What Is a Decimal?

Decimals, special shorthand for fractions of powers of 10, are actually decimal fractions or fractions that have a denominator of 10, 100, 1000, or any multiple of the power of 10. Decimals appear to be whole numbers, but actually the decimal value is always less than 1. Decimal numbers may include a whole number, a decimal point, and the decimal fraction. The metric system, the most frequently used measurement system in the medical field, is based on the use of decimals. Using a decimal is simpler to read than fractions and is easier to use when making mathematical computations. Examples of decimals include $0.1 = \frac{1}{10}$, $0.01 = \frac{1}{100}$, or $0.001 = \frac{1}{1000}$.

IMPORTANT SAFETY TIP

To avoid errors in the medical field, a decimal should never stand on its own but should be preceded by a "0" if a whole number is not before the decimal point. For example, .25 should be shown as 0.25, or .5 as 0.5. A medical professional should never write ".25" because the decimal could get lost in the prescription or the physician's order, and the amount of medication prescribed could be inaccurate. Such an inaccuracy of a highly increased dosage could be deadly to the person taking the medicine. (In the case of the example, the patient would receive 100 times the ordered amount of medication.)

When using the decimal system, think of the decimal point as the division between whole numbers that appear to the left of the decimal point and the decimal fraction that is found to the right of the decimal point. In the example 25.65, 25 is the whole number and 65 is 65 parts of 100 or $^{65}/_{100}$. (The decimal number is made into a fractional mixed number of 25 65/100.) With decimals, the numerator is the number following the decimal point. This number is placed over a number consisting of 1 followed by the number of zeros found in the number of the numerator. Thus 3.7 is $3^{7}/_{10}$. With decimals, zeros may be added to or deleted from the end of the decimal without changing the actual value of the number. Thus 3.7 is the same value as 3.70 or 3.700. Likewise 5.050 is the same value as 5.05.

Decimal Line

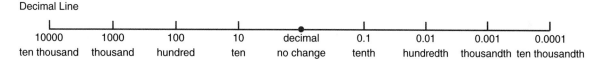

| 10000 | 1000 | 100 | 10 | decimal | 0.1 | 0.01 | 0.001 | 0.0001 |
| ten thousand | thousand | hundred | ten | no change | tenth | hundredth | thousandth | ten thousandth |

To write decimals using word names, the number to the left will be a whole number and the decimal point becomes the word "and," with the number to the right of the **decimal place** followed by the place values of the decimal ending with "th." For example, 3.47 would be three and forty-seven hundredths. Another example: 1.250 would be one and two hundred fifty thousandths; 4.5006 would be four and five thousand six ten thousandths.

Three	the number to the left of the decimal point
and	the decimal point
Forty-seven	the number to the right of the decimal point
Hundredths	the place value of the decimal

AND

One	the number to the left of the decimal point
and	the decimal point
Two hundred fifty	the number to the right of the decimal point
Thousandths	the place value of the decimal

TECH NOTE

The decimal line may be extended to the right of the decimal point as needed to meet the needs for the decimal places.

Practice Problems H

Write the following decimals into word names.

1. 4.34 _____

2. 3.5 _____

3. 6.750 _____

4. 90.54 _____

5. 954.6 _____

6. 0.0035 _____

7. 4.02 _____

8. 0.26 _____

9. 0.780 _____

10. 0.175 _____

To convert fractions to decimals, divide the numerator by the denominator. For example, ½ is 1 ÷ 2, or 1.0 ÷ 2, because 2 will not divide into 1. Thus 1.0 ÷ 2 = 0.5. Likewise, ¾ is 3 ÷ 4, or 3.0 ÷ 4. Thus 3 ÷ 4 = 0.75 is a decimal answer.

TECH NOTE
Remember that in both of these problems you must place a zero ("0") in front of the decimal point to prevent errors in reading the answer.

To convert a decimal to a fraction, the decimal number becomes the numerator of the fraction and the denominator is a 1 followed by zeros for the number of places to include the decimal and the numbers behind the decimal. For example, 0.25 would be 25 (the decimal number)/100 (a 1 followed by 2 zeros or a zero for the number of places behind the decimal point). Thus 0.25 can be converted to the fraction $\frac{25}{100}$.

TECH NOTE
Decimals are used in calculations of doses and dosage in the metric system and for calculation of dollars/cents in business math.

Practice Problems I

Change the following decimals to fractions. Do not reduce.

1. 0.125 = _____   2. 0.55 = _____   3. 0.33 = _____

4. 0.525 = _____   5. 0.625 = _____   6. 0.05 = _____

7. 0.150 = _____   8. 0.95 = _____   9. 0.1244 = _____

10. 0.042 = _____

Comparing Decimals

To compare a decimal, the decimal amounts must be aligned at the decimal point and zeros should be added so that the numbers behind the decimal point contain the same number of decimal places. This is important in the comparison of medications in the metric system of measurement. Compare 0.125, 0.25, and 0.5. At first glance 0.125 appears to be the largest number, but when the numbers are aligned and the proper zeros are added for numbers to have equal decimal places to the right of the decimal point, this proves to be incorrect.

0.125	one-hundred twenty-five thousandths
0.250	two-hundred fifty thousandths
0.500	five hundred thousandths

The largest number is really 0.5 and not 0.125, which might not seem apparent without the added zeros. Also note that the decimals do not have a whole number to the left of the decimal point, so a zero was added to ensure that the decimal point was not overlooked. The addition of the zero is important to prevent possible confusion and to avoid errors in calculating medication doses.

Rounding Decimals

When figuring dosage calculations, decimals may need to be carried only to a certain number value following the decimal point. Accuracy in calculating dosages to certain decimal places may be necessary in some acute care settings, while, at the same time, **rounding** or approximating a decimal to a certain placement on the value line may be acceptable (see the decimal line in the "What Is a Decimal?" section). Rounding of numbers must never include the whole number to the left of the decimal point. Usually numbers are rounded to tenths or hundredths, either by adding to or subtracting from the decimal. Rounding to a specific place value makes it easier to measure a drug or to compare decimals in stock medicines to medication orders. For example, a calculation for a medication shows that 3.99 mg of a medication should be given to the patient and the drug is available in 4-mg tablets. In this case the patient would receive a tablet by rounding the decimals; 3.99 would be rounded to the whole number 4.

TECH NOTE

Step 1: Underline the digit in the place for rounding.

Step 2: Look at the digit to the right of the underlined digit. If it is greater than or equal to 5, round to the next highest number. If it is less than 5, leave all digits to the right of the underlined digits.

Step 3: Drop all digits to the right of the underlined digit.

To round hundredths to tenths, the same rule of less than 5 and 5 or over applies, but the number being changed is the tenth value. In the previous example, 1.14 would be rounded to 1.1 while 1.15 would become 1.2.

Decimals may also be rounded to the next whole number by rounding from the tenths value (e.g., 3.4 would remain 3, whereas 3.5 would become 4). However, due to the degree of specificity often needed in medical dosing, rounding up or down in this manner is rarely done unless the number is within a small percentage of the next whole number, or, if a product's specific labeling indicates such rounding is preferred for ease of choosing a dosage form or for a measurable amount. It is more common to round dosages to the nearest tenth or hundredth.

For ease in adding decimals, use estimation to find the nearest tenth and add or subtract the rounded numbers. This will give an estimate of the desired answer. Then add the actual numbers; check that your answer is nearly equal to your estimate to be sure that it is reasonable.

Practice Problems J

Round to the nearest hundredth.

1. 2.356 = _____

2. 5.652 = _____

3. 36.445 = _____

4. 2.984 = _____

5. 0.1245 = _____

6. 8.2374 = _____

7. 3.3345 = _____

8. 6.116 = _____

Round to the nearest tenth.

9. 3.45 = _____

10. 3.64 = _____

11. 3.26 = _____

12. 12.14 = _____

13. 3.05 = _____

14. 12.4 mg = _____

15. 1.46 mg = _____

16. 2.54 mg = _____

Round the following to the nearest whole number.

17. 8.75 = _____

18. 9.64 = _____

19. 10.08 = _____

20. 14.16 = _____

21. 1.59 mg = _____

22. 2.55 qt = _____

23. 3.445 mg = _____

24. 1.4674 mg = _____

Adding and Subtracting Decimals

Adding and subtracting of decimals requires aligning whole numbers and decimal points, as you would do with whole numbers. After aligning the decimal points, add zeros at the end of the decimal fraction until all decimal numbers are to the same decimal place. Then just add or subtract as you would for whole numbers, remembering to correctly place the decimal point in the answer. The problem 3.4678 – 2.34, after alignment of the decimal, would look like the following:

$$
\begin{array}{r}
3.4678 \\
- \ 2.34 \\
\hline
\end{array}
$$

To make an equal number of decimal places in the numbers, add zeros behind the numbers following the decimal point.

$$
\begin{array}{r}
3.4678 \\
- \ 2.3400 \\
\hline
1.1278
\end{array}
$$

LEARNING TIP

Zeros may be added as the last number behind a decimal point and in front of the whole number without changing the value of the number. Whole numbers are understood to have a decimal point to the right of the number.

Practice Problems K

In the following problems, add or subtract decimals as indicated. Estimate your possible answer. Show all of your work. Round answers to the nearest hundredth. Be sure to indicate measurement as appropriate.

1. 2.35 + 3.1 + 4.678 = _____

2. 5.7 + 18.25 + 95.37 = _____

3. 2.38 + 14.7 + 1346 = _____

4. 6.002 + 3.23 + 9.1 = _____

5. 9.7 + 5.68 + 3.3 = _____

6. 5.75 + 4.678 + 2 = _____

7. 12.5 mg + 220.25 mg + 2.75 mg = _____

8. 6.75 mg + 125 mg + 4.25 mg = _____

9. $12.50 + $0.42 + $140.67 = _____

10. $5.67 + $136.99 + $89.09 = _____

11. 2.76 – 1.98 = _____

12. 4.8 – 1.987 = _____

13. 1.567 − 0.986 = _____   **14.** 75.3 − 16.95 = _____

15. 18.2 − 4.762 = _____   **16.** 125 − 0.125 = _____

17. $15.75 − $5.65 = _____   **18.** $17.49 − $5.05 = _____

19. 0.2 g − 0.02 g = _____   **20.** 12.5 mg − 10.5 mg = _____

21. 275 mg − 225.5 mg = _____   **22.** 65 mg − 45.5 mg = _____

23. A prescription costs $25.50. The customer gives you two $20 bills. How much change do you owe the customer? _____

24. A stock bottle of medication contains 500 mg of drug used in compounding other medications. You used 125 mg for one prescription and 62.5 mg for a second prescription, while the third prescription was for a child and only 25.25 mg were necessary. What quantity medication has been used? _____ What quantity of the original medication is left? _____

25. A customer has three prescriptions—one costing $35, the second costing $17.50, and the third costing $23.60. To pay for the prescriptions, the person gives you four $20 bills. Is this enough money for the prescriptions? _____ What is the total cost of the prescriptions? _____ If this is enough money, how much change do you need to return to the person? If you do not have enough money, how much more money is necessary to cover the costs? _____ Indicate if money is returned to the person or if more money is needed _____.

Multiplying Decimals

Multiplying decimals is similar to multiplying whole numbers. The alignment of the numbers is identical without having a relationship to the placement of the decimal. The difference is the proper placement of the decimal place after the product of the multiplication has been found. To multiply decimals, multiply the numbers after aligning calculations the numbers to the right and disregard the placement of the decimal. After the product of the multiplication of the multiplicand and the multiplier have been found, count the number of places to the right of the decimal points in both the multiplicand and the multiplier. Finally, place a decimal point in the product by counting from the right to left the number of decimal places found in both elements of the problem. An example follows.

```
    37.25  (2 decimal places)      OR          12.5  (1 decimal place)
 ×    1.5  (1 decimal place)             ×     3.75  (2 decimal places)
   18625                                        625
    3725                                        875
   55875  (move 3 decimal places to left)      375
                                              46875  (move 3 decimal places to left)
   OR
                                                OR
   55.875
                                              46.875
```

Zeros may be removed from the right end of a decimal number (to the right of the decimal point) without changing the value of the number; therefore if the multiplier has zeros at the end, remove the zeros and then multiply. This step simplifies the multiplication. For example, if multiplying 7.350 × 0.20, cancel the zeros (7.35Ø ×0.2Ø) so that the problem now looks like 7.35 × 0.2 or an answer of 1.470. The zero in the answer should then be canceled (1.47Ø) to give the final answer of 1.47.

If the multiplier is 10 or a multiple of 10 (e.g., 100, 1000, etc.), a shortcut in multiplying is to just move the decimal places as many places to the right as there are zeros in the multiplier, or 12.2×10 = 122.Ø, or just move the decimal point one space to the right in the 12.2. or 122. If the multiplier is 100, then the decimal would be moved 2 places; with 1000, 3 places, etc.

Practice Problems L

Calculate the following, being sure to show your calculations. Estimate the answer prior to figuring the final answer. Cancel zeros as appropriate in the final answer and round to hundredths. Be sure to indicate measurement as appropriate.

1. 65.3 × 10 = _____

2. 13.2 × 100 = _____

3. 4.25 × 10 = _____

4. 0.004 × 100 = _____

5. 0.2 × 1000 = _____

6. 16.5 × 0.5 = _____

7. $23.52 \times 0.5 =$ _____

8. $0.35 \times 0.45 =$ _____

9. $59.5 \times 39.99 =$ _____

10. $2.5 \text{ mg} \times 1.5 \text{ mg} =$ _____

11. $1.25 \text{ mg} \times 5 \text{ mg} =$ _____

12. $2.5 \text{ mL} \times 30 \text{ mL} =$ _____

13. $\$0.50 \times \$10.00 =$ _____

14. $2.5 \text{ qt} \times 0.75 \text{ qt} =$ _____

15. $18.5 \text{ mg} \times 15 \text{ mg} =$ _____

16. $35 \text{ g} \times 12.5 \text{ g} =$ _____

17. $0.005 \text{ mg} \times 1 \text{ mg} =$ _____

18. A physician orders 2.5 mg of a drug that is to be taken daily for 10 days. What is the total amount of the drug the patient will be taking? _____

19. A mother will give her child 2.5 mL of an antipyretic every 4 hours for fever. If the child is given the medication six times during the day, how many milliliters of medication will the child receive in a day? _____

20. You have a stock bottle of medication that contains 12.25 mg of medication. You have five bottles of the medication available. How many total milligrams of medication are available for dispensing? _____

Dividing Decimals

Dividing decimals is much like dividing whole numbers. Write the problem as for long division, such as the following:

$$\text{divisor}\overline{)\text{dividend}}^{\text{quotient}}$$

For example, if 2.50 is to be divided by 1.25, the problem should appear as $1.25\overline{)2.50}$. If a decimal appears in the divisor, move the decimal to the right until the divisor is a whole number. Then move the decimal point in the dividend the same number of places to the right. For example, in the previous example, the problem would appear as $125\overline{)250}$ when the decimals in the divisor and dividend are both moved ($1.25\overline{)2.50}$). Place a decimal point on the quotient (answer) line directly above the decimal point in the dividend and add zeros behind the decimal point in the dividend if more places are necessary for dividing. The answer is then 2. For example, $1 \div 5$ would be $5\overline{)1}$. In this problem, 5 cannot be divided into 1, so the problem must become $5\overline{)1.0}$ or 0.2 by placing the decimal point directly over the decimal point in the dividend and then dividing. Remember that if a whole number is not in front of the decimal point, a zero must be added to prevent medication errors. Another example would be $40.44 \div 0.4$, which, when placed in the long division format, would be $0.4\overline{)40.44}$. Next, move the decimal in the divisor to the whole number 4 and move the decimal in the dividend to 404.4. For $4\overline{)404.4}$, the answer is 101.1. Be sure to fill in the 0 in the quotient when the number cannot be divided by the divisor, as in the "0" in 101.1.

In some cases the division does not come out even, such as when 3 is divided into 1. The answer will be $0.333\overline{3}$ to the number of places that zeros are added to the dividend. In these cases, the number may be shown with a 3 with a line over the 3, meaning $\overline{3}$ is a repeating number. In this case in the medical field, the 3 should be rounded to the hundredth place or 0.33. Again, remember to place the 0 in front of the decimal point.

Practice Problems M

Calculate the following problems. Show your work. Be sure to indicate measurement as appropriate.

1. $268.4 \div 4 =$ _____

2. $125 \div 0.25 =$ _____

3. $1.5 \div 0.3 =$ _____

4. $19.95 \div 10.5 =$ _____

5. $33.03 \div 0.03 =$ _____

6. $15.66 \div 0.44 =$ _____

7. $25.5 \text{ mg} \div 15 \text{ mg} =$ _____

8. $2.5 \text{ g} \div 0.5 \text{ g} =$ _____

9. $\$24.68 \div \$0.40 =$ _____

10. $\$24.65 \div \$0.15 =$ _____

11. $10.50 ÷ $0.10 = _____

12. 120 mg ÷ 100 mg = _____

13. 2500 mL ÷ 100 mL = _____

14. 2.5 L ÷ 0.5 L = _____

15. 12.5 g ÷ 50 g = _____

16. 1.25 mg ÷ 5 mg = _____

17. $124.80 ÷ $4.40 = _____

18. 1.174 L ÷ 0.33 L = _____

19. A pharmacist has a stock bottle of medication containing 12.5 mL. To use this with prescriptions, the pharmacist will need to divide the medication into five equal parts. How many milliliters will be in each? _____

20. A customer comes to the pharmacy to obtain an expensive medication that contains 250 mg/25 mL. This medication can be divided into several prescriptions for ease of payment. She states that the total amount of medication, which costs $255.30, needs to be divided into five equal dispensing units. How many milligrams of medication will be dispensed each time? _____. How many milliliters of medication will be dispensed? _____. How much will the customer pay for each prescription? _____

POINTS TO REMEMBER

DECIMALS

- Always place a zero before a decimal if no whole number is present.
- If dividing decimals and the number is a repeating one in the quotient, round to the nearest hundredth (e.g., $1.66\overline{6}$ would be 1.67).
- When adding or subtracting decimals, always align decimal points and add zeros behind the decimal point if necessary to have decimal places the same length. Adding zeros behind the last decimal number does not change its value.
- When multiplying decimals, multiply the numbers together and then count the number of decimal places in the numbers multiplied and place the decimal point in the product (answer) to the left of the total number of places counted.
- To divide decimal fractions, form a whole number in the divisor by moving the decimal point to the right, then move the decimal point in the dividend (number to be divided) the same number of decimal places to the right that has been moved in the divisor. Place the decimal point in the quotient (answer) directly over the decimal point in the dividend and divide as if the numbers are whole numbers.

- When multiplying by 10 or multiples of 10 (e.g., 100 or 1000), the only step necessary is to move the decimal point in the product (answer) to the right by the number of zeros in the multiplier.
- To divide by 10 or a multiple of 10, the decimal point in the quotient (answer) may be moved to the left by the number of zeros in the divisor.

PERCENTAGES

TECH NOTE

In pharmacology, percentages are used to find the volume of solute in the solvent when preparing liquid medications, to find the amount of medication that has been administered over a given amount of time, discounts, and inventory control.

Converting a Decimal to a Percentage

A percentage is actually a part of 100 in fractions or hundredths in decimals. To express a fraction as a percent (%), the denominator is 100 and the numerator is the part of 100 found within the percent. For example, 5% would be $\frac{5}{100}$ or 5 parts of 100.

To convert a decimal to a percentage, multiply by 100 (which results in the decimal place being moved). The decimal point is moved two places to the right, and a percent sign is added. To convert 0.50 to a percentage, move the decimal two places to the right (0.50) by multiplying by 100 and add the % sign. So 0.50 is equal to 50%. If the decimal does not have two places to the right of the decimal point, you must add a zero so that the decimal point can be moved two places because two decimal places are needed to multiply by 100; 0.5 would need a zero added (0.50) and then the decimal point should be moved two places (0.50) so that 0.5 becomes 50%. Finally, if the number is a whole number such as 5, two zeros must be added to the number to find the percentage. Thus 5, when multiplying by 100, two zeros would be added (5.00), and 5 would become 500%.

LEARNING TIP

To remember the direction in which to move the decimal point when changing from a decimal number to a percentage or vice versa think of the alphabet: A-Z. D stands for decimal point while P stands for percent. To get from D to P in the alphabet you move to the right (D → P). So to change a decimal number to a percent, move the decimal point to the right. If you want to change a percentage number to a decimal number move from P to D (D ← P). To change from a percent to a decimal move decimal point from right to left.

Practice Problems N

Convert the following decimals to percentages. Show your calculations.

1. 0.25 = _____ %   **2.** 0.68 = _____ %   **3.** 0.025 = _____ %

4. 0.6 = _____ %   **5.** 0.555 = _____ %   **6.** 5.56 = _____ %

7. 0.7 = _____ %   **8.** 6 = _____ %   **9.** 10.4 = _____ %

10. 23.67 = _____ %   **11.** 12.1 = _____ %   **12.** 13 = _____ %

13. 105 = _____ %   **14.** 2.3 = _____ %   **15.** 21.50 = _____ %

16. 3.45 = _____ %   **17.** 1.025 = _____ %   **18.** 4.67 = _____ %

19. 0.467 = _____ %   **20.** 46.7 = _____ %

Converting Percentage to a Decimal

Remember that % actually means parts per 100. To convert a percentage to a decimal, drop the percent sign and divide the number by 100 (the dividend being the number in the percentage and the divisor being 100). This can actually be accomplished by moving the decimal point two places to the left. (This was discussed in dividing by multiples of 10 in the section on dividing decimals.) For example, 25% would become 0.25 by removing the % sign and moving the decimal (.25). An example is 25% = $^{25}/_{100}$ (or 25 ÷ 100) = 0.25. Remember, to prevent errors, always place a zero in front of the decimal place if no whole number is present. As with changing a decimal to a percentage, zeros may be added in front of the number as needed so that the two decimal places may be moved (e.g., 8% would become 0.08 [0.08] in decimals or 8/100).

If the number is already a decimal percentage, adding two zeros in front of the decimal point will allow the change to a decimal; for instance, 0.8% would need two zeros to become a decimal. In this problem, 0.8% would be 0.008 (0.008 or 0.8 divided by 100).

Finally, if the percentage is more than 100%, a whole number will be apparent in front of the decimal places (e.g., 255 is actually 255.0 in the decimal system, so moving the decimal to percentage would be 25500% [25500.0]). The moving of the decimal point is the same as with numbers less than 100%. If 155% is converted to a decimal, drop the percent sign and move the decimal two places to the left, or 155% = 1.55 (1.55).

Practice Problems ○

Convert the following percentages to decimals. Show your calculations.

1. 60% = _____

2. 3% = _____

3. 78% = _____

4. 128% = _____

5. 1.3% = _____

6. 325% = _____

7. 0.05% = _____

8. 0.3% = _____

9. 32% = _____

10. 7% = _____

11. 8.2% = _____

12. 1245% = _____

13. 56% = _____

14. 362.5% = _____

15. 14.6% = _____

16. 0.06% = _____

17. 12.5% = _____

18. 3.5% = _____

19. 0.78% = _____

20. 0.5402% = _____

Converting a Fractional Percentage to a Decimal

To change a fractional percentage to a decimal, first convert the fraction to a decimal and round to the nearest hundredth, leaving the percent sign as part of the number. Then convert the percentage to a decimal as you would with other percentages to decimal numbers. For example, ½% would first need to be converted to 0.5% (1 ÷ 2 = 0.5). Then convert the 0.5% to a decimal by moving the decimal two places to the left while adding the necessary zeros, or ½% = 0.005 (0.005). Remember that the calculation is actually dividing by 100.

Practice Problems P

Convert the following fractional percentages to decimals. Show your calculations. Round to the nearest 10000th.

1. $\frac{1}{3}\%$ = _____

2. $\frac{1}{4}\%$ = _____

3. $\frac{3}{4}\%$ = _____

4. $\frac{1}{8}\%$ = _____

5. $\frac{5}{6}\%$ = _____

6. $1\frac{1}{4}\%$ = _____

7. $2\frac{1}{4}\%$ = _____

8. $\frac{4}{5}\%$ = _____

9. $2\frac{1}{8}\%$ = _____

10. $\frac{3}{7}\%$ = _____

11. $3\frac{1}{3}\%$ = _____

12. $\frac{1}{7}\%$ = _____

13. $5\frac{1}{3}\%$ = _____

14. $\frac{3}{5}\%$ = _____

15. $3\frac{5}{6}\%$ = _____

16. $\frac{3}{8}\%$ = _____

17. $4\frac{2}{5}\%$ = _____

18. $1\frac{5}{6}\%$ = _____

19. $\frac{7}{8}\%$ = _____

20. $\frac{1}{5}\%$ = _____

Converting a Fraction to a Percentage

Remember that the denominator in a percentage is always 100 (because percent is a part of 100) and the number beside the % sign becomes the numerator. To convert a fraction to a percentage, multiply the fraction by 100 or by $^{100}\!/_1$ (the fraction for 100) and add the percent sign (%). This is the same step that was used to convert a fraction to a decimal. If the division is not even, round to ten-thousandths before converting the decimal to a percentage.

EXAMPLE 2-10

$$\frac{1}{5} = \underline{\hspace{2cm}}\% \qquad \frac{1}{\cancel{5}_1} \times \frac{\cancel{100}^{20}}{1} = \frac{20}{1} \qquad \frac{1}{5} = 20\%$$

If the fraction is a mixed number, change the mixed number to an improper fraction and then multiply by 100. For example, $2\frac{3}{5} = 5 \times 2 + \frac{3}{5}$ or $\frac{13}{5}$. Then multiply by 100:

$$\frac{13}{5} \times \frac{100}{1} \quad \text{or} \quad \frac{1300}{5}$$

$$\frac{\cancel{1300}^{260}}{\cancel{5}_1} = 260$$

Now divide this answer by 100 to change to decimal: $260 = 2.60\%$ (2.6% after rounding)

Remember that "0" at the end of a decimal is dropped.

TECH NOTE

Conversions of fractions to percentage may also be calculated using ratio and proportion such as $a:b::x\,(\%):100$. This is discussed in the next section of the chapter under ratio and proportion.

Practice Problems Q

Convert the following fractions and mixed numbers to percentages. Show your calculations. Round to hundreths as appropriate.

1. $\frac{1}{6} = \underline{\hspace{2cm}}\%$ **2.** $\frac{3}{7} = \underline{\hspace{2cm}}\%$ **3.** $\frac{2}{5} = \underline{\hspace{2cm}}\%$

4. $\frac{5}{9} = \underline{\hspace{2cm}}\%$ **5.** $\frac{11}{12} = \underline{\hspace{2cm}}\%$ **6.** $\frac{5}{22} = \underline{\hspace{2cm}}\%$

7. $\frac{2}{3} = \underline{\hspace{2cm}}\%$ **8.** $2\frac{1}{3} = \underline{\hspace{2cm}}\%$ **9.** $6\frac{4}{5} = \underline{\hspace{2cm}}\%$

10. $\frac{9}{40} = \underline{\hspace{2cm}}\%$ **11.** $5\frac{5}{6} = \underline{\hspace{2cm}}\%$ **12.** $\frac{3}{8} = \underline{\hspace{2cm}}\%$

13. $5\frac{1}{4} = \underline{\hspace{2cm}}\%$ **14.** $\frac{7}{8} = \underline{\hspace{2cm}}\%$ **15.** $1\frac{2}{3} = \underline{\hspace{2cm}}\%$

16. $\dfrac{5}{6}$ = _____%

17. $4\dfrac{1}{6}$ = _____%

18. $6\dfrac{1}{8}$ = _____%

19. $7\dfrac{2}{3}$ = _____%

20. $\dfrac{4}{5}$ = _____%

Converting a Percentage to a Fraction

To convert a percentage to a fraction, drop the % sign and write the number over 100 (or the percentage number becomes the numerator). The denominator will always be 100. Finally, reduce the fraction to its lowest terms. For example, to change 16% to a fraction, 16% becomes $^{16}/_{100}$ when changed to a fraction. This will reduce to $^{4}/_{25}$. Remember if the fraction is not reduced to the lowest term, it may be considered incorrect.

If the percentage is written as a mixed number, the mixed number becomes the numerator and 100 is the denominator. The mixed number must be changed to an improper fraction placed over 100. For example, to change $2\frac{2}{5}$% to a fraction, first change the mixed number to the improper fraction $^{12}/_{5}$. Remember that when dividing in percentage, you are actually dividing by 100. The fraction is now $^{12}/_{5} \div 100$. To divide fractions, the fraction must be inverted so that the divisor becomes the dividend and the dividend becomes the divisor; thus the equation now is as follows:

$$\dfrac{\cancel{12}^{3}}{5} \times \dfrac{1}{\cancel{100}_{25}} = \dfrac{3}{125} \quad \text{The fraction answer then is } ^{3}/_{125}.$$

Practice Problems R

Convert the following percentages to fractions. Reduce fractions. Show your calculations.

1. 12% = _____

2. 60% = _____

3. $1\dfrac{1}{4}$% = _____

4. $7\dfrac{1}{5}$% = _____

5. 125% = _____

6. 33% = _____

7. $\dfrac{2}{3}$% = _____

8. 75% = _____

9. $1\dfrac{1}{20}$% = _____

10. 80% = _____

11. 0.25% = _____

12. 0.5% = _____

13. 12.5% = _____

14. $4\frac{1}{2}\%$ = _____

15. 0.66% = _____

16. $\frac{1}{4}\%$ = _____

17. 4% = _____

18. $33\frac{1}{3}\%$ = _____

19. 0.025% = _____

20. $\frac{3}{8}\%$ = _____

RATIOS

Expressing Numbers as Ratios

Ratio indicates the relationship of one number to another or a whole. As with fractions, a ratio is expressed as numerators and denominators separated by a colon (:) rather than a division line found in fractions. Numerators are to the left of the colon with denominators to the right, such as 1:2. The colon is the traditional way to write a division sign in a ratio and is representative of "of," "per," "to," or "in." For example, ¾ as a fractional expression would be 3:4 when written in ratio. Like a fraction, a ratio is the relative size of two quantities and should be reduced to lowest terms. Because of the relationship of the numbers in a ratio, the value of the ratio will not be changed if both the numerator and denominator are multiplied or divided by the same number. Multiplication and division are the only numeric operations that can be performed on a ratio without changing its value.

TECH NOTE

A ratio may be written as a fraction, and a fraction may be written as a ratio because each has a numerator and denominator (2:3 or ⅔).

When numbers are expressed in ratios, numbers that designate a quantity must be expressed in the same units of measure. For example, if the numerator of the ratio is expressed in inches, the denominator must also be expressed in inches. So to establish a ratio of 3 inches:1 foot, the 1 foot must be changed to 12 inches (12" = 1 foot). Now the ratio has the same unit of measure in inches and the ratio is 3":12", or the ratio is reduced to 1:4. Thus 3 qts:1 gal (1 gal = 4 qt) becomes 3 qt:4 qt, or the ratio 3:4. Conversions within and among units of measure will be presented in Chapters 3 and 4.

To express a percentage as a ratio, the denominator will always be 100. For example, 30% = ³⁰⁄₁₀₀ = 30:100.

To change a decimal to a ratio, multiply the decimal by 100 or move the decimal point two places to the right and 100 will become the denominator. For example, 0.09 would be 9:100, 0.675 would be 67.5:100, and 0.0008 would be 0.08:100.

Ratios may also be shown as fractions, such as 3:4 would be ¾ or 20:100 would be ²⁰⁄₁₀₀, which will reduce to ⅕ by dividing both the numerator and the denominator by 20.

TECH NOTE

Ratios and ratio and proportion are used for dose/dosage calculations, such as number of tablets when the exact dosage for an order is not available or if the strength of drug per volume of medication is needed. This is also used for conversions between units of measure and in inventory control, but it may be very useful with other calculations and in checking math calculations.

POINTS TO REMEMBER
RATIO

- A ratio is a fraction that shows the relationship of one number to another.
- To convert using a ratio, both quantities must be in the same unit of measure.
- If the quantities are not in the same unit of measure, the problem cannot be solved until the quantities are changed to the same units (see Chapters 3 and 4).
- When converting percentages to ratio, the denominator or second number in the equation will always be 100.

Practice Problems S

Change the following to ratios, being sure that the ratio is expressed in the same unit of measure and is reduced to the lowest term. Show your calculations.

1. 2 is to 7 = _____

2. 6 is to 9 = _____

3. 5 is to 25 = _____

4. 36% = _____

5. 125% = _____

6. 95% = _____

7. $\dfrac{7}{8}$ = _____

8. $\dfrac{5}{9}$ = _____

9. $\dfrac{75}{125}$ = _____

10. $3\dfrac{1}{4}\%$ = _____

11. 0.04% = _____

12. 0.08 = _____

13. 0.36 = _____

14. 0.04 = _____

15. 0.1 = _____

16. 2 mg : 8 mg = _____

17. 6 ft : 3 yd = _____

18. 12 oz : 2 lb = _____

19. 6 in : 4 ft = _____

20. 50¢ : $3.50 = _____

21. 75¢ : $8.25 = _____

22. 4 pt : 16 pt = _____

23. 0.25 in : 25 in = _____

24. 0.2 mL : 5 mL = _____

25. 50 mg : 1000 mg = _____

Expressing Ratios as Proportions

True **proportion** is the expression of equality between two ratios that have an equal relationship or an equation formed between two equal ratios such as 4:6 and 8:12. In these pairs of numbers, the relationship between 4 and 8 is that 8 is twice as much as 4 and 12 is twice as much as 6. So these numbers are equally proportional to each other, although the numbers are not the same. The proportion in each is 2, or the second number in the proportion is twice as much as the first number in the proportion. We can place this in a proportional equation, $4:8::6:12$ or a fractional equation $\frac{4}{8} \times \frac{6}{12}$. When the fractions are cross-multiplied $\frac{4}{8} \times \frac{6}{12}$ both answers will be 48, or the products will be equal.

When writing the proportional equation of $\frac{4}{a} : \frac{8}{b} :: \frac{6}{c} : \frac{12}{d}$, we will multiply the two outside numbers (numbers a and d) or the **extremes**, and the two inside numbers (numbers b and c), or the **means**, so 4×12 and 6×8, with both answers being 48. The product of the means will always equal the product of the extremes in a true proportion. The computation of the problem can be checked by placing the answer into the unknown (x) and multiplying the means and extremes, checking that the answers are the same.

TECH NOTE

The equality of the proportions after calculation is important for ensuring patient safety and should be calculated with each use of ratio and proportion.

$$\frac{4}{8} \times \frac{6}{12} \qquad 4 \times 12 = 6 \times 8$$

LEARNING TIP

Multiply the outside numbers, "outsies," and then the inside numbers, "insies," to figure proportion. Think of "outsies" versus "insies" rather than extremes and means respectively, for ease of learning.

POINTS TO REMEMBER
PROPORTIONS

- When multiplying means and extremes, the products of the multiplication must be equal in a true proportion.
- If the product of the means is divided by one extreme number, the answer must be the other extreme number.
- If the product of the extremes is divided by one mean number, the answer must be the other mean number.

Practice Problems T

Which of the following are true proportions? Mark with either a yes or a no.

1. $3:9::9:27$ _____

2. $5:25::10:250$ _____

3. $4:12::6:18$ _____

4. $10:90::1:9$ _____

5. $15:3::5:2$ _____

6. $22:88::10:40$ _____

7. $\$1.50:\$7.50::\$0.25:\$1.25$ _____

8. $2 \text{ mg}:4 \text{ mg}::8 \text{ mg}:16 \text{ mg}$ _____

9. $2":12"::6":24"$ _____

10. $32 \text{ mg}:64 \text{ mg}::5 \text{ mg}:10 \text{ mg}$ _____

In the health care field, the concepts of ratio and proportion are often used to calculate different quantities of medication or to calculate dosages. If an amount of medication in a ratio is known and a new quantity of a substance is necessary, proportion may be used to obtain the new amount of medication that is required by multiplying the means and extremes. Proportional equations are therefore used to find the missing or unknown amount, often signified by "x." Knowing three of the four parts of the proportion is necessary for the proportion to be formed. When writing the proportion, like units of measure must be in positions a and c as well as in positions b and d when the proportion is designated in the following manner—a : b :: c : d or 1 mL : 1 L :: 6 mL : 6 L. Notice that positions a and c are in milliliters and b and d are in liters.

Remember that proportion can also be shown as a relationship between two fractions and then cross-multiply to solve for the unknown or to prove the computation is correct. The unknown (x) should always be placed on the left side of the equation.

TECH NOTE

Tips for working with proportions follow:

When three terms of a proportion are known, the fourth term may be found by making the fourth term an "x" and then simply calculating for the x in the equation by cross-multiplication or multiplying "insies" and "outsies." The mathematical problem that is formed can then be solved.

Each side of an equation may be multiplied or divided by the same nonzero number to reduce or simplify the equation and to isolate "x", such as in the problem $2x = 24$ x can be isolated by using 2 as the denominator.

$$\frac{2x}{2} = \frac{24}{2} \quad \text{or} \quad x = 24 \div 2 \quad \text{or} \quad 12$$

A proportion may be proved by adding the found answer into the "x" position in the previous problem and calculating the problem to prove both sides of the equation are equal in the proportional equation. In the example $1:2::x:24$ with the above calculation: $1:2::12:24$ or $24 = 24$. So the calculation is correct. This is an important step for patient safety.

Practice Problems U

With the unknown as "x," solve the following problems creating proportions as needed. Remember that the ratio components may be written as fractions and then you may cross-multiply. Indicate the measurement as appropriate.

1. $4:x::3:12 = $ _____

2. $x:2::14:7 = $ _____

3. $20:x::5:10 = $ _____

4. $7:x::6:12 = $ _____

5. $x:160::7:140 = $ _____

6. $7:x::35:125 = $ _____

7. $x:11::2:2.2 =$ _____

8. $5:x::2.5:125 =$ _____

9. $0.22:x::0.33:6.6 =$ _____

10. $\$0.20:x::\$1.00:\$25 =$ _____

11. $24 \text{ mg}:x::16 \text{ mg}:12 \text{ mg} =$ _____

12. $2 \text{ g}:24 \text{ g}::x:36 \text{ g} =$ _____

13. $x:36 \text{ tab}::6 \text{ tab}:8 \text{ tab} =$ _____

14. $\$20:\$15::\$100:x =$ _____

15. $18\#:12\#::12\#:x =$ _____

16. $20 \text{ mg}:24 \text{ mg}::18 \text{ mg}:x =$ _____

17. $\$1.20:\$4::x:\$9 =$ _____

18. $2 \text{ qt}:6 \text{ qt}::x:48 \text{ qt} =$ _____

19. $5 \text{ tab}:35 \text{ tab}::x:28 \text{ tab} =$ _____

20. $5 \text{ mL}:x::15 \text{ mL}:9 \text{ mL} =$ _____

21. $0.16 \text{ g}:x::0.4 \text{ g}:0.15 \text{ g} =$ _____

22. $14 \text{ mL}:2 \text{ L}::21 \text{ mL}:x =$ _____

23. John knows that Mr. Smith needs 14 tablets for a week's supply of an antiinflammatory drug. Mr. Smith is going on vacation and needs a 4-week supply. How many tablets does John need to fill the prescription? Show your work.
_____

24. Periactin liquid is labeled as 5 mg/5 mL. How many mg would be in 25 mL? Show your work. _____

25. An antilipidemic agent contains 5 mg of the medication per tablet. How many tablets would be necessary to supply 35 mg per dose? Show your work. _____

26. A cough medication contains 50 mg of active ingredient per mL. The physician desires 100 mg per dose. How many mL would each dose contain? Show your work. _____

27. Dr. Jones writes a prescription stating that he wants the patient to take 75 mg of a medication three times a day. The stock bottle shows 37.5 mg per tablet. How many tablets should the patient take at a time? How many tablets should the patient take in a day? Show your work. _____

28. A physician orders a 250 mg dose of an antibiotic for a child. The pediatric liquid medication contains 125 mg per 5 mL. How many milliliters should the child take with each dose? _____

29. If the physician wants the child to take the previously mentioned medication three times a day, how many milligrams of the medication will the child take in 1 day? _____

30. How many milliliters of the medication will the child take in 1 day? _____

QUANTITIES

Determining the Percentage of a Quantity

In dosage calculation, computation of a given percentage or part of a quantity may be figured to ascertain the part of a whole quantity that is in question. If a percentage of a whole quantity is in question, the known percentage is multiplied by the whole quantity to provide the needed information. The equation for finding the percentage follows:

Percentage (amount of the whole quantity) = Percent number × Whole number (base)

To find a percentage of a whole number, the term "of" means to multiply the number by the percentage: What is 3% of 42? First change the % to a decimal by dividing by 100 or moving the decimal point 2 places to the left or 0.03. Then multiply 42 × 0.03 = 1.26. So 1.26 (what) is 3% of 42.

Dividing percentage answers the question of "what." For instance, 15 is what percentage of 45? Set up the part number (15) over the whole number (45) and then complete the division.

$$\frac{15}{45} = \frac{1}{3}$$

Finally, convert 1/3 to 33% by dividing 1 by 3 and multiplying by 100%. Or use the following ratio and proportion:

$x(\%) : 15$ (whole number) :: $100\% : 45$ (whole number)

TECH NOTE
Remember, 100 is always the denominator in %.

As a review of determining the percentage of one number to another, make a fraction with the numbers. The denominator will be the number following the word "of" with the other number in the problem being the numerator. Consider the question, 10 is what percentage of 75? Place the 75 as the denominator and the 10 as the numerator or 10/75 or 10 ÷ 75 = 0.13 or 13% after changing answer to percentage.

TECH NOTE
Percentage of a quantity is used in strengths of medications as well as finding discounts for customers and pricing of medications.

The fraction may be found in three ways:

1. Finding the percentage, as in "What is 50% of 15?"

   Percentage or whole quantity (x) = percent number (50%) × whole number (15)

2. Find the whole quantity, as in "15 is 60% of what number?"

   Percentage or whole quantity (15) = percent number (60%) × whole number (x)

3. Finding the percent number, as in "5 is what percent of 15?"

   Percentage or whole quantity (5) = percent number (x) × whole number (15)

LEARNING TIP

A few tips on working with percentages of quantities are as follows:
- "what" is translated to the unknown, or x
- "of" translates to "times" or a whole number
- "is" translates to "=" or part of a number
- % represents percentage

For example, what is 50% of 15?

$$x = 50\% \times 15, \quad \text{or} \quad x = 0.5 \times 15, \quad \text{or} \quad 7.5$$

Answer: 50% of 15 is 7.5.

- "x" as the unknown should always be placed on the left side of the equation
- When finding what percentage one number is of another number, the number following the word "of" is the denominator of a fraction and the other number is the numerator of the fraction. Then change the decimal to a percent by moving the decimal two places to the right (multiply by 100).

For example: What percent of 15 is 5?

$$x = \frac{5}{15} \quad \text{or} \quad x = \frac{1}{3}, \quad 1.000 \div 3 \quad \text{or} \quad 3\overline{)1.000} \quad \text{or} \quad 0.333, \quad \text{or} \quad 33.3\%$$

Answer: 5 is 33.3% of 15

- When finding a given percentage of a number, write the percent as a decimal and multiply by the number.

For example: What is 75% of 200?

$$x = 200 \times 75\%$$

NOTE: 75% = 75/100 or 0.75

$$x = 200 \times 0.75$$

$$
\begin{array}{r}
200 \\
\times \quad .75 \\
\hline
1000 \\
1400 \\
\hline
150.00
\end{array}
$$

OR

$$
\begin{array}{r}
.75 \\
\times \quad 200 \\
\hline
150.00
\end{array}
$$

75% of 200 = 150

As a short cut, remember that you may set up a problem containing zeros at the end of a number by making that number (containing zeros) the multiplier and adding the zeros to the end of the product prior to multiplying the remaining number.

TECH NOTE

When working with medications, the higher the percentage of the active ingredient in a medication, the greater the strength of the medication within the whole.

Practice Problems V

Solve the following problems by translating them using the hints described earlier. Show your work, and round answers as appropriate. Indicate measurement as appropriate.

1. What percentage of 105 is 35? (Round to tenths.) _____

2. 25 is what percentage of 200? _____

3. 90% of 50 is what? _____

4. 105% of 0.9 is what? _____

5. 250 is what percentage of 75? (Round to a whole number.) _____

6. What percentage of 750 is 15? _____

7. What percentage of 49 is 11? (Round to hundredths.) _____

8. What is 45% of 180? _____

9. What percentage of 3 is ⅓? (Round to a whole number.) _____

10. Four is what percentage of 240? (Round to hundredths.) _____

11. What is 15% of $25.40? _____

12. What is 64% of 8 oz? _____

13. If you have 25 tablets, what is 5%? _____

14. What percentage of 40 tablets is 22 tablets? _____

15. What is ¼% of 48 mg? _____

16. If a discount of 15% is expected on a purchase of $25, what is the amount of the discount? _____

17. If a patient wants 60% of a prescription that is written for 60 tablets, how many tablets will be dispensed to the patient? _____

18. A physician orders 150% of a prescription that is written for 8 oz. How many ounces will be dispensed? _____

19. 40 tablets is what percentage of 90 tablets? (Round to hundredths.) _____

20. 35% of 70 tablets is what? _____

21. Six inches is what percentage of 24 inches? _____

22. 3¼ teaspoons are 20% of what total number of teaspoons? _____

23. 125 tablets is what percent of 1500 tablets? (Round to hundredths.) _____

24. 60% of 12 oz is what? _____

25. What is 3% of 1200 mL? _____

Posttest

Before taking the Posttest, retake the Pretest to check your understanding of the materials presented in this chapter.

Solve the following problems as indicated. Round to the nearest hundredth on the second line when appropriate. Indicate measurement as appropriate. As always, show your calculations.

1. $13 + 24.6 + 36.72 + 0.45 =$ _____   _____

2. $15.87 - 5.2 =$ _____   _____

3. $26.45 + 4.792 + 120.005 + 3.202 =$ _____   _____

4. $12.76 \times 5.2 =$ _____   _____

5. $25.01 \times 10.10 =$ _____   _____

6. $25 \div 0.25 =$ _____   _____

7. $16.82 \div 4.02 =$ _____   _____

8. $2 - 1.75 =$ _____   _____

Posttest, cont.

Solve the following fractional equations and reduce to the lowest term.

9. $\dfrac{1}{2} + \dfrac{3}{4} + \dfrac{3}{8} =$ _____   _____

10. $\dfrac{5}{6} + \dfrac{7}{12} + \dfrac{5}{8} =$ _____   _____

11. $\dfrac{11}{12} - \dfrac{3}{4} =$ _____   _____

12. $2\dfrac{2}{3} - 1\dfrac{5}{6} =$ _____   _____

13. $\dfrac{1}{5} \times \dfrac{3}{8} =$ _____   _____

14. $\dfrac{8}{9} \times \dfrac{3}{8} \times \dfrac{1}{2} =$ _____   _____

15. $9\dfrac{1}{4} - 5\dfrac{6}{11} =$ _____   _____

16. $8\dfrac{2}{3} \times \dfrac{1}{3} =$ _____   _____

17. $6\dfrac{2}{3} \div 2\dfrac{1}{4} =$ _____   _____

Continued

Posttest, cont.

18. $1\dfrac{1}{5} \div \dfrac{6}{7} =$ _____   _____

19. $\dfrac{3}{4} \div \dfrac{3}{8} =$ _____   _____

20. $7\dfrac{1}{2} \div 2\dfrac{2}{3} =$ _____   _____

Convert the following fractions to decimals. Round to the nearest hundreth.

21. $\dfrac{5}{9} =$ _____   22. $2\dfrac{1}{3} =$ _____   23. $\dfrac{16}{25} =$ _____

24. $5\dfrac{14}{15} =$ _____   25. $1\dfrac{5}{6} =$ _____

Convert the following decimals to fractions. If improper fractions are calculated, convert to a mixed number. Reduce as appropriate.

26. $0.44 =$ _____   27. $1.64 =$ _____   28. $5.33 =$ _____

29. $0.86 =$ _____   30. $10.8 =$ _____

Express the numbers in ratio expressions.

31. A medication container has 50 tablets in it for dispensing. _____

Posttest, cont.

32. A 4-oz medication bottle contains 1½ oz cough syrup. _____

33. To reconstitute a liquid, 250 mL of water is necessary for 500 mg. _____

34. An antibiotic contains 250 mg in 5 mL of medication. _____

35. Two capsules contain 1000 mg of penicillin. _____

Express the following in proportional equations and solve the unknown as appropriate. Be sure to show your calculations. Reduce as appropriate. Indicate measurement as appropriate.

36. A bottle of medication contains 75 tablets. How many tablets would be found in five bottles of medication? _____

37. A physician orders medication to be given at 250 mg per dose. What quantity of medication will be given in a day if the medication is given four times a day? _____

38. John has a prescription for medication to be taken one tablet twice a day. How many tablets of medication will John need to take as prescribed for 2 weeks? _____

39. The pharmacist wants a stock of medication for at least 10 patients available at all times. The medication usually requires a prescription of 24 tablets. How many tablets will need to be in stock each day? _____

Continued

Posttest, cont.

40. If the medication mentioned in the previous problem comes in bottles of 50 capsules per bottle, how many bottles of medication are necessary for inventory requirements? _____

41. Dr. Smith calls and wants the dispensing of 3 months supply of medication for hypertension. The usual dispensing amount for 1 month is 60 tablets. How many tablets do you need to count for the physician's order? _____

42. Mary comes into the pharmacy with a prescription for 90 tablets for a 30-day supply. She does not have the money to buy the complete prescription but wants to buy half today and will get the remainder next week when she has more money. How many tablets do you need to give her for a 2-week supply? _____

Solve the following quantity percentage problems using equations.

43. Three tablets are what percent of 90? (Round to hundredths.) _____

44. 45% of 1500 mL is what? _____

45. What is 15% of 60 tablets? _____

46. 250 mg is what percent of 1000 mg? _____

47. A prescription is for 120 tablets. What is 40% of that prescription? _____

Posttest, cont.

48. Jesse wants to know what 5% of his prescription of 125 mL is. _____

49. Juan is to take 25% of 24 tablets. How many tablets will Juan take? _____

50. What percent of 125 tablets is 25 tablets? _____

REVIEW OF RULES

Fractions

- To change an improper fraction to a mixed number, divide the numerator by the denominator.

- To change a mixed number to an improper fraction, multiply the denominator by the whole number and then add the numerator to the product obtained. This number then becomes the numerator for the fraction, and the denominator of the fraction retained is the original denominator.

- To reduce a fraction to the lowest term, divide both the numerator and denominator by the greatest common factor.

- To add or subtract fractions with a common denominator, add or subtract the numerators as indicated. Then write the sum or difference as the numerator for the fraction, and the common denominator becomes the denominator for the fraction. Reduce this fraction to the lowest term or change to a mixed number as indicated.

- For fractions with an uncommon denominator, the least common denominator must be found. The number that will divide exactly into the denominators must be found, and then the numerators of each fraction must be multiplied by the common number. After finding the common denominator, the mathematical calculation of adding or subtracting may be performed. When adding or subtracting fractions with uncommon denominators, add or subtract the numerators as indicated and then reduce to lowest terms or to the mixed number.

- To multiply fractions, multiply the numerators and multiply the denominators, with the product of the numerators being the new numerator and the product of the denominators being the new denominator. Reduce the fraction or change to a mixed number as indicated.

- To multiply mixed numbers, change the mixed number to an improper fraction and then multiply, as mentioned earlier with fractions.

- To divide fractions, invert the fraction that is the divisor and multiply the dividend by the inverted fraction—the remainder of the problem is actually like multiplying fractions. Reduce to the lowest term.

- To divide mixed numbers, change the mixed number to a fraction and then proceed as if the problem were a fractional unit. Reduce the fraction as needed or change to a mixed number as indicated.

Decimals

- To read a decimal, the number to the left of the decimal is a whole number, "and" is used to represent the decimal point, and the number to the right of the decimal point is read as a whole number value of the number farthest to the right including the decimal point as a number space, with "th" added to the number space. For example, 2.34 would be 2 and 34 hundredths.

- To round a decimal place to a certain place or determined number, begin at the farthermost right digit. If that number is 5 to 9, the second digit to the right will be increased by one (i.e., 1.567 would become 1.57). If the farthermost number is 0 to 4, the second number will remain the same. After determining the number of digits to remain, delete the excess numbers using the previous rule to the correct place (e.g., if 8.78934 is to be rounded to hundredths, the answer would be 8.79).

- To add or subtract decimal numbers, align the numbers, being sure that the decimal points are aligned. Add zeros at the end of the decimal fraction until all decimal numbers are the same length. Then add or subtract as for whole numbers, being sure the decimal point is correctly aligned in the answer. Whole numbers are understood to have a decimal point to the right of the number.

- To multiply decimal numbers, multiply the numbers as if the numbers are whole numbers, then count the numbers to the right of the decimal points and finally add a decimal point in the product so that there are as many decimal points in the product as in the numbers being multiplied.

- To divide a decimal number by a whole number, place the decimal point in the quotient directly above the decimal point in the dividend.

- To divide a decimal number by a decimal number, count the number of digits to the right of the decimal in the divisor; place a decimal point at the end of the same number of places in the dividend, moving the decimal point in place and adding zeros as needed; and then place the decimal point at that place in the quotient directly above the decimal point in the dividend. Divide the numbers as if the divisor is a whole number.

- To change a fraction to a decimal, divide the numerator by the denominator.

- To change a decimal to a fraction, place the decimal number as the numerator with the denominator being 1 plus the number of zeros as found in the decimal number and the decimal point (i.e., 0.01 would be $\frac{1}{100}$). Reduce the fraction as appropriate.

Ratio, Proportion, and Percentages

- If two fractions are equivalent, the cross-products will be equal. If the cross-products in a proportional equation are equal, the fractions are equivalent or the proportion is true.

- If each member of an equality is multiplied by the same number, the products will be equal.

- If each member of an equality is divided by the same number, the quotients will be equal.

- To multiply or divide in %, first change the percentage to a decimal and then do the calculation.

- To change a percentage to a decimal form, multiply by 0.01 or move the decimal point two places to the left. To change decimal to percent, move the decimal point two places to the right. Think of the alphabet placement of "D" and "P."

- To solve an unknown proportion, multiply the means or "insies" and the extremes or "outsies," setting the equation with the unknown on the left being equal to the quotient numbers on the right. Then solve for the unknown.

- To solve a percent proportion, the "what" translates to the unknown or a letter, "of" translates to times or "×," "is" translates to equal or "=," and "%" may be either $\frac{1}{100}$ or 0.01 for multiplication of the percentage. Read the problem and insert the translation, then solve the unknown.

Estimating of Answers

- Estimation is the best check of a reasonable mathematical calculation. To estimate a number, mentally round of to a slightly larger or smaller number containing fewer significant figures (Example: 59 would be estimated to 60). Then do the calculation mentally knowing that the mental answer will be slightly higher or lower than the actual calculation but will be close to the desired answer.

- After estimating the answer, calculate the answer and then check against the estimated answer.

SECTION II

Measurements Used in Health Care and Conversions among Measurement Systems

CHAPTER 3

Conversion of Clinical Measurements of Numbers, Time, and Temperature

OBJECTIVES

- Express Arabic numbers in Roman numerals
- Express Roman numerals in Arabic numbers
- Convert time between standard time and military (or universal) time
- Convert temperature between Fahrenheit and Celsius

KEY WORDS

Arabic numerals The numbers 1, 2, 3, and the like

Celsius (Centigrade) System of measuring temperature with 0° being the freezing point and 100° being the boiling point of water

Fahrenheit System of measuring temperature with 32° being the freezing point and 212° being the boiling point of water

Military time (International Standard Time) System of time that recognizes a 24-hour notation of hours and minutes

Roman numerals Numbers that use Roman letters such as I for 1, V for 5, and the like

75

Pretest

Follow the directions below and show all of your calculations as appropriate. Remember that this is a pretest to judge your current knowledge of the materials presented in this chapter.

Change the following to Roman numerals.

1. 21 _____   2. 16 _____   3. 54 _____   4. 122 _____

5. 44 _____   6. 95 _____   7. 68 _____   8. 75 _____

Change the following to Arabic numbers.

9. viii _____   10. xix _____   11. lxiv _____   12. xcvii _____

13. ix$\overline{ss}$ _____   14. xvii$\overline{ss}$ _____   15. xxxvii$\overline{ss}$ _____   16. xxiv _____

17. xxiv$\overline{ss}$ _____   18. xliv$\overline{ss}$ _____   19. xciii$\overline{ss}$ _____   20. lxxxvi$\overline{ss}$ _____

Change the following to universal, or 24-hour, time.

21. 7:30 AM _____   22. 5:32 PM _____   23. 12:01 AM _____   24. 11:59 AM _____

25. 1:59 PM _____   26. 1:46 AM _____   27. 8:42 PM _____   28. 9:08 PM _____

Pretest, cont.

Change the following to 12-hour time.

29. 1102 _____   30. 0520 _____   31. 0052 _____   32. 2357 _____

33. 0001 _____   34. 0648 _____   35. 1645 _____   36. 1235 _____

37. 0412 _____   38. 1308 _____

Change the following temperatures as indicated. Round to the nearest tenth.

39. 98.6° F = _____ C   40. 104.6° F = _____ C   41. 38.6° C = _____ F

42. 29.6° C = _____ F   43. 100.4° F = _____ C   44. 41.8° C = _____ F

45. 41.8° F = _____ C   46. 102.6° F = _____ C   47. 0° F = _____ C

48. 10° C = _____ F   49. 10° F = _____ C   50. 110.6° F = _____ C

51. 95.6° F = _____ C   52. 32.2° C = _____ F   53. 92.5° F = _____ C

54. 212° F = _____ C   55. 100° C = _____ F

INTRODUCTION

Whether in the hospital setting or in the community pharmacy, time, temperature, and the ability to read numbering systems are essential so the correct amount of medication will be given at the correct time and at the correct temperature if that is essential. A pharmacy technician will use both **Arabic numerals**, such as 1, 2, 3, and so on, and **Roman numerals**, such as I, V, X, and so on, when interpreting physicians' orders. As citizens of the Western Hemisphere, we are familiar with Arabic numbers, which are used daily, and numbers that are related to the English system of measurement. These numbers are used for steps in our daily lives from writing a check to looking at a page number in a book. Numbers in the preface of a book, however, are usually written in Roman numerals.

Most of you probably have not used Roman numerals for many years, but these numerical symbols will be used daily in the medical field. In the same manner, in our daily world we use the standard clock whereas in patient settings we often use **military time** to prevent misinterpretation of the medicinal order. Finally, temperature is read and recorded in **Fahrenheit** in our daily lives, using 32° as the freezing point of water and 212° as boiling, such as 95° F outside on a hot day. The **Celsius** thermometer, where water freezes at 0° and boils at 100°, is used in some medical settings that prefer metric measurements. The Celsius thermometer is used in many clinical teaching locations, with the normal body temperature being 37° instead of the 98.6° found in the Fahrenheit scale. When the patient information is used internationally for study, the Celsius or centigrade scale is often used.

ARABIC NUMBERS AND ROMAN NUMERALS

Medication orders or prescriptions are written in both Arabic and Roman numerals, depending on the amount of medication ordered or the prescriber's preference. Arabic numerals are those most common such as 2 for whole numbers, ⅛ as fractional numbers, or 0.53 as a decimal number.

Roman numerals, which date back to the ancient Roman Empire, use letters to represent numerical amounts. The following are the numbers depicted by Roman numerals.

> **ROMAN NUMERALS**
> $\overline{ss}$ = 1/2
> I, i, or $\dot{\overline{i}}$ = 1
> V, v, or $\overline{v}$ = 5
> X, x, or $\overline{x}$ = 10
> L = 50
> C = 100
> Other numerals: D = 500, M = 1000

TECH NOTE

Roman numerals are often used when writing prescriptions because these alphabetic symbols that indicate quantity are harder to alter than Arabic numerals.

Roman Numeral Use

The rules for using Roman numerals are as follows:

- When a numeral is repeated, the value of the number is the number of times for the repetition to provide the needed number (e.g., III = 3).
- A numeral may be repeated up to three times in succession and no more (e.g., IIII as 4 is incorrect; the correct way to express 4 is IV).

- The letters V, L, and D are not repeated (e.g., VV is incorrect for 10).
- When a numeral of lower value is placed following a larger numeral value, the smaller numeral is added to the larger numeral (e.g., XI = 11, VI = 6). Only I, X, or C can be used in this manner.
- If the smaller numeral value is placed before the larger numeral value, the smaller value is subtracted from the larger numeral value (e.g., IV = 5 – 1, or 4). Again, only I, X, or C may be used in this manner.
- Only one smaller number may be placed either before a larger number (e.g., IIX is not 8; rather, 8 is expressed as VIII).
- The subtracted number must be no less than one tenth of the value of the number from which it is subtracted (e.g., X may be placed before a C or an L but cannot be used with M or D. Thus 49 must be stated as XLIX rather than IL).
- Use the largest value numerals possible (e.g., 15 is XV, not VVV or XIIIII).
- Use I before V and X (the next two higher numerals). The numeral X may be used before L and C (the next higher numerals). Although seldom used, C may be used before D and M.
- $\overline{ss}$ is used as an abbreviation for one-half.
- Medical notations of Roman numerals are usually written in the lower case with a line drawn over the numerals to prevent misinterpretation. The lowercase "i" has the line usually with the dot above the line, not below as commonly written.

Converting Arabic Numbers to Roman Numerals

An example of changing Arabic numerals to Roman numerals is as follows:

EXAMPLE 3-1

Change 24 to Roman numerals: 20 is 10 + 10, or XX, whereas 4 is 5 – 1, or IV (subtract 1 from 5), so 24 is written as XXIV.

Practice Problems A

Convert the following Arabic numbers to Roman numerals, using the correct medical notation to prevent misinterpretation.

1. 6 _____

2. 11 _____

3. 21 _____

4. 56 _____

5. $7\frac{1}{2}$ _____

6. 9 _____

7. $54\frac{1}{2}$ _____

8. $17\frac{1}{2}$ _____

9. 75 _____

10. 101 _____

11. 66 _____

12. 35 _____

13. $1\frac{1}{2}$ _____   14. 49 _____   15. $33\frac{1}{2}$ _____

16. 18 _____   17. 61 _____   18. 126 _____

19. 90 _____   20. 42 _____

Converting Roman Numerals to Arabic Numbers

To change Roman numerals into Arabic numbers, divide the entire Roman numeral into the groups of letters that indicate a number, such as XIV where X = 10 and IV = 4. So the Roman numeral XIV = 14.

An example of changing Roman numerals to Arabic numbers is as follows:

EXAMPLE 3-2

Change XLVII to an Arabic number. Divide the number into XL and VII. XL means to subtract 10 (X) from 50 (L) or 40, whereas VII is 5 (V) + 1 (I) + 1 (I), or 7. When the numbers are placed together, XLVII (XL + VII) is 47.

Another example for changing Arabic numbers to Roman numerals follows:

EXAMPLE 3-3

Remember that $\overline{ss}$ is the same as ½. Change $xix\overline{ss}$ into an Arabic number by first dividing the Roman numeral into separate parts. Thus $xix\overline{ss}$ is xix, or 10 (x) + 9 (ix) (10 − 1) + $\overline{ss}$ (½), or 19½. To change an Arabic number to a Roman numeral, 16½ would be x (10) + v (5) + i (1) + $\overline{ss}$ (½), or $xvi\overline{ss}$

Practice Problems B

Convert the following Roman numerals to Arabic numbers.

1. viii _____   2. ix _____   3. xix _____

4. xxxix _____   5. xliv _____   6. lxvi _____

7. cxxv _____   8. $xxv\overline{ss}$ _____   9. xcv _____

10. viiss̄ _____   11. ixss̄ _____   12. xxxviiss̄ _____

13. xxv _____   14. lxiii _____   15. xcix _____

16. civ _____   17. xxviiiss̄ _____   18. xxss̄ _____

19. xlivss̄ _____   20. iiss̄ _____

CONVERSION BETWEEN 12-HOUR AND UNIVERSAL (MILITARY OR 24-HOUR) TIME

Because traditional time can be misinterpreted when using AM and PM with the same numbers to indicate the time of day for medication administration, many hospitals and other health care facilities use 24-hour, or military, time, also called universal time. This time will reduce the chance of errors when time is a necessary indicator in medication administration. The differentiation of time is not dependent on just the initials AM or PM but is expressed as different numbers of time from 0001 to 2400.

In universal time, all time is expressed in four-digit numbers beginning at 1 minute past midnight, or 0001 hours. The time is stated in hundreds of hours with 1 AM being 0100 hours and said as "zero one-hundred hours." Ten in the morning is the first time that a double digit precedes the hour with 10 o'clock being said as "ten hundred hours." Noon is 1200 hours and said as "twelve hundred hours." One o'clock in the afternoon becomes 1300 hours, or "thirteen hundred hours." Midnight then becomes 2400, or "twenty-four hundred hours," or at some sites it is read as 0000, or "zero hundred hours." Figure 3-1 shows an example of a military time clock. The AM (ante meridian, or before noon) readings are found on the inside of the clock face, whereas the PM (post meridian, or after noon) readings are found on the outside of the clock face.

TECH NOTE

If seconds are needed in military time, the number becomes a six digit number with seconds being the last two digits. For example, 1 minute and 10 seconds past midnight would be 000110.

LEARNING TIP

To change time after noon or PM time, the number of the hour past 12 noon can be added to 12 to obtain the hour in military time (e.g., 3 PM would be 0300 + 1200, or 1500 hours).

Minutes in military time are written as the last two digits in the time line (e.g., 2:59 AM would be expressed as 0259). The minutes are just converted to the last digits in the time behind the hour of time. If the time is 4:46 PM, it would be read as "sixteen forty-six hours," or 1646 hours.

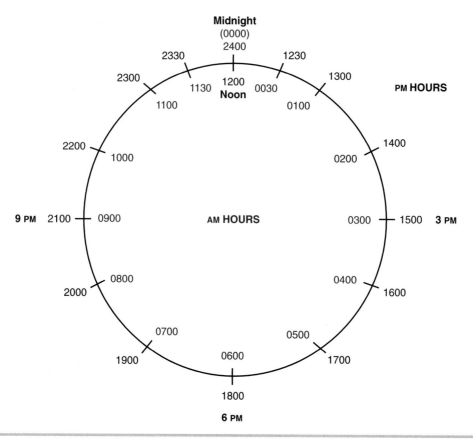

FIGURE 3-1 Military time clock.

POINTS TO REMEMBER

CHANGING TO 24-HOUR, OR INTERNATIONAL, TIME

- Traditional and universal time have the same numerical meaning from 1:00 AM (0100 hours) to 12:59 PM (1259 hours).
- Minutes after midnight and before 1:00 AM (0100 hours) will be written with 00 with the number of minutes, such as 0010 (12:10 AM).
- Midnight will be written as either 0000 or 2400 hours.
- Hours between 1:00 PM through 12:00 AM are the time plus 12 added to the hour, for instance, 5:35 PM would be 1735 hours.

Practice Problems C

Convert the following 12-hour times to 24-hour times.

1. 12:35 AM _____   2. 2:45 PM _____   3. 6:15 AM _____

4. 6:20 PM _____   5. 12:05 AM _____   6. 3:45 AM _____

7. 12 AM _____   8. 12 PM _____   9. 6:55 AM _____

10. 7:25 PM _____   11. 2:15 PM _____   12. 8:20 PM _____

13. 9:05 AM _____   14. 11 AM _____   15. 9 PM _____

16. 8:06 AM _____   17. 10:45 PM _____   18. 6:04 PM _____

19. 11:59 PM _____   20. 12:03 PM _____

Convert the following 24-hour times to 12-hour times. Be sure to indicate morning and evening.

21. 1130 _____   22. 0354 _____   23. 1201 _____

24. 0030 _____   25. 1425 _____   26. 1615 _____

27. 0830 _____   28. 2345 _____   29. 0705 _____

30. 2145 _____   31. 0404 _____   32. 2020 _____

33. 1020 _____   34. 0330 _____   35. 0945 _____

36. 2244 _____   37. 0006 _____   38. 2306 _____

39. 0202 _____   40. 1515 _____

CONVERSION BETWEEN FAHRENHEIT AND CELSIUS TEMPERATURE

In the United States, Fahrenheit temperature (F) is the measurement most commonly used. In countries where the metric system is used, Celsius (C) or centigrade temperature measurement is the most commonly used scale. In the Fahrenheit scale, water boils at 212°, whereas in Celsius water boils at 100°. Likewise, the freezing points are not the same; Fahrenheit is 32°, whereas Celsius is 0°. Figure 3-2 provides a comparison of the scales. As you can quickly see, the Fahrenheit scale has 180° between the freezing and boiling points, whereas the Celsius scale contains only 100°. The formulas for conversion between the two scales have been developed with these differences as the basis. The conversion equations are shown below.

If the differences in Fahrenheit to Celsius could be placed into a fractional unit, the fraction for changing to the Celsius scale would be that for each Celsius degree in temperature, the Fahrenheit difference would be $\frac{180}{100}$. Another way of looking at it is that the Celsius degree is 1.8 Fahrenheit degrees after the difference of 32° has been subtracted from the Fahrenheit temperature. If we want the number of Celsius degrees in the Fahrenheit scale, the Celsius scale would be that $\frac{100}{180}$, or $\frac{5}{9}$ of the Celsius degree is found in one Fahrenheit degree. So the following conversion formulas may be used to change from one temperature scale to the other.

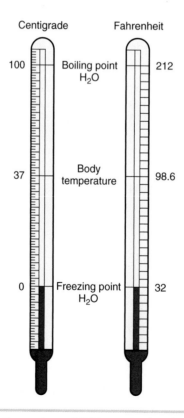

FIGURE 3-2 Comparison of Celsius and Fahrenheit thermometers.

Converting Fahrenheit Temperature to Celsius Temperature

Two methods are available to convert a temperature in Fahrenheit to the equivalent Celsius temperature:

$$\text{(A) } C^\circ = \frac{F^\circ - 32}{1.8} \quad \text{or} \quad \text{(B) } C^\circ = (F^\circ - 32) \times \frac{5}{9}$$

In the first method (A), subtract 32 from the Fahrenheit temperature and divide by 1.8. In the second method (B), subtract 32 from the Fahrenheit temperature and multiply that answer by 5. Then divide by 9. In either case, the remainder should be rounded to tenths as appropriate.

EXAMPLE 3-4

Convert 96.5° F to C°.

$$\text{(A) } C^\circ = 96.5 - 32 \ (64.5) \div 1.8 = 35.833 \text{ or } 35.8^\circ$$

OR

$$\text{(B) } C^\circ = 96.5 - 32 \ (64.5) \times 5 \ (322.5) \div 9 = 35.8333 \text{ or } 35.8^\circ$$

Converting Celsius Temperature to Fahrenheit Temperature

To convert Celsius temperature to Fahrenheit temperature, you can also use two methods:

$$\text{(A) } F^\circ = 1.8 \ C^\circ + 32 \ (1.8 \times C^\circ + 32) \quad \text{or} \quad \text{(B) } F^\circ = \frac{9 \times C^\circ}{5} + 32$$

In the first method (A), multiply the Celsius temperature by 1.8 and add 32. In the second method (B), multiply the Celsius temperature by 9 and divide that answer by 5. Then add 32 to the answer.

EXAMPLE 3-5

Convert 65° C to F° using F° = 1.8° C + 32.

$$F^\circ = 65^\circ \times 1.8 \ (117) + 32 = 149^\circ F$$

OR

Using $F^\circ = \dfrac{9 \times C^\circ}{5} + 32$, the formula would look like the following:

$$F^\circ = 585 \ (9 \times 65^\circ) \div 5 + 32 = 117 + 32 = 149^\circ F$$

Alternate Formula for Converting between Celsius and Fahrenheit

This formula may be used for conversions for both systems:

$$9C^\circ = 5F^\circ - 160$$

EXAMPLE 3-6

Convert 65° C to F°.

Hint: When crossing the equal sign, the mathematical signs are reversed and those numbers subtracted on one side become added on the other, as shown here:

$$9 \times 65 = 5F - 160$$

$$5F = 9 \times 65 + 160$$

$$5° F = 585 + 160 \text{ or } 745$$

$$F° = 745 \div 5$$

$$F° = 149°$$

EXAMPLE 3-7

Convert 96.5° F to C°.

$$9 \ C = 96.5 \times 5 - 160$$

$$9 \ C = 482.5 - 160$$

$$9 \ C = 322.5$$

$$C° = 322.5 \div 9$$

$$C° = 35.8°$$

Learn the formula that is easiest for you. Notice that the answers obtained using this formula are identical to those using the formulas earlier.

! TECH ALERT

If an electronic thermometer is used in the clinical area, most of these devices automatically convert between Celsius and Fahrenheit. The machine may have to be manually changed between the different scales. Each thermometer would have directions from the manufacturer to accomplish the change.

Practice Problems D

Convert the following temperatures using the appropriate formulas. Round to tenths as appropriate.

1. 1° F = _____ C   **2.** 35° C = _____ F   **3.** 35° F = _____ C

4. 19° C = _____ F   **5.** 112° F = _____ C   **6.** 34° C = _____ F

7. 36.5° C = _____ F   **8.** 102.6° F = _____ C   **9.** 98.6° F = _____ C

10. 99.2° F = _____ C   11. 37.2° C = _____ F   12. 100.2° F = _____ C

13. 10.2° C = _____ F   14. 130.6° F = _____ C   15. 48.2° C = _____ F

16. If a serum is to be stored at a temperature cooler than 40° F, what is the temperature for storage in a refrigerator on a Celsius thermometer? _____

17. Mrs. Jones is to receive an antibiotic if her temperature is above 103.8° F. What is the Celsius conversion? _____

18. A parenteral medication is to arrive through the mail. The label on the box states that the medication cannot be exposed to temperatures higher than 47.8° C. The current outdoor temperature is 100.2° F. Can the medication be safely used? _____ What is the converted temperature? _____

19. If a bottle of medication must be stored at a temperature cooler than 45° F, what is the Celsius temperature at which the medication must be stored? _____

20. A bag of fluids must be given at body temperature of 98.6° F. What is that temperature in the Celsius measurement? _____

Posttest

Before taking the Posttest, retake the Pretest to check your understanding of the materials presented in this chapter.

Complete the mathematical calculations as needed. Always show your work so that you can verify the results.

Change the following to either Arabic numbers or Roman numerals as appropriate.

1. xxvii$\overline{\text{ss}}$ _____

2. xliv _____

3. xciii$\overline{\text{ss}}$ _____

4. ccl _____

5. 45 _____

6. $36\frac{1}{2}$ _____

7. 46 _____

8. 59 _____

9. 75 _____

10. viii$\overline{\text{ss}}$ _____

11. lxviii _____

12. cxxv _____

13. xii _____

14. 78 _____

15. 165 _____

Change the following to either 24-hour time or 12-hour time as appropriate.

16. 0530 _____

17. 8:30 AM _____

18. 1625 _____

19. 2:30 PM _____

20. 1325 _____

21. 0045 _____

22. 12:05 AM _____

23. 9:30 PM _____

24. 12:10 PM _____

Posttest, cont.

25. 0010 _____

26. 1755 _____

27. 3:26 PM _____

28. 1455 _____

29. 5:30 PM _____

30. 0635 _____

Convert the following temperatures. If Fahrenheit is listed, change to Celsius; if Celsius is given, change to Fahrenheit. Round to tenths.

31. 124° F _____

32. 49.2° F _____

33. 36.5° C _____

34. 234° F _____

35. 12.4° C _____

36. 99.6° F _____

37. 38.6° C _____

38. 86° F _____

39. 180° F _____

40. 94.2° F _____

41. 103° F _____

42. 100° C _____

43. 32° F _____

44. 2° F _____

45. 2° C _____

Answer the following questions in mathematical terms.

46. The room temperature in the pharmacy is 68° F. What is the temperature in Celsius?
_____

Continued

Posttest, cont.

47. A medication cannot be frozen. The refrigerator is set for 5° C. What is the temperature in Fahrenheit? _____ Will the medication freeze? _____

48. A patient has a temperature of 38.6° C. What is the temperature in Fahrenheit? _____ Should the medical professional be concerned about this body temperature? _____

49. A refrigerator in the pharmacy department shows a temperature of 35.2° C. Should the pharmacy technician be concerned about any medications that must be stored below 50° F? _____ What is the temperature in Fahrenheit? _____

50. A physician writes an order for xxiv tablets. How many tablets should be dispensed? _____

51. An order shows to dispense xc number of tablets. How many tablets will be dispensed? _____

52. When writing a prescription, the physician wants grains viiss to be dispensed as a tablet dose. How many grains of medication will be given as the dose? _____

53. An order states to give medications at 0800, 1200, and 2000. What times are the medications to be given in 12-hour time? _____ _____ _____

Posttest, cont.

54. A physician wants medication to be given every 6 hours beginning at 6:00 AM. Write the universal time for every 6 hours. _____ _____ _____ _____

55. A chart reads that the patient had pain medication at 5:35 PM. The medication can be taken every 6 hours. At what time in universal time could the next dose of medicine be given? _____

56. A medication order is to dispense xlviii tablets. How many tablets is this in Arabic numbers? _____

57. You supply a medication to the floor at 4:30 PM. You must chart the supply in universal time. What is the time of delivery? _____

58. The temperature in a patient's room is 37.6° C. What is the temperature in Fahrenheit? _____

59. If a medication is to be stored below 45° F, what would be the temperature on a Celsius thermometer in a refrigerator? _____

60. If a medication must be frozen at all times and the label states that it should be stored below 27° F, what would you need the refrigerator temperature to be in Celsius? _____

REVIEW OF RULES

Roman Numerals and Arabic Numerals

- When a Roman numeral is repeated, the value of the number is the number of times of repetition. The numeral may be repeated up to three times.

- The letters V, L, and D are not repeated.

- When a numeral of a lower value is placed following a larger numeral value, the value of the smaller numeral is added to the larger numeral.

- If a numeral of a lower value is placed before a larger numeral, the value of the smaller numeral is subtracted from the larger numeral. Only one smaller numeral may be placed in front of a larger numeral to indicate the decrease in the larger numeral.

- The numeral subtracted from a larger numeral can be no less than one tenth of the value of the number from which it is subtracted.

- Use the largest numerals possible for the number.

Military Time and 12-Hour Time

- Military and traditional time have the same meaning from 1 AM to 12:59 PM.

- Minutes after midnight may be written either as 0000 or 2400 hours depending on the policy of the employment site.

- Minutes after midnight and before 1:00 AM are written with 00 followed by the number of minutes.

- The hours between 1 PM and 12 AM are the time plus 12 added to the hour.

- If time requires seconds, the military time will include 6 numerals. Add two digits to the right of the minutes.

Celsius and Fahrenheit Temperature

- To convert Fahrenheit to Celsius: $C° = \dfrac{F° - 32}{1.8}$ or $C° = (F° - 32) \times \dfrac{5}{9}$

- To convert Celsius to Fahrenheit: $F° = 1.8\,C° + 32$ or $F° = 9 \times C° \div 5 + 32$

- The following formula may be used to convert from Celsius to Fahrenheit or from Fahrenheit

- to Celsius: $9\,C° = 5\,F° - 160$

CHAPTER 4

Comparisons of Measurement Systems

OBJECTIVES

- Know standard abbreviations for the household, metric, and apothecary systems used in the medical field
- Identify, convert, and calculate using household measurements of length, weight, and volume found in the medical field
- Identify, convert, and calculate using International System of Units (SI), or metric, measurements of length, weight, and volume found in the medical field
- Identify, convert, and calculate using apothecary system measurements of weight and volume found in the medical field

KEY WORDS

Apothecary system One of the oldest measurement systems used to calculate drug orders using measurements such as grains and minims

International System of Units (SI) (or metric system) Internationally accepted system of measurement of mass, length, and time based on international units

U.S. customary system (household system) System of measurement based on common kitchen measuring devices

Viscosity Thickness of a substance

Pretest

Identify the following abbreviations related to systems of measurement used with prescriptions.

1. mg _____

2. mcg _____

3. g _____

4. gr _____

5. kg _____

6. " _____

7. oz _____

8. ʒ _____

Continued

Pretest, cont.

9. mEq _____

10. ʒ _____

11. gtt _____

12. tsp _____

13. tbsp _____

14. ♍ _____

Show your calculations as you complete the following conversions. When calculating in U.S. Customary System, use ounce and pound conversions as found in that system.

15. 15 gtts = _____ tsp

16. 6 tbsp = _____ oz

17. 15 tsp = _____ tbsp

18. 1 mcg = _____ mg

19. 6 kg = _____ mg

20. 3 viii = ʒ _____

21. 4 c = _____ oz

22. 6 pt = _____ qt

23. 3 tbsp = _____ oz

24. 250 mg = _____ g

25. 0.125 mg = _____ mcg

26. 1.56 g = _____ mg

27. 5.6 kg = _____ g

28. 3 ii = ʒ _____

29. 2.5 g = _____ mg

30. 60″ = _____ ′

Pretest, cont.

31. 2′ = _____ ″

32. 5 kg = _____ mcg

33. 44# = _____ oz

34. $\text{ʒ} \frac{3}{4} = \text{ʒ}$ _____

35. 6 tbsp = _____ tsp

36. 2.5 g = _____ kg

37. 60 gtts = _____ tsp

38. ʒ iv = ʒ _____

39. 6 c = _____ oz

40. 6 c = _____ pt

INTRODUCTION

Three measurement systems are presently used in the medical field to calculate drug amounts in weight, length, or volume, although length is not as commonly used in the pharmaceutical field as in other medical disciplines. One of the three systems is used in the United States on a daily basis—the household measurement, or **U.S. Customary system**. This system uses measurements such as cups, teaspoons, and pints. The **International System of Units** (abbreviated SI from the French, Système International d'Unités), or the metric system, is used in most of the remaining world. Its measurements are milligrams, grams, milliliters, and so on. The **apothecary system**, which uses grains and drams, is an older system that has been used in pharmacy for many years but is used less frequently today. Knowledge of these three systems is absolutely necessary so you can interpret medication orders or prescriptions and to advise patients in administration of drugs as needed. To administer the correct amount of the medication on a consistent basis, the pharmacy technician must understand how to use the medication that was probably written on an order, whether a prescription or chart, in the metric, U.S. Customary, or apothecary system. The conversion of values from one system to another is discussed in the next chapter, but this chapter is designed to ensure that you have basic knowledge of the measurements, their abbreviations, and the system in which each occurs.

All three systems—household, metric, and apothecary—have units of measure for weight and volume. In the household system, weight is in pounds and ounces with volume in quarts, pints, cups, teaspoons, tablespoons, and the like. The metric system is based on grams for weight and liters for volume. Length is found in the household as yards, feet, and inches and in metric systems as meters. But length is not found in the apothecary system. The apothecary units of interest are grains for weight with drams and ounces for liquids.

Metric weight is the measurement used most often in pharmacy to show a dosage unit. Most medications are ordered and supplied by the weight of a drug in solid, liquid, or gaseous amounts such as milligrams or grains per tablet or per liquid amount such as milliliters. Household units of weights are usually seen in conversions for individual dosing at home and are found by volume rather than actual weight. We do not use pounds and ounces in dosage administration. Start thinking about metric units of weight—milligrams and grams—and remember that these weight measurements are most often used in the medical field because of accuracy and ease of the system based on units of 10. Other weight measurements include pounds and ounces in household weights, kilograms and micrograms in the metric system, and grains for the apothecary system.

Volume is capacity or how much a container of liquid medication holds. Amounts of medications per teaspoon or tablespoon would be the weight of medication found in the liquid measurement or dosage per volume. Volume measurements include milliliters, liters, quarts, pints, teaspoons, tablespoons, and minims or drops.

Length is used in household and metric systems to measure height or body circumference as well as length of a suture line. In pharmacy, length is only used to measure medications that require application to the body that must be measured in inches or centimeters or millimeters. In this case, the means of application is usually premarked on a dispensing paper for ease in ensuring that the correct amount of medication is being administered, such as with nitroglycerin ointment. Another pharmaceutical use of length is in finding body surface area (BSA) in which height and weight are compared for dosage calculation (BSA is discussed in Chapter 10). Length measurements also include inches, feet, centimeters, meters, kilometers, yards, and miles.

Some of the previously mentioned measurements are those you use daily, whereas others may be foreign and need explanation. This chapter covers the basic measurements per system, which are essential for learning conversions in Chapter 5.

HOUSEHOLD OR U.S. CUSTOMARY SYSTEM

The household or U.S. customary system of measure is being introduced first because much of it is already familiar. From elementary school to the present, these measurements have been taught and used in your daily life, such as with cooking. Measurements are based on the English system of measures, which had its beginnings with the Greeks and Romans. These measurements will most likely be used in the home setting for administration of medications, although use of a measurement device that is provided with the medication increases patient safety. Therefore, you must be familiar with this system, although it is the least accurate of the measurement systems. In a hospital setting, these measurements would not be as appropriate.

Household measurements are expressed in Arabic numbers with the abbreviation for each following the number, such as 5 tsp or 2½ pt. Table 4-1 provides the basic household measurements for weight accompanied by abbreviations and equivalents as appropriate.

Some medication labels include household measurements as well as metric measurements as seen on the label for Retrovir (Figure 4-1).

Table 4-2 gives the measurements of length often seen in the medical setting. A mile is also a measurement of length but is not used in pharmaceutical calculations.

Table 4-3 shows the household measurements of volume or liquid used most frequently in the home and in pharmaceutical calculations. Always remember that the size of a drop is totally dependent on the size of the opening in the dropper and **viscosity** of the liquid; therefore the 60 drops per teaspoon often found in measurement tables for household measurements is only an approximation. Drops used with intravenous therapy are stated in invariable amounts in the metric system as will be seen in later chapters. Also, household utensils are not necessarily accurate, so the amounts measured in these utensils should be considered only approximations.

TABLE 4.1 Household Measurements of Weight

MEASUREMENT UNIT	ABBREVIATION	EQUIVALENT
Ounce	oz	—
Pound	lb, #	16 oz
Ton	T	2000#

TABLE 4.2 Household Measurements of Length

MEASUREMENT UNIT	ABBREVIATION	EQUIVALENTS
Inch	in, "	—
Foot	ft, '	12 inches
Yard	yd	36 inches, 3 feet

TABLE 4.3 Household Measurements of Volume

MEASUREMENT UNIT	ABBREVIATION	EQUIVALENTS
Drops	gtts	—
Teaspoon	tsp, Tsp, t	60 drops (depending on the size of the dropper and the viscosity of the medication)
Tablespoon	tbsp, Tbsp, tbs, T	3 teaspoons
Ounce	oz	2 tbsp or 6 tsp
Cup	C, c	8 oz
Pint	pt	2 c, 16 oz
Quart	qt	2 pt, 4 c, 32 oz
Gallon	gal	4 qt, 8 pt, 16 c, 128 oz

TECH ALERT

A teaspoon is a smaller measurement used in household measures, so the abbreviation is "t." A tablespoon is larger and is often abbreviated with a "T."

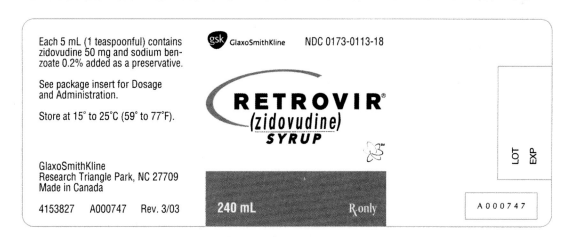

FIGURE 4-1 Label for Retrovir.

TECH ALERT

Learn the conversion presented as an appropriate equivalency table may not be available each time you need to make a conversion.

! TECH ALERT

In oral medications drops vary in size depending on the dropper opening and the viscosity of the medication. In general with oral medications, drops should not be used for measuring drugs unless using the specific dropper available for the medication (preferably a calibrated dropper).

TECH NOTE

The household system of measurement also uses fractions for expressing parts of a whole, such as $\frac{1}{2}$, $\frac{2}{3}$, or $\frac{3}{4}$. For example, a teaspoon and a half would be expressed as $1\frac{1}{2}$ tsp. You will later learn that the apothecary system also uses fractions, whereas the metric system uses decimal values.

Using Ratio and Proportion for Finding Equivalency with Household System

POINTS TO REMEMBER

STEPS FOR SOLVING THE UNKNOWN USING PROPORTION
1. Identify the unknown unit of measurement.
2. Find the known equivalent for the problem to be solved.
3. Write the known equivalent on the left side of the proportion.
4. Write the unknown desired on the right side of the proportion with the identical measurements in the same positions in the equation (i.e., inches : feet :: inches : feet; tsp : tbsp :: tsp : tbsp; inches : feet :: inches : feet).
5. Solve the equation by cross-multiplication of means and extremes or use "insies" and "outsies."

EXAMPLE 4-1

4 ft = x inches

A known factor is 1 ft = 12 inches. Use ratio and proportion to calculate the number of inches in 4 feet.

Known   Unknown

1 ft : 12 in :: 4 ft : x

After cross multiplying the equation will be as follows:

$1x = 48$ in

NOTE: *ft* may be cancelled because both equivalents of the same measurement are known and appear on both sides of the fractional equation.

So, 4 ft = 48 inches because the "x" is asking for inches.

EXAMPLE 4-2

In this example the known factor is 3 tsp = 1 tbsp. Using ratio and proportion the fractional equation is as follows:

4 tbsp = _____ tsp

Known   Unknown

3 tsp : 1 tbsp :: x tsp : 4 tbsp

$1x = 12$ tsp

NOTE: *tbsp* may be cancelled because both equivalents of the same measurement are known and appear on both sides of the fractional equation.

TECH ALERT

When calculating using ratio and proportion, be careful to place the designated measurement in the same position in each ratio. Place the known equivalents on the left side of the equation with the unknown on the right side of the equation. This will assist in being sure placement of the measurements is the same in each ratio.

Using Fractional Method for Finding Equivalency in Household Measurements

POINTS TO REMEMBER
STEPS FOR SOLVING THE UNKNOWN USING FRACTIONS AND CROSS MULTIPLICATION

1. Identify the unknown unit of measurement.
2. Find the known equivalent for the problem to be solved.
3. Write the known equivalents in a fraction on the left side of the equation.
4. Write the unknown desired equivalent in a fraction on the right side of the equation using x as the indication of the unknown.
5. Cross-multiply the numerators and denominators to solve for the unknown.

Another method of solving the unknown is to place the known equivalent and unknown equivalent into fractions and cross-multiply, as follows:

4 ft = _____ in (Unknown equivalent) 1 ft = 12 in (Known equivalent)

$$\frac{\text{Known}}{\text{Known}} \diagup\!\!\!\!\diagdown \frac{\text{Unknown}}{\text{Unknown}} \qquad \frac{4\ \text{ft}}{1\ \text{ft}} \diagup\!\!\!\!\diagdown \frac{x\ \text{in}}{12\ \text{in}}$$

NOTE: *ft* may be cancelled because both equivalents of the same measurement are known on the functional equation.

x in $= 12 \times 4$ or   48

Therefore, 4 ft = 48 in

OR

4 tbsp = _____ tsp (Unknown equivalent)   3 tsp = 1 tbsp (Known equivalent)

$$\frac{\text{Unknown}}{\text{Known}} \diagup\!\!\!\!\diagdown \frac{\text{Unknown}}{\text{Known}} \qquad \frac{3\ \text{tsp}}{1\ \text{tbsp}} \diagup\!\!\!\!\diagdown \frac{x\ \text{tsp}}{4\ \text{tbsp}}$$

NOTE: *tbsp* may be cancelled because both equivalents of the same measurement are known.

x tsp $= 3 \times 4 = 12$ tsp

Therefore, 4 tbsp = 12 tsp.

EXAMPLE 4-3

An infant is measured at 2′ 1½″. What would this be in inches? (1 ft = 12 inches)

To set up this problem, use a proportion as follows:

Known   Unknown
1 ft : 12″ :: 2 ft : x inches

1 ft : 12″ :: 2 ft : x inches

$$x \times 1 \text{ ft} = 12'' \times 2 \text{ ft}$$

$$x = 24 \text{ inches}$$

Now add $1\frac{1}{2}''$ to the 24″ as indicated in the problem.

So the infant's length is $25\frac{1}{2}''$.

OR

Known   Unknown

$$\frac{1 \text{ ft}}{12 \text{ in}} \diagdown\!\!\!\diagup \frac{2 \text{ ft}}{x \text{ in}}$$

$$1 \times x \text{ in} = 2 \times 12 \quad \text{or} \quad x = 24 \text{ in}$$

$$24 \text{ inches} + 1\frac{1}{2} \text{ inches} = 25\frac{1}{2} \text{ inches}$$

EXAMPLE 4-4

Sally needs to take a teaspoon of medication. The only measuring spoon available is a tablespoon. How much medication should Sally place in the tablespoon for an approximation of each dose?

Known   Unknown

$$1 \text{ tbsp} : 3 \text{ tsp} :: x : 1 \text{ tsp}$$

$$1 \text{ tbsp} : 3 \text{ tsp} :: x : 1 \text{ tsp}$$

$$3 \text{ tsp} \times x \text{ tbsp} = 1 \text{ tbsp} \times 1 \text{ tsp}$$

$$3x \text{ tbsp} = 1 \text{ tbsp}$$

$$x = \frac{1}{3} \text{ tbsp}$$

OR

Known   Unknown

$$\frac{1 \text{ tbsp}}{3 \text{ tsp}} \diagdown\!\!\!\diagup \frac{x}{1 \text{ tsp}}$$

$$x \times 3 \text{ tsp} = 1 \text{ tbsp} \times 1 \text{ tsp}$$

$$3x = 1 \text{ tbsp}$$

$$x = \frac{1}{3} \text{ tbsp}$$

! TECH ALERT

The use of household measurement utensils provide only an approximation of a needed dose and may result in either an overdose or too little of the medication. When an approximate dose is given, therapy may be varied and may not provide the therapeutic results desired.

POINTS TO REMEMBER

THE HOUSEHOLD SYSTEM
- The household system uses fractions and Arabic numerals.
- Teaspoon and tablespoon are common measures in household measures.
- For patient safety, household utensils should not be used except when absolutely necessary. Household utensils are only approximations. For correct dosing use the measuring device provided with the medication.

Practice Problems A

Calculate the following conversions. Show all of your calculations. Use the tables as provided in this section of text, using the correct indications for parts of a number if the answer is not a whole number.

1. 9 tsp = _____ tbsp

2. 39″ = _____ ft _____ ″

3. 2 qt = _____ gal

4. 3 tbsp = _____ oz

5. 6 oz = _____ c

6. 5 c = _____ oz

7. 15 tsp = _____ tbsp

8. 75 gtts = _____ tsp

9. 24 tbsp = _____ c

10. $4\frac{1}{2}$ oz = _____ tsp

11. 4 c = _____ pt

12. 20 oz = _____ #

13. 4′ 6″ = _____ ″

14. 6′ 1″ = _____ ″

15. $3\frac{1}{2}$ # = _____ oz

16. 5′ 10″ = _____ ″

17. $\dfrac{1}{2}$ tbsp = _____ tsp

18. $\dfrac{1}{2}$ tbsp = _____ gtts

19. 3 pt = _____ qt

20. 6 qt = _____ gal

21. 3 tsp = _____ gtts

22. 45 gtts = _____ tsp

23. 30 oz = _____ # (use decimal places to hundredths for this problem)

24. 24 oz = _____ c

25. 10 c = _____ oz

Practice Problems B

Patients will often use calibrated medication cups or oral syringes at home to take medications; however, these utensils may not be provided or may be misplaced so the pharmacy technician must have an understanding of conversions within household measurements. Convert the following problems to easier-to-use household measurements.

1.   The physician orders 4½ tsp of amoxicillin.

How many tablespoons would the patient take? _____

2.   The physician orders 1 oz of milk of magnesia.

How many tablespoons are ordered? _____

3. The physician orders 120 gtts of Rondec DM for a child.

   How many teaspoonfuls would you give the child? _____

4. A patient is to take 1 quart of Go-Lytely in preparation for x-rays.

   How many ounces of the medication should the patient drink? _____

5. The physician tells the patient to drink at least 24 additional ounces of water a day.

   How many cups of additional water would the patient need to drink to follow the physician's order? _____

LEARNING TIP

When using ratio and proportion to convert either within the same measurement system or when converting between two measurement systems, place your known measurements first and then be sure to place the unknown measures in the same order.

METRIC SYSTEM OF MEASUREMENT

The metric system of measurement is the most widely used throughout the world and is the most commonly used system for measuring medications and dosage. Most prescriptions are written in the metric system, and most liquid drugs are administered using this system. The *U.S. Pharmacopeia* names the metric system as the appropriate system for use on drug labels. The Metric Conversion Act of 1975 stated that the United States would convert to the use of the metric system, but the date for the completion of the conversion was not given. Transition to the metric system is evident in gauges, road signs, car speedometers, and other commercial products, but members of the U.S. public have not converted their thinking to the metric system in all areas such as height, weight, and length.

The metric system is based on units of 10 and uses decimals to move within the system. The basic measurements are gram for weight, liter for volume, and meter for length. In this system, prefixes for the base measurements are used to indicate the multiples or submultiples of the base that is being described, such as milli- (one thousandth of the base), micro- (one millionth of the base), and kilo- (1000 base units). These are the prefixes most commonly used, whereas centi- is one hundredth of a base and is the most commonly used with length. Deci- equals one tenth of the base, deka- is 10 times the base, and hecto- is 100 times the base.

TECH NOTE

A gram is about the weight of two large sized paper clips.

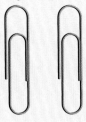

A liter is about the size of a quart container.

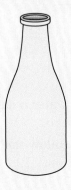

A meter is a little longer than a yardstick.

Inches

Centimeters

TECH NOTE

A grain is the approximate mass or size of a grain of rice. It is approximately $\frac{1}{2}$ inch long and less than $\frac{1}{8}$ inch in diameter. Fifteen grains make one gram.

Labels in the metric system are shown in the appropriate metric unit. However, some labels still contain abbreviations that are found on The Joint Commission "Do Not Use" List, such as μg for microgram as found on the label for Lanoxin in Figure 4-2.

See Figure 4-3 for basic metric units with their prefixes and Tables 4-4 and 4-5 for a summary of the metric system and its equivalents.

! TECH ALERT

Be careful to distinguish between mg (weight) and mL (volume) to prevent medication errors. Also, although μg (mcg) is on the "Do Not Use" list, it is still found on medications and should not be confused with mg. An error by 1000 times too much or too little will occur if there is confusion.

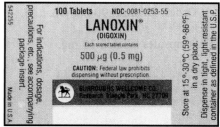
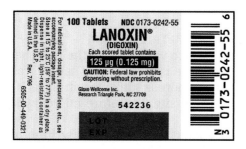

FIGURE 4-2 Label for Lanoxin.

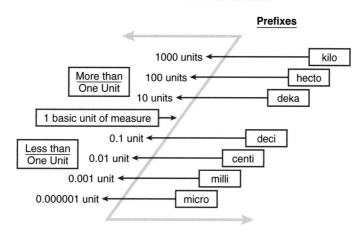

FIGURE 4-3 The basic units of measure—gram, liter, and meter—with prefixes indicating larger or smaller measures.

TABLE 4.4 Metric System of Measurements

UNIT	WEIGHT	VOLUME	LENGTH
Basic unit	gram (G, g, gm, Gm)	liter (L, l)	meter (M, m)
1000 units	kilogram (kg, kG)	*kiloliter*	*kilometer (km)*
100 units	*hectogram**	*hectoliter*	*hectometer*
10 units	*dekagram*	*dekaliter*	*dekameter*
1/10th unit	*decigram*	*deciliter*	*decimeter*
1/100th unit	*centigram*	*centiliter*	centimeter (cm)
1/1000th unit	milligram (mg, mG)	milliliter (ml, mL)	millimeter (mm)
1/1,000,000th unit	microgram (mcg)	*microliter*	*micrometer (mcm)*

*The measurements found in italics are those that are not commonly used in calculating pharmaceutical dosages in heights, weights, or volumes. Measurements with abbreviations are those that are commonly used in pharmacology.

TABLE 4.5 Equivalents in the Metric System

TYPE OF SUBSTANCE	ABBREVIATION	UNIT OF MEASURE	COMMON EQUIVALENTS
Volume/Liquid	L, l	liter	1000 mL, 1000 cc*
	mL, ml, cc*	milliliter, cubic centimeter*	0.001 L
Weight	G, g, gm, Gm	gram	1000 mg, 0.001 kG
	kG, kg	kilogram	1000 g
	mG, mg	milligram	0.001 gm, 1000 mcg
	mcg	microgram	0.000001 gm, 0.001 mg
Length	M, m	meter	100 cm, 1000 mm
	cm	centimeter	0.01 m, 10 mm
	mm	millimeter	0.001 m, 0.1 cm

*A cubic centimeter (cc) is another way to express a milliliter. A cubic centimeter is the amount of space that is required to hold a milliliter of liquid. The abbreviation "cc" is found on the "Do Not Use" list but is often still used in ambulatory care.

POINTS TO REMEMBER

RULES FOR CALCULATING EQUIVALENTS WITHIN THE METRIC SYSTEM

- The metric system is actually a system of "place values" with the base being the unit of measure from which the value place is measured. That is, gram, meter, and liter are at place "1" or base site, whereas kilos are at place 10^3 or 1000 site and millis are 10^{-3} or one thousandth site. Therefore micros would be 10^{-6} or one millionth site.
- When using the metric system of measurement, the numeral is written before the abbreviation for the quantity with a full space between the number and abbreviation (e.g., 10 mg, 2.5 mm, 1.5 L).
- Another rule with the metric system is that all fraction parts are written as a decimal number (e.g., 1.5 mL, 2.5 gm, or 2.75 m).
- A zero should always be placed before a decimal point when the number is less than a whole to prevent confusion and a possible error in calculating dosage For instance, .25 mg might be misread as 25 mg if the metric number had not been written 0.25 mg. The potential error would be 100 times too much medication being administered to a patient. **ALWAYS BE SURE THAT ANY METRIC NUMBER WITH A DECIMAL NUMBER HAS EITHER A "0" OR A NUMBER PRECEDING THE DECIMAL POINT.**
- Any unnecessary, or trailing, zeros should be eliminated from the number (e.g., 2.50 mg should read as 2.5 mg, 1.500 L should read as 1.5 L). Remember, zeros found at the end of a number behind the decimal point may be removed without changing the value of the number.

Converting from Larger Metric Numbers to Smaller Metric Numbers

The metric system is easy for conversions from one unit to the next because multiples of 10 are the base for the system. The placement of the decimal point is based on moving from the different powers of 10 by moving the decimal point. When moving from a larger metric unit to a smaller one, move the decimal point to the right the number of times that the unit is larger than the smaller unit or multiply by the number of zeros in the equivalent (large to small → multiply). See Examples 4-5 and 4-6.

EXAMPLE 4-5

1.2 L = _____ mL

A liter is larger than a milliliter, so we must move the decimal from left to right. A milliliter has three decimal places to the right, so we want to move the decimal three places to the right or multiply by 1000.

1.2 L becomes 1.2 0 0. or 1200 mL

$$\begin{array}{r} 1.2 \\ \times\ \ 1000 \\ \hline 1200.0 \end{array}$$

1.2 L = 1200 mL

LEARNING TIP

To go to the **S**maller number, move the decimal to the **R**ight. "R" and "S" are next to each other in the alphabet.

EXAMPLE 4-6

5.4 kg = _____ mg

5.4 kg becomes 5.4 0 0 0 0 0.   5.4
                ⌣⌣⌣⌣⌣⌣   ×   1000000
                ──────────→   ──────────
                                    5,400,000.0̸

5.4 kg = 5,400,000 mg

Converting from a Smaller Metric Number to a Larger Metric Number

If the movement is from a smaller to larger unit, move the decimal point to the left the number of times the unit is smaller or divide by the number of zeros found in the desired equivalent (small to large ← divide). To change a kilogram to a milligram, a kilogram is larger than a milligram, so we must move the decimal to the left. A kilogram has six zeros when moving to a kilogram, so we want six places behind the decimal point. See Examples 4-7 and 4-8.

> **LEARNING TIP**
>
> To move from the smaller number to a **Larger** number, move the decimal to the **Left**. Both "Larger" and "Left" begin with "L".

EXAMPLE 4-7

5 mg = _____ g

A milligram is smaller than a gram, so we move the decimal to the left by the number of zeros between a gram and a milligram (1 gram is equal to 1000 mg) or divide 5 mg by 1000 units.

5 mg is the same as 0.0 0 5 g or 5 ÷ 1000
                        ⌣⌣⌣
                      ←
                        5 mg = 0.005 g

> **TECH NOTE**
> Remember to always place a "0" in front of the decimal point if no number is otherwise present.

EXAMPLE 4-8

500 g = _____ kg

A gram is smaller than a kilogram, so the decimal moves to the left. A kilogram is equal to 1000 grams or three zeros to the left of a gram.

500 g is the same as 0.5 0 0 kg or 500 ÷ 1000
                         ⌣⌣⌣
                      ←

Because the zeros behind a decimal that are not followed by a number or trailing zeros can be dropped, the problem answer is as follows:

500 g = 0.500 kg = 0.5 kg

Using a Mnemonic to Convert Within the Metric System

An easy way to calculate within the metric system is to use a mnemonic in which the first letters in the mnemonic is the first letter of a metric unit. This allows the moving of decimal places from the known unit to the desired unit without having to remember whether to multiply or divide for the correct answer.

To use Figure 4-4, circle the two letters on the metric line that are stated in the desired conversion. Place the given amount on the metric line with the decimal point in the correct place on the line. (Remember that the decimal point in a whole number follows the number.) Now place a decimal point directly behind the letter on the line for the desired placement value and add zeros under each letter of the metric scale using the mnemonic until the desired metric unit is reached. See Figure 4-3 for the basic units of measure.

K	H	D	B	D	C	M	–	–	M
Kilo	Hecto	Deka	Base	Deci	Centi	Milli			Micro
0	0	0	•	0	0	0	–	–	0
Kids	Hate	Dogs	Because	Dogs	Chase	Mailmen	(many)	(many)	Mailmen
1000	100	10	Base	0.1	0.01	0.001			0.000001
Thou-sand	Hun-dred	Ten		Tenths	Hun-dredths	Thou-sandths			Thousand-thousandths

FIGURE 4-4 An easy way to find the equivalents in the metric system, using a mnemonic.

RULES FOR CONVERTING WITHIN THE METRIC SYSTEM USING THE MNEMONIC
- Using the mnemonic, construct the horizontal metric line from kilo- to micro- (K H D B D C M _ _M).
- Circle the known metric unit and the desired metric unit that are found in the problem.
- Place the decimal point of the known number in the correct place on the metric line.
- Place the decimal point of the unknown number in the correct place on the metric line.
- Fill in the spaces between the decimal points on the metric line with zeros.
- Avoid using decimals when whole numbers can be used (e.g., 0.5 g would be better expressed as 500 mg).

EXAMPLE 4-9

500 g = _____ kg

```
K H D B.D C M _ _ M          K H D B.D C M _ _ M
  5 0 0.                       0.5 0 0
                                  ᴗ ᴗ ᴗ
                                  ←
  5 0 0. gm       =             0.5 kg
```

Hint: Remember that gram is a base unit.

(Move the decimal to the left to behind the kilogram unit and add a zero under the kilograms because grams are smaller than kilograms. The zeros are dropped because trailing zeros should be removed or mistakes in calculations and administration may occur.)

EXAMPLE 4-10

5.4 kg = _____ mg

K.H D B D C M _ _ M   K.H D B D C M _ _ M
5.4   5. 4 0 0 0 0 0
                                             ‿ ‿ ‿ ‿ ‿ ‿
                                             ⟶

5.4 kg   =   5, 4 0 0,0 0 0 mg

(Move the decimal to the right to behind the milligram unit because kilograms are larger than milligrams. Then add zeros under each unit that the decimal has been moved.)

EXAMPLE 4-11

0.1 mg = _____ gm

K H D B D C M._ _ M   K H D B D C M._ _ M
        0.1   0.0 0 0 1
                                             ‿ ‿ ‿
                                             ⟵

0.1 mg   =   0.0 0 0 1 gm

(Move the decimal to the left from behind the milligram to the gram. Notice that the decimal is behind the 0 in milligram and in front of the 1 because the unit is 0.1 mg. After placing the number correctly on the unit line and placing the decimal at the base for gram, add the proper number of zeros in front of the one for the number of units between the decimal points.)

Practice Problems C

Complete the following problems by either using the number line of the mnemonic or by multiplying or dividing for the conversions within the metric system.

1. 2 L = _____ mL   2. 2.5 mg = _____ mcg

3. 4 kg = _____ g   4. 450 g = _____ kg

5. 0.5 L = _____ mL

6. 0.5 mg = _____ mcg

7. 0.5 mg = _____ g

8. 2.5 mL = _____ L

9. 50 mL = _____ L

10. 5.5 L = _____ mL

11. 1.5 g = _____ mg

12. 2.5 cm = _____ mm

13. 6.54 kg = _____ mg

14. 450 mm = _____ m

15. 25 mcg = _____ mg

16. 50.6 kg = _____ g

17. 10 L = _____ mL

18. 500 mL = _____ L

19. 3500 mL = _____ L

20. 0.0045 kg = _____ g

21. 0.3 mg = _____ mcg

22. 5 mL = _____ L

23. 58,400 mL = _____ L   24. 505 mL = _____ L   25. 300 mg = _____ mcg

26. A container of IV fluids contains ½ liter. How many milliliters is this? _____

Hint: Change ½ to a decimal first.

27. Amoxicillin is available as 250 mg/capsule.

How many grams of amoxicillin does each capsule contain? _____

28. A tablet of digoxin contains 250 mcg.

How would this be written in mg? _____

29. A physician orders 1 g of Cipro.

How many mg would the physician expect to be administered to the patient?

_____

30. A physician orders a thyroid replacement, Synthroid 0.175 mg.

How many micrograms would be given to the patient? _____

APOTHECARY SYSTEM OF MEASUREMENT

Less often used and used only with pharmacology, the apothecary system is one of the oldest systems of measurement. First used by an apothecary (precursor to a pharmacist), this system is gradually being replaced with the metric system. As long as prescriptions are written in this system, the health care worker must be aware of its notations and rules.

The metric system is the preferred measurement system; however, the apothecary system can still be found on rare occasions, especially with older medications, such as Nitrostat as seen in Figure 4-5. Other places where apothecary measurements are found are syringes, such as minims (ℳ); drams (ℨ) are found on medication-dispensing cups even though the use of these items and measurements are discouraged. These apothecary abbreviations are also found on the "Do Not Use List."

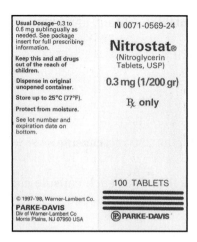

FIGURE 4-5 Label for Nitrostat.

TABLE 4.6 Equivalents in the Apothecary System

TYPE OF SUBSTANCE	ABBREVIATION	UNIT OF MEASURE	COMMON EQUIVALENTS
Volume/Liquid	♏	minim	—
	fl₃	fluid dram	♏ lx (60)
	fl℥	fluid ounce	₃ viii (8)
Mass/Weight	gr	grain	—
	₃	dram	gr lx (60)
	℥	ounce	₃ viii (8)
	#	pound	℥ xii (12)*

*Note that in the apothecary system a pound is only 12 ounces, but this not used on a regular basis in pharmacy calculations.

In the apothecary system, lower case Roman numerals are used for expression of numbers below 10, rather than Arabic numerals found in the metric and household systems. The Roman numerals should be expressed with lines placed over numerals to tie these together such as ī, īī, īīī, īv̄, v̄, and x̄, Arabic numerals may be used for numbers higher than 10, except with 20 ($\overline{xx}$) and 30 ($\overline{xxx}$), for which Roman numerals are required. Over the years, the use of the line over the Roman numeral has gradually diminished, but using it is the correct notation. The proper abbreviation is written first with Roman numerals placed to the right of the unit of measure—the opposite placement as found with metric and household. Most fractions are written using Arabic numbers such as ¼ or ⅙, except ½, which is abbreviated as s̄s̄. The abbreviation s̄s̄ actually means "semis." Also of importance is that decimals are not used with the apothecary system.

In ancient times, a minim (drop) of water was considered to weigh the same as a grain of wheat. Therefore the basic unit of liquid in the apothecary system is a minim (♏) and the basic unit of weight is a grain (gr). See Table 4-6 for equivalents in the apothecary system.

! TECH ALERT

Care should be taken that gr (grain) and g or gm (gram) are not confused. These measurements have different weights and are in two separate measurement systems.

LEARNING TIP

Notice that the ounce is larger than a dram, and the ounce symbol has one more loop than the dram symbol.

When notated in the apothecary system, the measurement is abbreviated and the amount drug always follows or is to the right (or behind) the abbreviated symbol (e.g., 5 oz would be written ℥ v, or 10 drams would be ℨ x).

As with household measurements, the use of ratio and proportion or fractional components can be used to make the conversion within the system.

> **! TECH ALERT**
>
> When using pound (#) abbreviations, be sure to determine whether it is in the household or apothecary system. The household pound is 16 ounces to a pound; the apothecary system is 12 ounces to a pound. In most modern uses, the household pound (16 oz) will be the correct conversion.

EXAMPLE 4-12

℥ ii = ℨ _____

Known   Unknown

℥ i : ℨ viii :: ℥ ii : x

℥ i : ℨ viii :: ℥ ii : x

$1x = 8 \times ℨ 2$

$x = ℨ 16$,   so   ℥ i(1) : ℨ viii(8) :: ℥ ii(2) : ℨ xvi(16)   or   ℥ ii(2) = ℨ xvi(16)

NOTE: Remember that the apothecary system is written in Roman numerals, although you may decide to convert to Arabic numbers to compute the problem.

OR

Known   Unknown

$$\frac{℥\ i}{ℨ\ viii} \quad \frac{℥\ ii}{x}$$

$1x = 8 \times ℨ 2$

$x = ℨ 16$,   so $\dfrac{℥\ i}{ℨ\ viii} = \dfrac{℥\ ii}{ℨ\ xvi}$ or   ℥ ii = ℨ xvi

POINTS TO REMEMBER
RULES FOR CONVERTING WITHIN THE APOTHECARY SYSTEM
- The quantity should be expressed in lower case Roman numerals with a line placed over the entire numeral, but this is not commonly seen today. (The line over the Roman numerals is often not added.)
- If the amount is greater than 10 and is not 20 or 30, the number may be written in Arabic numbers.
- Decimals are not used when writing numbers in the apothecary system.
- Numbers less than a whole are written as fractions, except 1/2, which is written s̄s̄.
- The symbol or abbreviation is written before the quantity of medication that is ordered.
- When using the symbols dram (ℨ) and ounce (℥), be sure to count the loops on the symbol for accuracy in measurements.

Practice Problems D

Practice your skills in the apothecary system, using the correct numerals for this system in the following problems. Show all of your calculations.

1. fl℥ vi = ℨ _____

2. fl℥ xii = ℨ _____

3. gr iv = ℨ _____

4. gr xxx = ℨ _____

5. gr x = ℨ _____

6. fl℥ v = fl℥ _____

7. fl℥ ii = fl℥ _____

8. fl℥ iii = fl℥ _____
drams 3

9. fl℥ vi = ℥ _____
drams 6

10. fl℥ xx = fl℥ _____

REVIEW

Three measurement systems are used in practicing pharmacology. The household system is the most commonly used on a daily basis in our homes and is also the system used for giving liquid medications at home if the appropriate dispenser is not provided. However, using the household system provides only approximate measurements because of the difference in utensils; it may cause an inaccurate dose when used for administering medication. The metric system is used as a standard unit of measure throughout the world and is structured on base 10 or multiples of 10. Most medications are designated in the metric system today. The final system, rarely used today but found with some medications, is the apothecary system, which is based on grains for weight and minims, drams, and ounces for volume. Although this system is not popular and its use is being discouraged, these measurements are still seen occasionally with some medications. Because of the three systems, the measurements for length, weight, and volume must be learned for conversions that are discussed in the next chapter, where conversions among systems are often approximate conversions and not exact conversions as found in this chapter.

Ratio/proportion may be used for the calculation of changes within a system. With the metric system, the decimal may be moved to make the necessary conversion. Use the method that is best for you and use it consistently.

Posttest

Before taking the Posttest, retake the Pretest to check your understanding of the materials presented in this chapter.

Using the appropriate system of measurement, figure the equivalents found in this posttest. Be sure to show all of your calculations. Round to hundredths appropriately unless otherwise indicated.

1. 36 kg = _____ g

2. 5.4 g = _____ mg

3. 3 tsp = _____ gtts

4. 4 tbsp = _____ tsp

5. gr v = 3 _____

6. fl℥ x = fl℥ _____

7. 6 pt = _____ qt

8. 125 mcg = _____ mg

9. 12.5 mg = _____ g

10. 0.5 mL = _____ cc

11. 1.75 L = _____ mL

12. 2 qt = _____ gal

13. 1 tsp = _____ gtts

14. 2 tbsp = _____ oz

15. 4 oz = _____ c

16. 4 c = _____ pt

17. 0.4 mg = _____ mcg

18. 1.3 kg = _____ mg

19. 1 tbsp = _____ oz

20. 4 oz = _____ tsp

21. fl℥ xvi = fl℥ _____

22. fl℥ xx = fl℥ _____

23. 40.5 mg = _____ g

24. 40.5 mg = _____ mcg

Continued

Posttest, cont.

25. 3.75 L = _____ mL   26. 12 c = _____ qt   27. 250 mg = _____ g

28. 0.25 g = _____ mg   29. 75 mL = _____ L   30. 250 mL = _____ L

31. 2 tsp = _____ tbsp   32. 8 tbsp = _____ oz   33. 32 oz = _____ c

34. 64 oz = _____ pt   35. 24 tsp = _____ oz   36. 1.2 mg = _____ mcg

37. ℈ xxiv = ℥ _____   38. ℥ viii = ℈ _____   39. ℥ iii s̄s̄ = ℈ _____

40. 4 c = _____ oz   41. 9 tsp = _____ tbsp   42. 55 mg = _____ g

43. 600 mg = _____ g   44. 650 mcg = _____ mg   45. fl℥ 1 1/4 = ℈ _____

46. 15 tbsp = _____ oz   47. 15 tsp = _____ oz   48. 0.05 g = _____ mg

49. 0.0025 g = _____ mg   50. 2.5 kg = _____ g

Posttest, cont.

51. A physician orders digoxin 0.125 mg tablet.

How many micrograms of medication should be provided with each tablet to the patient? _____

52. An order is given for amoxicillin 250 mg.

How many grams would this be? _____

53. A physician writes a prescription for Benadryl flℨ viii.

How many flℨ would that be? _____

54. An order is written for ranitidine 0.075 g.

How many mg is that? _____

55. A patient is given a prescription for sulfamethoxazole 2000 mg.

How many gm would be necessary? _____

56. An order is written for a patient with hypertension for hydralazine 25 mg tablets.

How many grams would be in each tablet? (Do not round.) _____

57. A physician asks a patient to take an ounce of Mylanta every 4 hours.

How many tablespoons would need to be taken with each dose? _____

58. A child is to take 1/2 tbsp of amoxicillin suspension.

How many teaspoons would the parent give the child? _____

Continued

Posttest, cont.

59. A physician orders Carafate Suspension 2 tbsp to be taken 30 minutes before meals. How many teaspoons would this be with each dose? _____

60. Because of hyperlipidemia, a patient is given a prescription for Zetia 0.01 g. How many milligrams would this be? _____

REVIEW OF RULES

Steps for Solving the Unknown Using Proportion

- Identify the unknown unit of measurement.
- Find the known equivalent for the problem to be solved.
- Write the known equivalent on the left side of the proportion.
- Write the unknown desired on the right side of the proportion with the identical measurement indicators in the same positions in the equation as was found in the known measurement equivalents (i.e., inches : feet :: inches : feet or tsp : tbsp :: tsp : tbsp).
- Solve the equation by cross-multiplication of means and extremes, or "insies" and "outsies."

Steps for Solving the Unknown Using Fractions and Cross-Multiplication

- Identify the unknown unit of measurement.
- Find the known equivalent for the problem to be solved.
- Write the known equivalents in a fractional unit on the left side of the equation.
- Write the unknown desired equivalent on the right side of the equation in the same position as the known equivalent using x as the indication of the unknown. Be sure to keep measurement indicators in the same positions.
- Cross-multiply numerators and denominators to solve for the unknown.

Rules for Calculating Equivalents within the Metric System

- The metric system is actually a system of "place values" with the base being the unit of measure from which the place value is measured. That is, gram, meter, and liter are at place value "1," kilos are at place 10^3 and millis are 10^{-3}. Therefore micros would be 10^{-6}.

- When using the metric system of measurement, the numeral unit is written before the abbreviation such as 10 mg, 2.5 cc, or 1.5 L.

- All fractions are written as decimals such as 1.5 mL, 2.5 gm, or 2.75 m.

- A zero should always be placed before a decimal point when the number is less than a whole number to prevent confusion and a possible error in calculating dosage. For example, .25 mg might be misread as 25 mg if the metric number had not been written 0.25 mg. The potential error would be 100 times too much medication being given to the patient. **ALWAYS BE SURE THAT ANY METRIC NUMBER WITH A DECIMAL NUMBER HAS EITHER A "0" OR A NUMBER PRECEDING THE DECIMAL POINT.**

- Any unnecessary or trailing zeros should be eliminated from the number (e.g., 2.50 mg should read as 2.5 mg, 1.500 L should read as 1.5 L). Remember, zeros found at the end of a number behind the decimal point may be removed without changing the value of the number.

- Avoid using a decimal number if a whole number can be used (e.g., 0.5 g would be better expressed as 500 mg).

Rules for Using the Metric Mnemonic for Conversions

- Write the metric scale (K H D B D C M _ _ M).

- Circle the two units found in the conversion.

- Count the number of metric units between the two circled units (the known and the unknown units) and add zeros under the units on the metric scale.

- Move the decimal point from behind the known amount to behind the unknown amount in the direction noted by the movement on the scale.

- Drop any unnecessary or trailing zeros that are found in front of or behind the decimal point.

Rules for Using the Apothecary System

- Numbers in the apothecary system are written in Roman numerals for those less than 10 and for 20 and 30. Other numbers may be written in Arabic numbers.

- Fractions are written as fractional units except 1/2, which is written as "s̄s̄."

- Numbers below 10 should be written with a line over them, although this line is not used as often as it used to be.

- When writing in the apothecary system, the measurement is abbreviated and the numeral unit follows or is placed to the right of (behind) the abbreviated symbol (e.g., 5 oz would be written ℥ v).

CHAPTER 5

Conversions among Measurement Systems

OBJECTIVES

- Convert among metric, household, and apothecary systems using ratio and proportion
- Convert among metric, household, and apothecary systems using dimensional analysis

KEY WORDS

Avoirdupois system English system of weights in which values range from 1 pound equals 16 oz to 7000 grains equals 1 pound

Dimensional analysis Mathematical means of manipulating units or the dimension given to numbers to cancel unwanted units when converting unit equivalency; an advanced form of ratio and proportion

Measurable amount The quantity of medication that can be most accurately measured and the utensil available

> **! TECH ALERT**
>
> When making conversions between two measurement systems, the answers will usually not be exact, and the accepted difference between the measurement systems is in the range of 10% either above or below the actual calculated amount. Other factors in calculating approximate measurements do exist, such as the viscosity of the medication and the size of the utensils that will be used to provide the medication. In this text, please be sure that your conversion is as close to an exact amount as possible, so use the conversion factor that will give you an answer that can be administered with the utensil available. For example, in some cases a teaspoon may be 4 milliliters, but in others, when calculating a teaspoon, the conversion may be 5 milliliters. In these cases, you will need to complete the problem using both conversions to find the answer that is measurable. You always want to find the **measurable amount** for the ease of administration. For example, if your answer from the conversion indicates 4.4 milliliters is to be administered and this medication will be given with a utensil holding either 4 or 5 milliliters, such as a dosespoon, you would indicate that 4 milliliters would be given; however, if this is being given with a teaspoon that holds 5 milliliters, measuring 4.4 milliliters would not be possible, so you would state to administer a teaspoon of medication. Finally, if the dosespoon or other measurement utensil is found in 0.01-milliliter increments, the exact amount may be administered. This concept is difficult to understand, but as you go through this chapter, please use the conversion factor that supplies the approximate dose that is measurable. Also remember that some of the conversions used in the mathematical calculations in this chapter are based on the materials presented in Chapter 4. This text builds on previously learned materials, and materials in previous chapters will be important for use starting with this chapter on conversions among measurement systems.

Pretest

Be sure to use the correct numerical system when solving the problems in the Pretest. Show your calculations and round to the nearest hundredth. Remember that in this chapter you are converting among measurement systems and not within the measurement system. In converting drops to milliliters, you will have two answers based on the commonly used conversions of drops to milliliters. The two lines are provided for the problems needing two answers.

1. 20 mL = _____ gtts _____ gtts

2. 4 tsp = ℨ _____

3. 15 tbsp = _____ oz

4. 2 oz = _____ tsp

5. 6″ = _____ cm

6. 16 oz = _____ pt

7. 8 c = _____ qt

8. ♏ xxxii = _____ mL

9. ♏ vi = _____ gtts

10. gr $\frac{1}{4}$ = _____ mg

11. 88# = _____ kg

12. 120 mg = _____ gr

13. ♏ viii = _____ mL

14. 8 kg = _____ mg

15. 15 gtts = ♏ _____

16. 6 tbsp = _____ oz

17. 15 tsp = ℨ _____

18. gr xv = _____ mg

19. gr v = _____ mg

20. 60 mL = ℨ _____

21. 4 c = ℨ _____

22. 25 cm = _____ ′

Continued

Pretest, cont.

23. 3 tbsp = ℥ _____

24. 250 mg = gr _____

25. 0.125 mg = _____ mcg

26. gr $\frac{1}{6}$ = _____ mg

27. gr xxx = _____ mg

28. gr viiss̄ = _____ mg

29. 4.56 g = _____ mcg

30. 60″ = _____ ′

31. 2′ = _____ cm

32. 5 kg = _____ #

33. 44 # = _____ kg

34. gr $\frac{3}{4}$ = _____ mg

35. ʒ vi = _____ tsp

36. ℥ xv = _____ tbsp

37. gr iiss̄ = _____ mg

38. 156 # = _____ kg

39. ℥ vi = _____ tbsp

40. ʒ viiss̄ = _____ tsp

INTRODUCTION

In the previous chapter you learned the basic measurements found in the household, metric, and apothecary systems of measurements. Each of these is used today in prescribing and administering medications. Another measurement system, **avoirdupois,** is also available, but this system is not normally found in calculations or conversions. In this system, 16 ounces = one pound (7000 grains = one pound). Two other measures are used in dosage calculations—milliequivalents and units—that will be discussed in Chapter 6.

The household measures are those that use common measuring tools found in most homes. Therefore for the person taking medication to be able to use utensils available, you must convert any orders written in apothecary or metric systems to the household measurements for ease of drug administration. If a physician writes an order in the apothecary system and the medication is available in a metric dose, you must convert the apothecary dose to an approximate metric equivalent to ensure the patient receives the correct amount of medication. As the metric system becomes more widely accepted, the need for conversion will decrease, although the need to calculate a dose in the household measure will remain as long as the United States is measuring in household equivalents.

Conversions among the systems are only necessary if the two factors needed for calculation are not found within the same measurement system. If both factors are already in the metric system, then moving within the system is all that is necessary, as seen in Chapter 4. This is likewise true for the apothecary and household measurements. However, if one factor is in one system, such as the metric system, and the other factor is in another system, such as household, proportional equations are used to find the unknown approximation.

Either ratio and proportion or an advanced system of ratio and proportion, called **dimensional analysis,** may be used.

Both systems are presented in this chapter so you can decide which method is easier for your personal use. Find the system with which you feel comfortable and use it regularly to perfect its use. Only through practice will this become a skill that is easy for you to use for making pharmaceutical calculations.

One further hint is necessary before beginning the process of converting measurements: Because the measurement systems are not identical, any conversions among them are approximate in the conversion. You cannot find an exact equivalent in most conversions; rather the number will be an approximate amount. An example is that a dram is often used as a symbol for a teaspoon when a dram is actually 4 mL and a teaspoon may be either 4 or 5 mL depending on the utensil. This conversion therefore becomes an approximate amount.

USING RATIO AND PROPORTION FOR CONVERSION OF UNITS

Ratio is the relationship of one quantity to another, whereas proportion is the relationship between two equal ratios. In ratio and proportion, an unknown is solved using "x" as the unknown. This provides a logical and systematic means of finding the equivalent unknown when knowns are used for calculations. Two equal ratio sets (or the relationship between two equivalents, such as a [extreme] : b [mean] :: c [mean] : d [extreme]) is indicated for calculating proportional equivalents. When one of the equivalents is unknown, an "x" is used to indicate the unknown. (See Chapter 2 if you need to review this material.)

TECH NOTE

When converting between two measurement systems, the conversion is an approximate amount, not an exact calculation. The final answer should always be one that is measurable in the system of the conversion, such as 1.7 tsp would be 1 3/4 tsp in household measurements, because 0.7 tsp cannot be measured.

EXAMPLE 5-1

A physician orders an antibiotic that is available as 250 mg/5 mL. The household measurement to be used is a teaspoon. To be able to change the metric amount of 5 mL to the household teaspoon, the proportion would appear as follows:

$$5 \text{ mL} : 1 \text{ tsp} :: 5 \text{ mL} : x \text{ tsp}$$

$$5 \text{ mL} : 1 \text{ tsp} :: 5 \text{ mL} : x \text{ tsp}$$

$$5x = 1 \times 5 \quad \text{or} \quad 5$$

$$x = 1 \text{ tsp}$$

In review, when calculating using ratio and proportion, a good rule of thumb is to place the known conversion ratio on the left side of the equation. The equal measurements must be placed in the same position in the both ratios. (If "x" and "y" are being used to identify specific units of a ratio, the "x" and "y" must remain in the same order in all ratios of the proportions. In other words, if the "x" is on the left of the first ratio, "x" must be on the left in the second ratio.)

Known		Unknown
$x : y$	$::$	$x : y$

When the ratios have been properly aligned into proportion(s), multiply the two inside numbers (means, or "insies") and the two outside numbers (extremes, or "outsies") and then solve for "x." Remember that what is done to numbers on one side of the equation must be done to numbers on the other side of the equation. If you need more review for ratio and proportion, refer to Chapter 2.

> **TECH NOTE**
>
> Placing "x" on the left side of the equation formed simplifies the solving of the problem because the known is now identified. Remember to use the number in front of the "x" to divide on both sides of the equation to find "x."

USING DIMENSIONAL ANALYSIS FOR CONVERTING AMONG UNITS

Dimensional analysis is actually ratio and proportion in multiple sections expressed as fractional forms written across one fractional equation.

EXAMPLE 5-2

To use dimensional analysis, take the example of a prescription to be prepared for 250 mg of an antibiotic. The available medication is 125 mg/5 mL. How many teaspoons of antibiotic should be administered? The formula appears asfollows:

$$x \text{ tsp} = \frac{250 \text{ mg}}{1 \text{ dose}} \times \frac{5 \text{ mL}}{125 \text{ mg}} \times \frac{1 \text{ tsp}}{5 \text{ mL}}$$

$$x \text{ tsp} = \frac{\overset{2}{250} \text{ mg}}{1 \text{ dose}} \times \frac{\overset{1}{5} \text{ mL}}{\underset{1}{125} \text{ mg}} \times \frac{1 \text{ tsp}}{\underset{1}{5} \text{ mL}}$$

$$\frac{2}{1 \text{ dose}} \times \frac{1}{1} \times \frac{1 \text{ tsp}}{1} = \frac{2 \text{ tsp}}{1 \text{ dose}} \quad \text{or} \quad 1 \text{ dose} = 2 \text{ tsp}$$

To use dimensional analysis, the system uses the multiplication of a series of fractions in which the numerator and denominator contain related conversion factors. Each factor has a number and unit of measurement. By using dimensional analysis, remembering multiple formulas to solve drug calculations is not necessary for drug dosages to be accurate and safe.

TECH NOTE
> The multiple conversion fractions allow a single conversion to lead to another conversion factor until the desired conversion is calculated.

Using dimensional analysis involves using a series of ratios or factors that are arranged as a fractional equation. Each factor is written as a fraction, and the factors must be related to each other and to the problem that is being solved. As with all fractions, each factor must have a numerator and a denominator. Each problem requires the use of only one equation to determine the answer. If the units are not in the same measurement system, the conversion to the system becomes part of the equation. If both quantities are in the same measurement system, the conversion among systems is not indicated.

Conversion factors are the equivalents between two measurements whether in the same system or not. Each conversion factor includes a value (numerical value) and a label (units of measurement). For example, 12 in = 1 ft. This is a conversion between feet and inches. It can be used to convert measurements for length within the U.S. system but not for direct analysis if the measurement is given in meters or centimeters found in the metric system. In that case, the factor for the metric system must be placed within the equation for the answer to be correct.

EXAMPLE 5-3

$$4' = \underline{\hspace{2cm}} \text{ cm}$$

The equation for dimensional analysis would be on the conversion 2.54 cm = 1″.

$$x \text{ cm} = \frac{4'}{1} \times \frac{12''}{1'} \times \frac{2.54 \text{ cm}}{1''}$$

$$x \text{ cm} = \frac{4\cancel{'}}{1} \times \frac{12\cancel{''}}{1\cancel{'}} \times \frac{2.54 \text{ cm}}{1\cancel{''}}$$

$$x \text{ cm} = \frac{4}{1} \times \frac{12}{1} \times \frac{2.54}{1} \qquad x = \frac{121.92 \text{ cm}}{1} \qquad x = 121.92 \text{ cm} \quad \text{or} \quad 4' = 121.92 \text{ cm}$$

To perform dimensional analysis, always start with what you are looking for, or the unknown (x). Place the x to the left of the equation so that you will not forget what you are solving for. As you work the problem, all matching symbols in the equation must be removed by identifying and canceling those identifying symbols/abbreviations that are alike in the numerators and denominators as the equation evolves.

There are six distinct steps in setting up a fractional analysis, or the fractional equation used in dimensional analysis. To illustrate these steps, the following example used the familiar household measurement system. A recipe calls for ¼ cup of an ingredient for a cake. At the time of baking, the only available measurement device is a tablespoon. How can you help the person baking the cake know the proper amount of the ingredient to be used when only a tablespoon is available? (¼ c = _____ tbsp)

1. Find the known, or given, quantity—¼ c.
2. What is the desired, or wanted, amount?—x tablespoons.
3. What are the conversion factors that are needed to make the necessary calculation? In this case, we need to know that 2 tablespoons equals 1 oz and 8 oz equals 1 c.
4. Set up the problem with factors that are available for conversion factors. You want to cancel out like factors by placing them in a numerator of the first fraction followed by the denominator in the next fraction as follows:

$$x \text{ tbsp} = \frac{1/4 \text{ c}}{1} \times \frac{8 \text{ oz}}{1 \text{ c}} \times \frac{2 \text{ tbsp}}{1 \text{ oz}}$$

5. Cross out the unwanted units. Just as with any other mathematical equation, if units appear in both the numerator and the denominator, you may cancel them to find the unit that is desired. In this case, the remaining unit is a tablespoon, which is the unit you are seeking.

$$x \text{ tbsp} = \frac{\frac{1}{4}\cancel{c}}{1} \times \frac{8 \cancel{oz}}{1 \cancel{c}} \times \frac{2 \text{ tbsp}}{1 \cancel{oz}}$$

6. Multiply the numerators, multiply the denominators, and divide the product of the numerators by the product of the denominators. This will give you the desired quantity that was originally your unknown factor.

$$x \text{ tbsp} = \frac{1/4 \times 8 \times 2 \text{ tbsp}}{1 \times 1 \times 1} \quad \text{or} \quad \frac{16/4 \text{ tbsp}}{1} \quad \text{or} \quad \frac{4 \text{ tbsp}}{1} \quad \text{or} \quad x = 4 \text{ tbsp}$$

So, after completing the problem:

$\frac{1}{4}$ c = 4 tbsp of the ingredient needed in the cake

Now let's look at other examples found within the same measurement systems.

EXAMPLE 5-4

5 kg = _____ mg

$$x \text{ mg} = \frac{5 \cancel{kg}}{1 \cancel{g}} \times \frac{1000 \cancel{g}}{1 \cancel{kg}} \times \frac{1000 \text{ mg}}{1 \cancel{g}}$$

$x = 5 \times 1000 \times 1000 \quad \text{or} \quad 5 \text{ kg} = 5,000,000 \text{ mg}$

! TECH ALERT

When using dimensional analysis, be sure the conversion factors follow each other in a related manner from the known quantity, through the needed conversions, and finally to the unknown quantity. Then cancel conversions as possible to simplify the problem.

EXAMPLE 5-5

6 mL = _____ L

$$x \text{ L} = \frac{6 \cancel{mL}}{1} \times \frac{1 \text{ L}}{1000 \cancel{mL}}$$

$$x = \frac{6 \cancel{mL}}{1000} \quad \text{or} \quad \frac{1 \text{ L} \times 6}{1000 \cancel{mL}}$$

$$x = \frac{6 \text{ L}}{1000} \quad \text{or} \quad \frac{(6 \text{ L} \times 1)}{(1000)}$$

$x = 0.006 \text{ L}$

POINTS TO REMEMBER
RULES FOR USING DIMENSIONAL ANALYSIS

- Use dimensional analysis for working with two quantities that are proportional to each other or that can be converted to find the proportional amounts.
- Use the common equivalencies or conversion factors to find the desired proportional amounts. Be sure the conversion factors used are in direct proportion to the previously used conversion factor.
- Always express the equation as fractional units.
- Cross out the common unwanted units before finding the products of the numerators and denominators.
- Complete the mathematical problem as you would any fractional equation.

TECH NOTE

Remember that ratio and proportion or dimensional analysis may be used for calculations. Use the method that is most comfortable for you, but use that method for all calculations to prevent mistakes.

CONVERSIONS BETWEEN HOUSEHOLD AND APOTHECARY SYSTEMS

The apothecary system has only a few significant measurements that, although not commonly used, do convert into household measurements. Of importance are minims to drops, drams to teaspoons, and ounces to tablespoons (Figure 5-1). Cups, pints, quarts, and gallons are used by both systems. Length is not found in the apothecary system, so the conversions are not included in Table 5-1. As the chapter unfolds, the metric system will be added to combined tables for conversions among measurement systems.

TABLE 5.1 Conversions between Apothecary and Household Systems of Measurement

PARAMETER	APOTHECARY UNITS	HOUSEHOLD UNITS	METRIC UNITS
Volume	♏ i (1 minim)	1 gtt (1 drop)	—
	ʒ i (1 dram, ♏ 60)	1 tsp (1 teaspoon)	—
	ʒ ss (½ ounce)	1 tbsp (1 tablespoon, 3 tsp)	—
	℥ i (1 oz)	2 tbsp (2 tbsp, 6 tsp)	—
	℥ viii	1 c (8 oz, 1 cup, ½ pint)	—
	1 pt (1 pint, 2 c, ℥ xvi)	1 pt (1 pint, 2 c, 16 oz)	—
	1 qt (1 quart, 2 pt, 4 c, ℥ 32)	1 qt (1 quart, 2 pt, 4 c, 32 oz)	—
	1 gal (4 qt, 8 pt, 16 c, ℥ 128)	1 gal (4 qt, 8 pt, 16 c, 128 oz)	—
Mass/Weight	℥ i (1 oz, 60 gr)*	1 oz	—
	1# (1 lb, ℥ xii)	1# or 1 lb (16 oz)*	—
Length	N/A	N/A	—

*Note that an apothecary pound contains only 12 oz, while a household pound contains 16 oz.

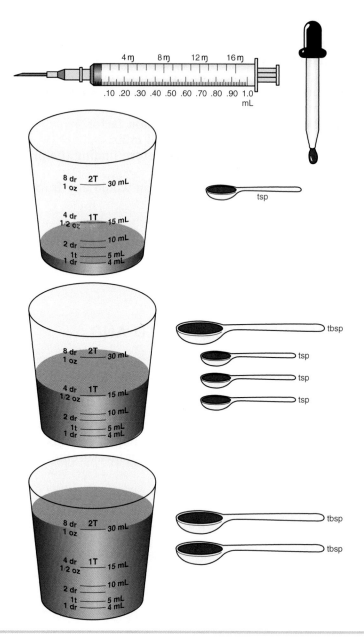

FIGURE 5-1 Equivalents between apothecary and household measurements.

TECH ALERT

Do not confuse the symbols for ʒ (dram) and ℥ (ounce).

TECH ALERT

When calculating between measurement systems, always be sure the answer is measurable and sensible for the system to be used. A person could not measure 1.1 tsp but could measure 1 tsp.

EXAMPLE 5-6

℥ iii = _____ tsp

Ratio and Proportion	Dimensional Analysis

Known   Unknown

℥ i : 1 tsp :: ℥ iii : x

$$℥\, x = \frac{℥\, iii}{1} \times \frac{1\ tsp}{℥\, i}$$

℥ i × x = ℥ iii × 1 tsp

$$℥\, x = \frac{(iii \times 1)\ tsp}{1}$$

x = 3 × 1 tsp, or 3 tsp, or ℥ iii = 3 tsp

$$x = ℥\, iii = 3\ tsp$$

EXAMPLE 5-7

4 oz = _____ tsp

Known   Unknown

1 oz : 6 tsp :: 4 oz : x tsp

$$x\ tsp = \frac{4\ \cancel{oz}}{1} \times \frac{2\ \cancel{tbsp}}{1\ \cancel{oz}} \times \frac{3\ tsp}{1\ \cancel{tbsp}}$$

(1 oz = 2 tbsp and 1 tbsp = 3 tsp)

1x tsp = 6 × 4 tsp

$$x\ tsp = \frac{(4 \times 2 \times 3)\ tsp}{1}$$

x = 24 tsp   or   4 oz = 24 tsp

4 oz = 24 tsp

Practice Problems A

Calculate the following problems using either ratio and proportion or dimensional analysis. Show all of your calculations. Be sure to use the correct numeral indicator for the measurement system of the unknown. Remember these answers may be approximates, NOT EXACT ANSWERS.

1. 6 tsp = ℥ _____

2. 2 tsp = ℥ _____

3. 16 gtts = ♏ _____

4. 4 tbsp = ℥ _____

5. ℥ s͞s = _____ tsp

6. 24 gtts = ♏ _____

7. ʒ v = _____ tsp

8. 75 gtts = _____ tsp

9. 3 tbsp = ʒ _____

10. 10 tsp = ʒ _____

11. 2 tsp = _____ gtts

12. 25 gtts = ℳ _____

13. ʒ vi = ʒ _____

14. 8 c = ʒ _____

15. ʒ xxiv = _____ c

16. 75 gtts = ʒ _____

17. 4 tsp = ʒ _____

18. 30 tsp = ʒ _____

19. 16 tbsp = ʒ _____

20. ʒ xxx = _____ tbsp

21. $ʒ \frac{3}{4}$ = ʒ _____

22. ℳ xxiv = _____ tsp

23. ʒ vi = ʒ _____

24. 15 tsp = _____ tbsp

25. 45 gtts = ℳ _____ = ʒ _____

26. A physician writes a prescription for ʒ ii of Robitussin cough medication q4h.

How much is this in household measures? _____

How often will the person take the medication? _____

27. The label on the bottle of Maalox reads that the medication may be taken ℥ iss every 3 to 4 hours as needed for indigestion.

How much is each dose in household measures, using tablespoons? _____

How often can this be taken? _____

28. A child is to take Tri-Vi-Sol ℳ viii daily.

How many drops would the parent place in a spoon? _____

29. A physician writes a prescription for MiraLax one capful in H2O ℥ viii.

How could you tell the patient to easily measure the water? _____

30. A physician instructs the parent to give a child 30 gtts of Benadryl for an allergy.

How many teaspoons would this be? _____

CONVERSIONS BETWEEN HOUSEHOLD AND METRIC UNITS

Now that the household system has been compared with the apothecary system, it is time to compare the household system with the metric system, which is more frequently used in drug measurements (Table 5-2). Recall that the metric system is formed on the base 10 for ease of conversion. Most conversions from metric to household, such as milliliters to teaspoons, or milliliters to ounces, are volume conversions, although length from inches to centimeters is used in the medical field. Also notice that conversions between household and metric measurements are most commonly found in volume, but length and weight are found minimally when converting between these two systems for pharmaceutical purposes (Figure 5-2).

TECH NOTE
Remember that answers are approximations not exact equivalents.

! TECH ALERT
The medicine dropper provided with the medication is the only dropper that will dispense the correct medication amount. All droppers do not dispense the correct size for the medication available.

TABLE 5.2 Conversions between Household and Metric Systems of Measurement

PARAMETER	APOTHECARY UNITS	HOUSEHOLD UNITS	METRIC UNITS
Volume	—	1 gtt (1 drop)	N/A
	—	15 or 16 gtts*	1 mL
	—	1 tsp (1 teaspoon)	5 mL or cc
	—	1 tbsp (1 tablespoon, 3 tsp)	15 mL
	—	2 tbsp (2 tablespoons)	30 mL
	—	1 oz (2 tbsp)	30 mL
	—	1 c (8 oz, 1 cup, ½ pint)	240 mL
	—	1 pt (1 pint, 2 c, 16 oz)	480 mL
	—	1 qt (1 quart, 2 pt, 4 c, 32 oz)	960 mL
	—	1 gal (4 qt, 8 pt, 16 c, 128 oz)	3840 mL
Mass/Weight	—	2.2#	1 kg
Length	—	1″	2.54 cm

*Remember that the equivalents are approximate and not exact when doing conversions.

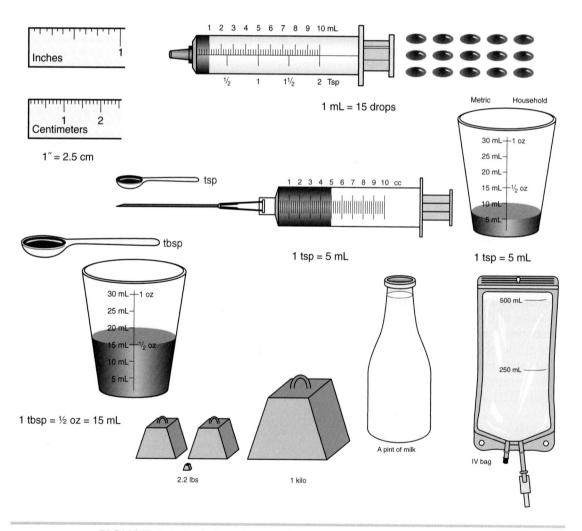

FIGURE 5-2 Equivalents between household and metric measurements.

EXAMPLE 5-8

4 tsp = _____ mL

Ratio and Proportion

Known   Unknown

1 tsp : 5 mL :: 4 tsp : x

$1x = 5\text{ mL} \times 4$

$x = 20\text{ mL}$ or   4 tsp = 20 mL

Dimensional Analysis

$x\text{ mL} = \dfrac{4\text{ tsp}}{x} \times \dfrac{5\text{ mL}}{1\text{ tsp}}$

$x\text{ mL} = \dfrac{(4 \times 5)\text{ mL}}{1\,x}$

4 tsp = 20 mL

EXAMPLE 5-9

60 mL = _____ oz

Ratio and Proportion

Known   Unknown

30 mL : 1 oz :: 60 mL : x

$30x = 60 \times 1\text{ oz}$

$30x = 60\text{ oz}$

$x = \dfrac{60\text{ oz}}{30}$

$x = 2\text{ oz}$

Dimensional Analysis

$x\text{ oz} = \dfrac{60\text{ mL}}{1} \times \dfrac{1\text{ oz}}{30\text{ mL}}$

$x\text{ oz} = \dfrac{(60 \times 1)\text{ oz}}{30}$

$\dfrac{60\text{ oz}}{30}$

60 mL = 2 oz

! TECH ALERT

When moving between metric and household measures, be sure the conversion is a measurable amount.

Practice Problems B

Calculate the following problems. Remember that the only time a conversion is neces-sary is when the units are not in the same measurement system. Also remember that all calculations in conversions are approximates and should be rounded to the nearest fractional number or hundredth as appropriate. Show all of your calculations.

1. 8 tsp = _____ tbsp

2. 16 oz = _____ mL

3. 8 kg = _____ #

4. 3 tsp = _____ mL

5. 2 pt = _____ mL

6. 5″ = _____ cm

7. 3 c = _____ mL

8. 90 mL = _____ oz

9. 6 tsp = _____ tbsp

10. ℥ iv = _____ tsp

11. ℥ ii = _____ tbsp

12. ♏ x = _____ gtts

13. 10 cm = _____ ″

14. 30 cm = _____ ft

15. 75 mL = _____ oz

16. 10 kg = _____ #

17. 720 mL = _____ pt

18. 720 mL = _____ qt

19. 10 tsp = _____ mL

20. 2 pt = _____ c

21. 500 mL = _____ qt

22. 6 tsp = _____ mL

23. 1.5 L = _____ pt

24. 3120 mL = _____ qt

25. 10 c = _____ L

26. 5 ft = _____ cm

27. A physician writes an order for an antihelmintic for a child weighing 35#. The dosage must be calculated in mg/kg body weight.

How many kilograms does the child weigh? _____

28. A physician writes a prescription for Rondec DM 15 gtts.

How many milliliters would this be on a dose syringe? _____

29. A physician writes a prescription for 5 mL of azithromycin liquid for a child.

How many teaspoons would you tell the parent to give the child? _____

30. A parent has an infant with colic. A bottle of Mylicon drops is available for relief of the pain. The label reads to give 15 drops for a child who is the age of the infant.

How many milliliters would you tell the parent to give using the dropper that came with the medication? _____

CONVERSIONS BETWEEN METRIC AND APOTHECARY SYSTEMS

Remember that the metric system uses grams, liters, and meters, whereas the apothecary system frequently uses grains, minims, drams, and ounces. Also remember that in converting between two systems of measure, the equivalents are approximate. This is important when converting between apothecary and metric systems. If the answer is a portion of a minim, you should round to the closest full amount because minims cannot be divided (e.g., if the calculation is for $4\frac{1}{2}$ minims, the amount should be rounded to 5 minims; if the calculation is $4\frac{1}{4}$ minims, the amount should be rounded to 4 minims). Portions of grains, milligrams, grams, and other measures can be expressed with fractional units. Again, with these conversions, ratio and proportion or dimensional analysis may be used, depending on the method that is most comfortable for you. Table 5-3 shows the equivalents between the apothecary system and the metric system.

The important conversions to remember are as follows and these are approximations as stated early in the chapter:

MASS	VOLUME
gr i = 60 mg (or 65 mg)	1 mL = ℥ xv or xvi (use the figure that will give you as close to a whole number as possible)
1 g = gr xv	ℨ i = 4 or 5 mL
	℥ i = 30 mL

TECH NOTE

Please remember that the numbers are approximations NOT EXACT NUMBERS so you need to use the conversion that will give you a measurable answer here and below.

A quick way to remember conversions between grains and milligrams is to use a clock as the basis for conversions. There are 60 minutes in an hour just as there are 60 mg to a gr. Figure 5-3 shows how this can be used.

TABLE 5.3 Conversions between Apothecary and Metric Systems of Measurement

PARAMETER	APOTHECARY UNITS	HOUSEHOLD UNITS	METRIC UNITS
Volume	℥ xv (15) (or xvi [16])*	—	1 mL
	ℨ i	—	4 or 5 mL *
	℥ ss	—	15 mL
	℥ i	—	30 mL
	℥ viii	—	240 mL
	℥ xvi or 1 pt	—	480 mL
	℥ 32 or 1 qt	—	960 mL
	℥ 128 or 1 gal	—	3840 mL
Mass/Weight	gr i	—	60 mg
	gr xv	—	1 g

*Remember that all equivalents are approximates when converting between measurement systems.

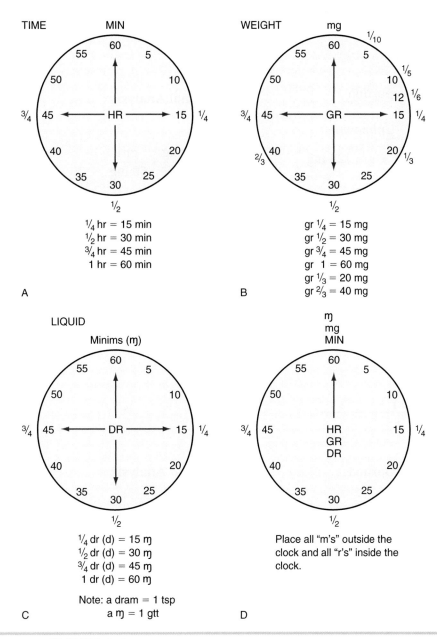

FIGURE 5-3 Conversion of apothecary and metric measurements.

If you use the clock as a basis for conversions, gr ¼ or ¼ hour is 15 milligrams or minutes; gr ½ is 30 milligrams, while ½ hour is 30 minutes; gr ¾ or ¾ hour equals 45 milligrams or hours; and finally gr i equals 60 milligrams, while 1 hour equals 60 minutes. This same clock can be used for 1/6, 1/3, and 2/3 grains or hours just as easily. See Figure 5-3, A and B.

The clock can also be used to convert drams to minims as shown in Figure 5-3, C. As with the other clock examples, drams can be converted to minims by keeping the minim on the outside of the clock and the drams on the inside.

As with previous conversions, ratio and proportion or dimensional analysis may be used for conversions as desired.

EXAMPLE 5-10

120 mg = gr _____

| Ratio and Proportion | Dimensional Analysis |

Known   *Unknown*

gr i : 60 mg :: x gr : 120 mg

$$x\ gr = \frac{120\ mg}{1} \times \frac{gr\ i}{60\ mg}$$

$60 \times x = 120 \times 1$

$$x\ gr = \frac{120 \times gr\ 1}{60 \times 1} \quad or \quad x = \frac{120\ gr}{60} \quad or \quad x = gr\ ii$$

$60x = 120 \quad or \quad 120 \div 60$

$x = 2$

120 mg = gr ii

EXAMPLE 5-11

10 g = gr _____

Ratio and Proportion   Dimensional Analysis

Known   *Unknown*

1 g : gr 15 :: 10 g : gr x

$$gr\ x = \frac{10\ g}{1} \times \frac{15\ gr}{1\ g}$$

$1 \times x = 10 \times gr\ 15$

$$gr\ x = \frac{(10 \times 15)\ gr}{1 \times 1} \quad or \quad gr\ 150$$

$1x = gr\ 150 \quad or \quad x = gr\ 150$

10 g = gr 150

Before beginning practice problems, remember the conversions are approximates and may not be exact equivalents. Also remember that a minim is the smallest unit that can be measured in the apothecary liquid measure, so round the amount as appropriate. Finally, remember that if you are using equivalents within the same measurement system, you do not need the conversions between measurement systems.

Practice Problems C

Calculate the following practice problems. Round as appropriate, being sure the answer is measurable; for instance, 1½ drop would be 2 drops because a drop cannot be divided for administration. Show all of your calculations.

1. gr ii = _____ mg

2. 5 mg = _____ mcg

3. ℳ xvi = _____ mL

4. 6 g = gr _____

5. ʒ iv = _____ mL

6. 45 mL = ʒ _____

7. 15 mg = gr _____

8. 60 mL = ʒ _____

9. 5 mL = ℳ _____

10. 1.5 mL = ℳ _____

11. gr viiss̄ = _____ g

12. 750 mL = ʒ _____

13. ʒ iv = ʒ _____

14. gr $\dfrac{1}{150}$ = _____ mg

15. gr s̄s̄ = _____ mg

16. 0.6 mg = gr _____

17. 15 cc = ʒ _____

18. 12 ℳ = _____ mL

19. 2 L = ʒ _____

20. 0.1 mg = gr _____

21. 16 mL = ʒ _____

22. 55 mL = _____ cc

23. gr $\dfrac{3}{4}$ = _____ mcg

24. gr $\dfrac{1}{600}$ = _____ mg

25. 4 mL = ♏ _____

26. ♏ 48 = ℥ _____

27. A physician orders a parent to give a young child 2 mL of amoxicillin suspension.

How many minims would the parent give the child? _____

28. A patient reads a prescription for Maalox 16 mL.

How many drams would you tell the patient to take? _____

29. A patient has a prescription for Seconal gr $\overline{\text{iss}}$. The available medication is Seconal 100 mg/capsule.

How many capsule would you use for dispensing? _____

30. A prescription is written for phenobarbital gr ¼. The medication stock bottle reads phenobarbital 30 mg per unscored tablet.

Is this the correct medication stock bottle for the prescription? _____

Show the mathematical calculation you used to determine the answer.

PUTTING IT ALL TOGETHER—METRIC, HOUSEHOLD, AND APOTHECARY MEASUREMENTS AND THEIR CONVERSIONS

Throughout this chapter you have converted between two measurement systems at a time. Now you need to put all of the conversions together. Table 5-4 is a combination of all tables previously shown in this chapter. Please remember that all conversions are approximations and could be changed depending on the conversion used for calculation, such as the number of mL in a dram. The conversion should always be made on the basis of a measurable dose.

Now add one last conversion to the clock (see Figure 5-3, D). Remember that you are now adding a liquid measure that should not be confused with the weight or solid measure.

Using the clock, the calculation of minims to drams can easily be accomplished by using 60 minims equals 1 fl dram. Again, remember to place all symbols or abbreviations ending in "r" in the center of the clock and all beginning with "m" on the outside of the clock. The fractional parts as seen with the grains and hours will again apply to fluid drams, such as 10 minims is 1/6 fluid dram.

> **TECH NOTE**
>
> Keep the symbols ending with "m" outside of the clock circle and those beginning with "r" within the clock. Remember that minutes are on the outside of the clock, and hours are on the inside of the clock; this should help you place the symbols correctly.

REVIEW

In this chapter the concepts of conversion among the metric, apothecary, and household systems have been shown. The conversions may be accomplished using either ratio and proportion, dimensional analysis, or in some cases the use of the clock. As a student, you should find one method with which you are the most comfortable and use it regularly. Although conversions are made, the fact that the conversion is not exact but is an approximation is an important concept to remember. Conversions are necessary only when more than one measurement system is presented in the problem. Remember that the more you use conversions and approximate equivalencies, more comfortable you will be with this concept.

TABLE 5.4 Conversions among Metric, Apothecary, and Household Systems of Measurement

PARAMETER	APOTHECARY UNITS	HOUSEHOLD UNITS	METRIC UNITS
Volume	ℳ i	1 gtt	N/A
	ℳ xv (or xvi)*	15 or 16 gtts	1 mL
	ʒ i	1 tsp	4 or 5 mL
	ʒ ss	1 tbsp or 3 tsp	15 mL
	℥ i	2 tbsp or 6 tsp	30 mL
	℥ viii	1 c (8 oz, ½ pt)	240 mL
	℥ xvi or 1 pt	1 pt (2 c, 16 oz)	480 mL
	℥ 32 or 1 qt	1 qt (2 pt, 4 c, 32 oz)	960 mL
	℥ 128 or 1 gal	1 gal (4 qt, 8 pt, 16 c, 128 oz)	3840 mL
Mass/Weight	gr i	N/A	60 mg
	gr xv	N/A	1 g
	℥ i (60 gr)	1 oz	4 g
	N/A	2.2#	1 kg
Length	N/A	1″	2.54 cm

*Remember that all equivalents are approximates when converting among measurements.

Posttest

Before taking the Posttest, retake the Pretest to check your understanding of the materials presented in this chapter. Be sure to use the correct numeral indications for each system. Also be sure the approximate calculation could be administered and makes a sensible dose.

Use either ratio and proportion or dimensional analysis to solve these problems. If two lines appear for an answer line, two conversions are possible for that answer based on the difference in the conversion factors. Round all answers to hundredths.

1. 3 tsp = ℥ _____

2. 6 tsp = _____mL

3. gr $\frac{3}{4}$ = _____ mg

4. ℈ v = _____mL _____ mL

5. 88 # = _____ kg

6. 0.6 mg = _____ gr

7. 1250 mL = _____ pt

8. 2.5 L = _____ mL

9. 2.5 mL = _____ gtts

10. 8 tbsp = _____ oz

11. 4 qt = _____ L

12. 5050 mL = _____ L

13. 45 mg = gr _____

14. ℥ 24 = _____ c

15. 15 tsp = _____ tbsp

16. 16 tbsp = ℥ _____

17. 16 tbsp = ℈ _____

18. 16″ = _____ cm

19. 46 # = _____ kg

20. 0.1 mg = gr _____

21. 2500 g = _____ #

22. 12 mL = _____ gtts

Posttest, cont.

23. 45 mL = ʒ _____

24. 45 mL = _____ tsp

25. gr $\frac{1}{200}$ = _____ mg

26. 430 mg = _____ g

27. 5 tbsp = ʒ _____

28. 4 tsp = ℳ _____

29. 10 kg = _____ #

30. 324 cm = _____ ″

31. 2000 mL = _____ pt

32. 12 mg = gr _____

33. 11 mL = ℳ _____

34. 28 mL = ʒ _____

35. 2 yd = _____ cm

36. 2784 mL = _____ L

37. 2784 mL = _____ cc

38. 35 mL = _____ tsp

39. gr 45 = _____ g

40. 0.6 kg = gr _____

41. gr xx = _____ mg

42. 2500 mL = _____ pt

43. A physician orders acetylsalicylic acid 325 mg. Available are gr v tablets. Show your work. Should this medication be used for the order? _____

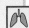

44. A young child is to receive Benadryl elixir 2 mL. How many gtts would you place on the prescription for the parent to administer to the child? _____

Continued

Posttest, cont.

45. An older sibling of the child mentioned in question 44 is to receive Benadryl elixir 7.5 mL. The parent needs to give this with a teaspoon.

How many teaspoons would you tell the parent to give with each dose?

_____

46. A physician orders codeine gr $\overline{\text{iss}}$ stat for pain.

How many milligrams of codeine would the person receive if the label on the stock

bottle is in milligrams? _____

47. A chemotherapeutic medication will be ordered by weight in kilograms. The patient weighs 166 #.

What is the weight in kilograms? _____

48. A child is measured in a teaching hospital in centimeters. The height is 104 cm.

How many inches tall is the child? _____

49. A physician orders atropine sulfate 0.4 mg as a preoperative order.

How many grains will the patient receive if the medication label is in grains?

_____

50. A prescription for amoxicillin must be reconstituted with ℥ iii of water.

How many milliliters of water must be added? _____

The final amount in the bottle is 150 mL. How many ounces of medication are in the

bottle after reconstitution? _____

REVIEW OF RULES

Rules of Conversion among Measurement Systems Using Ratio and Proportion

- Set up the conversion ratio with the known conversion units on the left of the equation.

- Set up the second ratio of the proportion with the conversion units for the unknowns.

- Label the units so that the like unit is placed in the same position within each ratio and proportion. This sets the ratios so that they are equal to each other.

- Solve for the unknown.

Rules for Using Dimensional Analysis to Solve Conversions

- Use dimensional analysis for working with two quantities that are proportional to each other or that can be converted to find the proportional amounts.

- Use the common equivalencies or conversion factors to find the proportional amounts that are desired. Be sure the conversion factors used are in direct proportion to the previously used conversion factor.

- Always express the equation as fractional units.

- Cross out the common unwanted units before finding the products of the numerators and denominators.

- Complete the mathematical problem as you would any fractional equation.

SECTION III

Medication and Prescription Orders and Their Calculations

CHAPTER 6

Interpretation of Medication Labels and Orders

OBJECTIVES

- Describe components of a prescription
- Interpret prescriptions and medication orders
- Interpret labels found on medication containers
- Use and understand units of measurement found in pharmacology

KEY WORDS

Auxiliary label Label added to prescriptions to provide supplementary instructions

Diluent Agent that dilutes a substance; in pharmacology, liquid added to a powder or crystals to change solid to a liquid or to dilute another liquid

Dosage (Dose) strength Weight of medication in a dose

Generic name Official nonproprietary name approved for a drug by the U.S. Food and Drug Administration (FDA)

Indication Reason to prescribe a medication

Inscription Part of prescription indicating name of drug, quantity, and dosage prescribed

Medication order Written or verbal direction for administration of medication in a health care setting

National Drug Code (NDC) Unique number on a drug product label that identifies the manufacturer, product, and size of container

Pharmacokinetics Processing of drugs and movement of drugs through the body; describing characteristics such as absorption, distribution, metabolism, and excretion

Pharmacotherapeutics Effects of drugs in treatment of conditions and diseases in the body

Prescription: Written order by a licensed health care professional for dispensing or administering medications

Pulvule Capsule filled with medication in powdered form

Reconstitution Process of adding **diluent** (fluid), such as water or saline, to a powdered or crystallized form of a drug, making a specific liquid dosage strength

Scheduled medications Classification of medications with potential for abuse and misuse

Signa (Sig) Part of prescription indicating how a medication is to be taken or applied

147

Superscription: Part of prescription designated with the symbol ℞

Toxicology Study of adverse toxic reactions or toxic levels of chemicals and drugs

Trade/Brand name Proprietary name given to a medication by the manufacturer

Pretest

Interpret the following orders. Remember that this is a pretest to check your level of knowledge. The first line presented is for interpretation of the prescription and the second line is for the directions found on a prescription label for the medication provided to the patient. The dosage given should be in the appropriate dosage form.

1. penicillin 250 mg po qid × 10 days

Prescription interpretation: _____

Label directions: _____

2. nitroglycerin 0.4 mg sl q5min × 3 doses prn

Prescription interpretation: _____

Label directions: _____

3. chlorothiazide 0.25 g i tab po qam prn swelling

Prescription interpretation: _____

Label directions: _____

4. Synthroid 0.025 mg po daily @ 8 am

Prescription interpretation: _____

Label directions: _____

Pretest, cont.

5. Phenergan 25 mg po q4-6h prn

Prescription interpretation: _____

Label directions: _____

6. Premarin 1.25 mg tab po daily × 21d

Prescription interpretation: _____

Label directions: _____

7. Benadryl El 3 s̄s̄ po q4h prn itching

Prescription interpretation: _____

Label directions: _____

8. meperidine 50 mg and promethazine 25 mg IM q4-6h prn pain

Prescription interpretation: _____

Label directions: _____

9. Zithromax 250 mg tab ii po stat, then tab i po daily on days 2-5

Prescription interpretation: _____

Label directions: _____

10. Lanoxin 0.25 mg tab po qam if P 60 or ↑

Prescription interpretation: _____

Label directions: _____

Continued

Pretest, cont.

Interpret the following prescriptions on the line provided.

11.

Lawrence Merry, M.D.
4th Street and Jones Ave.
Holly, GA 00111
phone# - 001-555-2176

Patient Name_____ Date _____
Address_____ Age _____

R̶x   Pen-V 250 mg
        #40
        Sig: i tab po q6h

_____ Refill _____
DEA#_____

_____

12.

Lawrence Merry, M.D.
4th Street and Jones Ave.
Holly, GA 00111
phone# - 001-555-2176

Patient Name_____ Date _____
Address_____ Age _____

R̶x   Thorazine 100 mg
        #100
        Sig: tab i po tid

_____ Refill _____
DEA#_____

_____

Pretest, cont.

13.

Lawrence Merry, M.D.
4th Street and Jones Ave.
Holly, GA 00111
phone# - 001-555-2176

Patient Name_____ Date _____
Address_____ Age _____

Rx   tetracycline 250 mg
      #120
      Sig: ii cap po qid x 2wk; i cap po bid x 2wk;
      then i cap po daily

_____ Refill _____
DEA#_____

_____

14.

Lawrence Merry, M.D.
4th Street and Jones Ave.
Holly, GA 00111
phone# - 001-555-2176

Patient Name_____ Date _____
Address_____ Age _____

Rx   furosemide 40 mg
      #30
      Sig: ss̄ to i tab po daily prn swelling

_____ Refill _____
DEA#_____

Continued

Pretest, cont.

15.

Lawrence Merry, M.D.
4th Street and Jones Ave.
Holly, GA 00111
phone# - 001-555-2176

Patient Name_____ Date _____
Address_____ Age _____

Rx   lovastatin 10 mg
         #30
         Sig: i tab po daily c̄ evening meal or at
         bedtime c snack for hyperlipidemia

_____   Refill _____
DEA#_____

16.

Lawrence Merry, M.D.
4th Street and Jones Ave.
Holly, GA 00111
phone# - 001-555-2176

Patient Name_____ Date _____
Address_____ Age _____

Rx   Humulin 70/30
         10 mL vial
         Sig: 22 units subcutaneously qam

_____   Refill _____
DEA#_____

Pretest, cont.

ENDO **17.**

Lawrence Merry, M.D.
4th Street and Jones Ave.
Holly, GA 00111
phone# - 001-555-2176

Patient Name_____ Date _____
Address_____ Age _____

℞   Reg Insulin
10 mL vial
Sig: 16 units subcutaneously qam and 20
units subcutaneously 30 min ac evening
meal

_____ Refill _____

DEA#_____

18.

Lawrence Merry, M.D.
4th Street and Jones Ave.
Holly, GA 00111
phone# - 001-555-2176

Patient Name_____ Date _____
Address_____ Age _____

℞   diazepam 10 mg
#30
Sig: $\overline{ss}$ — i tab po q4-6h prn anxiety or
muscle spasms

_____ Refill _____

DEA#_____

Continued

Pretest, cont.

19.

Lawrence Merry, M.D.
4th Street and Jones Ave.
Holly, GA 00111
phone# - 001-555-2176

Patient Name_____ Date _____
Address_____ Age _____

℞   Zoloft 50 mg
            #30
            Sig: i tab po qam

_____ Refill _____
DEA#_____

20.

Lawrence Merry, M.D.
4th Street and Jones Ave.
Holly, GA 00111
phone# - 001-555-2176

Patient Name_____ Date _____
Address_____ Age _____

℞   Robitussin DM syrup ℥viii
            Sig: 3 ii po q4-6h prn cough

_____ Refill _____
DEA#_____

INTRODUCTION

Medications are ordered by a physician either as a **medication order** in a patient medical record or on a written **prescription** for the patient to take to a pharmacy for dispensing. In whatever setting, the order must be read and interpreted exactly so the correct medication and its dosage can be provided for patient safety. Even if the order is a verbal order to a health care professional, the order must be transcribed into writing to create a medication record for legal purposes. Therefore, the ability to understand the components of the prescription, as well as the ability to interpret the order or prescription, is an essential skill for the health occupation professionals who work with medications on a daily basis.

Just as a reminder, because many drugs have similar-sounding or look-alike names, reading the prescription can become much like working a puzzle. If an order should be questioned in any way, the pharmacy technician should bring this to the attention of the pharmacist. The pharmacist is ultimately responsible for dispensing the medication as ordered. As a pharmacy technician, you must be sure that you stay current with new medications and new **indications** for older medications. As new precautions are found for medicines, you should keep these in mind. You should always remember that the highest level of patient safety is the most important aspect of dispensing medications.

Remember the knowledge of pharmacy includes the action of the medication in the body or **pharmacokinetics,** the therapeutic uses and effects or **pharmacotherapeutics,** and the adverse and toxic reactions or **toxicology**. Each of these must be considered as medications are dispensed to patients. As a pharmacy technician, you must be aware of the usual dosage of a drug and other possible medications being taken concurrently by the patient so that you may assist the pharmacist in attaining a high level of quality control and patient safety and help prevent drug interactions.

WHAT DOES A PRESCRIPTION INDICATE?

A prescription is a means for a physician or other health professional to provide the information needed by the pharmacist to dispense the desired medication for a patient in an outpatient setting. It is an order written for a specific person by a medical professional licensed to prescribe for a specific condition. The rules about who may prescribe vary from state to state, so the statutes of the state of practice determine the legalities of prescription writing. As a legal document, the prescription indicates the medication desired and the directions for its use to meet the health needs of the patient. The components of a prescription are included as a review of what is necessary for this legal document.

Figure 6-1 provides short descriptions of the parts of a prescription. The five major components are the **superscription, inscription, signa (Sig),** subscription and signature of the health care professional. Line A of Figure 6-1 is the preprinted name of the physician or group of physicians, the address, and phone number. Line B includes the patient's name, address, date of the prescription, and the patient's age if the patient is a child. Dating the prescription is important because prescriptions must be filled within 12 months of writing except with controlled substances or **scheduled medications,** and the refilling of prescriptions is dependent on the date. Line C is the superscription or the symbol ℞, meaning "recipe" or "take thou," from Latin. The inscription, which specifies the name of the medication, its strength, and quantity of drug to be dispensed, appears on line D. If the medication must be compounded or prepared, the ingredients would appear in this location. Line E is the "Sig," or signa, giving directions for taking the medication. The subscription, line F, tells the pharmacist the drug form, as well as how the medication is be taken. The physician's signature appears on line G, and the number of allowed refills on Line H. Finally, if the prescription is for a controlled medication, the physician must place his or her U. S. Drug Enforcement Administration (DEA) number either under or beside the signature.

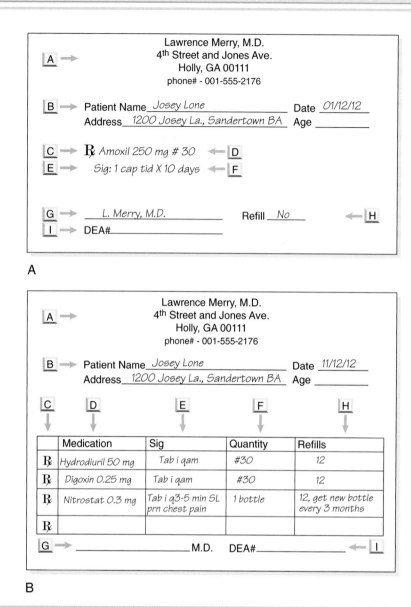

FIGURE 6-1 **Examples of prescription blanks and their components**. **A,** Single-line prescription.
B, Multiple-line prescription. The five major components of a prescription are the superscription (C);
the inscription (D); the signa (E); the subscription (F); and the signature (G). Use of multiple-line prescription
blanks is dependent on state statutes in the state of practice.

Prescriptions may be written or verbal (except with Schedule II medications, which
require a written signed prescription), but the legal implications are the same for both.
Both means of communicating a prescription must provide identification of the patient
who is to receive the medication and the amount of medicine to be received. It is the
responsibility of the pharmacy technician to follow the orders. When the orders are given
verbally, the order should always be repeated with the health care professional to verify
the drug, the amount, and the directions to avoid errors. If a question about the prescription or medication error is noted, clarification or corrections must occur before the medication is dispensed. This clarification will require further communication with the person
prescribing the drug.

TECH NOTE

Not all prescriptions are handwritten in the medical field today. They may be electronically submitted to the pharmacy for dispensing.

Abbreviations are often used in the writing of prescriptions. Only standard abbreviations should be used. Remember that a prescription is a legal document that could appear in a court case. In those instances, "local" or nonstandard abbreviations might become an area of concern for possible misinterpretation. Abbreviations are actually medical shorthand that is used to write clear and concise orders that will be used among health care professionals. For orders to be correctly written and interpreted, the health care professional and the person dispensing the medication must understand the meaning of each abbreviation used. For commonly accepted abbreviations, see the table on the inside front cover and Chapter 1.

TECH NOTE

As you work through prescriptions, an understood meaning is that if a tablet or capsule is ordered, the route of administration is by mouth (po) unless otherwise indicated.

Practice Problems A

Interpret the following prescriptions and write the sig that would appear on a prescription label.

1.

```
                Lawrence Merry, M.D.
               4th Street and Jones Ave.
                    Holly, GA 00111
                 phone# - 001-555-2176

   Patient Name_____  Date _____
   Address_____   Age _____

   R̥        atorvastatin 10 mg
            #30
            Sig: i tab po nightly at bedtime

   _____  Refill _____
   DEA#_____
```

Prescription interpretation: _I tab by mouth nightly at bedtime_

Label instructions: _Take 1 tab by mouth nightly at bedtime_

2. PA IN

Lawrence Merry, M.D.
4th Street and Jones Ave.
Holly, GA 00111
phone# - 001-555-2176

Patient Name_____ Date _____
Address_____ Age _____

℞   hydrocodone w/APAP 5/500
       #20
       Sig: i or ii tab po q6-8 prn pain

_____ Refill _____

DEA#_AM123321_____

Prescription interpretation: _____

Label instruction: _____

3. ⚥

Lawrence Merry, M.D.
4th Street and Jones Ave.
Holly, GA 00111
phone# - 001-555-2176

Patient Name_____ Date _____
Address_____ Age _____

℞   Premarin 0.625 mg
       #30
       Sig: i tab po daily at approximately
       same hour

_____ Refill _____

DEA#_____

Prescription interpretation: _____

Label instruction: _____

4.

Lawrence Merry, M.D.
4th Street and Jones Ave.
Holly, GA 00111
phone# - 001-555-2176

Patient Name_____ Date _____
Address_____ Age _____

℞   Zoloft 50 mg
     #30
     Sig: i tab po daily c̄ morning meal

_____ Refill _____
DEA#_____

Prescription interpretation: _____

Label instruction: _____

5. ENDO

Lawrence Merry, M.D.
4th Street and Jones Ave.
Holly, GA 00111
phone# - 001-555-2176

Patient Name_____ Date _____
Address_____ Age _____

℞   Prednisone 10 mg
     #40
     Sig: i tab po qid x 4 d ; i tab po tid x 4 d ; i tab
     po bid x 4 d ; i tab po daily x 4

_____ Refill _____
DEA#_____

Prescription interpretation: _____

Label instruction: _____

6.

Lawrence Merry, M.D.
4th Street and Jones Ave.
Holly, GA 00111
phone# - 001-555-2176

Patient Name_____ Date _____
Address_____ Age _____

Rx   Allegra 180 mg
          #30
          Sig: i tab po daily

_____ Refill _____
DEA#_____

Prescription interpretation: _____

Label instruction: _____

7.

Lawrence Merry, M.D.
4th Street and Jones Ave.
Holly, GA 00111
phone# - 001-555-2176

Patient Name_____ Date _____
Address_____ Age _____

Rx   ibuprofen 800 mg
          #100
          Sig: i tab po q8h

_____ Refill _____
DEA#_____

Prescription interpretation: _____

Label instruction: _____

8.

Lawrence Merry, M.D.
4th Street and Jones Ave.
Holly, GA 00111
phone# - 001-555-2176

Patient Name_____ Date _____
Address_____ Age _____

Rx   Norvasc 5 mg
            #30
            Sig: i tab po qam for ↑ B/p

_____ Refill _____

DEA#_____

Prescription interpretation: _____

Label instruction: _____

9.

Lawrence Merry, M.D.
4th Street and Jones Ave.
Holly, GA 00111
phone# - 001-555-2176

Patient Name_____ Date _____
Address_____ Age _____

Rx   furosemide 40 mg
            #30
            Sig: i tab po daily @ 10am

_____ Refill _____

DEA#_____

Prescription interpretation: _____

Label instruction: _____

10.

Lawrence Merry, M.D.
4th Street and Jones Ave.
Holly, GA 00111
phone# - 001-555-2176

Patient Name_____ Date _____
Address_____ Age _____

℞   Fosamax 70 mg
       #4
       Sig: i po on same d qwk

_____   Refill _____

DEA#_____

Prescription interpretation: _____

Label instruction: _____

11.

Lawrence Merry, M.D.
4th Street and Jones Ave.
Holly, GA 00111
phone# - 001-555-2176

Patient Name_____ Date _____
Address_____ Age _____

℞   diazepam 5 mg
       #100
       Sig: i po tid prn anxiety

_____   Refill _____

DEA# AM123321_____

Prescription interpretation: _____

Label instruction: _____

12.

Lawrence Merry, M.D.
4th Street and Jones Ave.
Holly, GA 00111
phone# - 001-555-2176

Patient Name_____ Date _____
Address_____ Age _____

℞   Neurontin 600 mg
            #50
            Sig: i po daily x 5 d ; i po bid x 5 d ;
            then i po tid

_____ Refill _____
DEA#_____

Prescription interpretation: _____

Label instruction: _____

13.

Lawrence Merry, M.D.
4th Street and Jones Ave.
Holly, GA 00111
phone# - 001-555-2176

Patient Name_____ Date _____
Address_____ Age _____

℞   ciprofloxacin 500 mg
            #20
            Sig: i po q12h until all med taken

_____ Refill _____
DEA#_____

Prescription interpretation: _____

Label instruction: _____

14. **EN DO**

Lawrence Merry, M.D.
4th Street and Jones Ave.
Holly, GA 00111
phone# - 001-555-2176

Patient Name_____ Date _____
Address_____ Age _____

Rx   Glucotrol XL 10 mg
          #30
          Sig: i tab po c̄ am meal

_____   Refill _____
DEA#_____

Prescription interpretation: _____

Label instruction: _____

15.

Lawrence Merry, M.D.
4th Street and Jones Ave.
Holly, GA 00111
phone# - 001-555-2176

Patient Name_____ Date _____
Address_____ Age _____

Rx   Prilosec 40 mg
          #30
          Sig: i po daily in am

_____   Refill _____
DEA#_____

Prescription interpretation: _____

Label instruction: _____

WHAT IS A MEDICATION ORDER?

A medication order is a method of providing the same information as found on a prescription given to the patient, but is used in an inpatient or physician's office environment (Figure 6-2). An exception with the medication order is that the order is written for either the number of doses or for the specific length of time for the medicine to be taken. With the medication order, the health care professional is told what drug or drugs should be administered, the strength of the medication, and the frequency to be taken. This order is a means of providing drugs at correct frequency in an inpatient setting. The medication order has six parts: date; patient name, which may appear on the patient record; medication name; dose or medication strength/form; route, time, and frequency of administration;

A

PHYSICIAN'S ORDERS				Patient, James A.

▶

DATE		ORDERS			TRANS BY
	Diagnosis:		Weight:	Height:	
	Sensitivities/Drug Allergies:				
1/12/07	0900	Lasix 80 mg. p.o. b.i.d.			
		Digoxin 0.125 mg. p.o. q.d.			
		Slow-K 10 mEq. p.o. b.i.d.			
		A. Physician, M.D.			

MEDICAL RECORDS COPY		**PHYSICIAN'S ORDERS**				**T-5**	
B-CLIN. NOTES	E-LAB	G-X-RAY	K-DIAGNOSTIC	M-SURGERY	Q-THERAPY	T-ORDERS	W-NURSING	Y-MISC.

B

Transcription of Med Sheet by: _____

Reviewed by: _____   Page _____ of _____

Initials	Signature
___	_____
___	_____
___	_____
___	_____
NJ	N. Jones R.N.
AN	A. Nurse R. N.

Allergies: ☑ NKDA   Injection Sites:

Special Notes:

Patient, James A.

☐ Inpatient   ☐ Outpatient

See Legend on Back

DATE	DRUG						DATES 1/12/07		1/13/07		1/14/07	1/15/07	1/16/07
1 1/12	Lasix						09 AN		21 NJ		09 AN	21 NJ			
	80 mg dose	p.o. route	b.i.d. interval	09	21								
2 1/12	Digoxin						09 AN				09 AN			
	0.125 mg dose	p.o. route	q.d. interval	09									
3 1/12	Slow-K						09 AN		21 NJ		09 AN	21 NJ			
	10 mEq dose	p.o. route	b.i.d. interval	09	21								
4													
	dose	route	interval										
5													
	dose	route	interval										

		MEDICATION PROFILE						
B-CLIN. NOTES	E-LAB	G-X-RAY	K-DIAGNOSTIC	M-SURGERY	Q-THERAPY	T-ORDERS	W-NURSING	Y-MISC.

FIGURE 6-2 Examples of physician's orders **(A)** and patient's medication administration record **(B)** with appropriate drug interpretations.

and signature of the prescribing professional. Medication orders may be verbally communicated, but for legal purposes, each order should be transcribed onto a written form by the health care professional who accepts the order and the order must be countersigned by the health care professional who communicated the order and is licensed to prescribe medications in the state of practice.

For the pharmacy technician, medication orders have usually been transcribed from the medication order form to a drug administration record and to an order that will be sent to the pharmacy to be filled for the patient. The order to the pharmacy is much like a prescription in that the pharmacist provides the needed medication to the inpatient floor for administration. In some instances medication orders are written in duplicate, and the duplicate copy is sent to the pharmacy for preparation of the medications. Using this type of transmittal of medication orders provides a double-check between the pharmacist and health care personnel on the floor. As with a prescription, the medication order must be written by a health care professional who is licensed to prescribe in the state of employment. Because medicines found in the inpatient setting often can be given by several routes of administration, the route of administration is also added so that the pharmacy provides the correct form of medication to be administered. A route of administration prescribed by the physician or other health care professional cannot be changed without the permission of the prescriber. Once the route has been specified, that route cannot be substituted without obtaining another order for the change by the prescriber.

> ❗ **TECH ALERT**
>
> For patient safety and even though an allied health care professional has interpreted a medication order, the pharmacy technician still has the responsibility to check the order for any inconsistencies, such as dosage ordered versus usual dosage, and report any concerns to the pharmacist for possible questioning of the health care provider.

Practice Problems B

Interpret the following as medication orders.

1.   Discontinue Zocor; Lipitor 10 mg tab i po hs*

    _____

2.   amoxicillin suspension 250 mg po tid until discontinued

    _____

3.   cephalexin 500 mg po q8h × 3 d

    _____

4.   Paxil-CR 12.5 mg po qam

    _____

*These abbreviations are found on the TJC Do Not Use List and ISMP's List of Error-Prone Abbreviations, Symbols, and Dose Designations due to medication safety issues. They should not be used. You are being tested on them here because these abbreviations may still appear in the pharmacy setting.

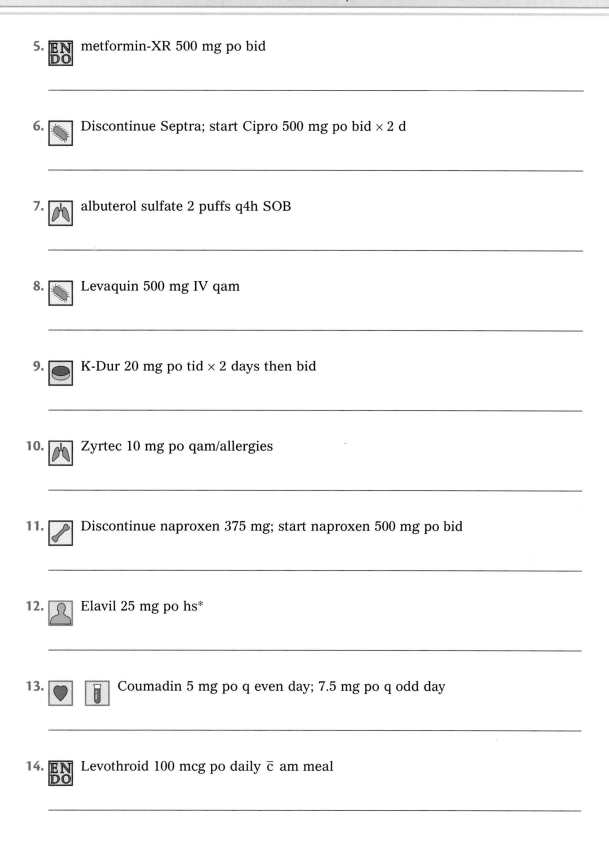

5. metformin-XR 500 mg po bid

_____

6. Discontinue Septra; start Cipro 500 mg po bid × 2 d

_____

7. albuterol sulfate 2 puffs q4h SOB

_____

8. Levaquin 500 mg IV qam

_____

9. K-Dur 20 mg po tid × 2 days then bid

_____

10. Zyrtec 10 mg po qam/allergies

_____

11. Discontinue naproxen 375 mg; start naproxen 500 mg po bid

_____

12. Elavil 25 mg po hs*

_____

13. Coumadin 5 mg po q even day; 7.5 mg po q odd day

_____

14. Levothroid 100 mcg po daily c̄ am meal

_____

*These abbreviations are found on the TJC Do Not Use List and ISMP's List of Error-Prone Abbreviations, Symbols, and Dose Designations due to medication safety issues. They should not be used. You are being tested on them here because these abbreviations may still appear in the pharmacy setting.

15. Advair Diskus 250/50 i puff bid

_____

16. diazepam 5 mg po tid prn anxiety

_____

17. hydrocodone/APAP 7.5/650 po q6h prn pain

_____

18. Flonase i spray each nostril bid

_____

19. Ambien 10 mg po hs prn sleep

_____

20. furosemide 40 mg po qam prn swelling

_____

WHAT DOES A MEDICATION LABEL INDICATE?

The label on the medication bottle is the identification of the drug within the container. It indicates the following important information needed to dispense the drug:

* The **generic name** is the official name that has been given to a medication when it is accepted by the FDA and is the name found in the *U.S. Pharmacopeia-National Formulary* (USP-NF).

> **TECH NOTE**
> Remember that the generic name begins with a lowercase letter, such as diazepam.

* The **trade** or **brand name** or the marketed name is the name assigned by the manufacturer for a given product. This name begins with a capital letter, such as Valium. Registered trade or brand medications are marked with ® to show that the name is registered.

> **TECH NOTE**
> If the medication is only in the generic form of the drug, a trade name will not be found on the label.

* The **National Drug Code** (NDC) number. This usually appears just above the drug name at the top of the label. The NDC identifies the manufacturer, the product, and the size of the container in which the medication is packed.

- The **dosage strength**, or the amount of active ingredient found in the medication per dosage form, found in the container, such as milligrams (mg), units (u), grams (g), milliliters (mL), grains (gr), or milliequivalents (mEq).
- The total quantity of medication as packed by the manufacturer.

TECH NOTE

Total number of tablets, capsules, ounces, or milliliters depends on the type of medication and the manufacturer's packaging quantities.

- The dosage form of the medication.

TECH NOTE

Tablets, capsules, liquids, suspensions, or suppository are some of the common medication dosage forms.

- The name of the company manufacturing the medication.
- Special instructions for mixing or compounding the medicine if indicated by the manufacturer.
- Storage requirements of the medication because of environmental factors.

TECH NOTE

Be sure the environmental factors have been followed for patient safety. Report any concerns about any medications that may not have been stored properly.

- Lot and batch numbers or control number of the medication that can be used for identification if the medication is recalled.
- Expiration date.
- Controlled substance indicators as appropriate.

TECH NOTE

Controlled substances are indicated by a large "C" with the schedule number in Roman numerals within the "C."

One of the most important aspects of patient safety is the careful reading of the medication label. To ensure that the proper medication has been provided for dispensing, the label (i.e., drug name, drug strength, drug form, expiration date, and the NDC number) should be read when taking the medication from the shelf, before preparing the medication, and finally, when returning the medication container to the shelf for storage. By reading medication labels carefully, you can prevent possible errors and avoid confusion, and the therapeutic potential of the drug is maximized. The pharmacy technician must be fully aware of the parts of the label and the information on the label including expiration dates and the need for **auxiliary labels** to ensure that the medicines dispensed, or the "recipe" (℞), are at the level of highest quality possible and are the exact medications that have been ordered by the health care professional.

 TECH ALERT

Always read medication labels at least three times before using to fill prescriptions. Read before removing from storage place; before counting when preparing the prescription; and finally, before returning the stock medication to the shelf if appropriate.

TECH NOTE

Check the NDC number when returning medications to the shelf to prevent possible errors in the future, such as number of tablets to be dispensed if an entire stock container of a drug is routinely dispensed.

Practice Problems C

Using the following labels, answer the questions that follow each label.

1.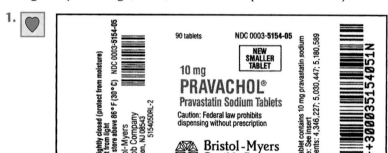

Who is the manufacturer of this medication? _____

What is the NDC number on this container? _____

What is the trade name for this medication? _____

What is the generic name for this medication? _____

The dosage strength is indicated on this label. What is the strength of this medication? _____

Before any medication has been dispensed, how many tablets are in the container?

_____

2.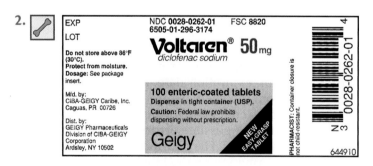

What is the NDC number on this container? _____

Who is the manufacturer of the medication? _____

Is this a controlled substance? _____

What is the amount of active ingredient in this medication? _____

What are the special storage conditions for the medication? _____

What is the trade name of this medication? _____

What is the generic name of this medication? _____

What is the form of this medication? _____

3.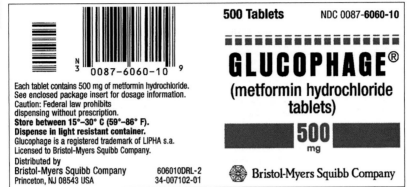

How many milligrams of medication are in each tablet? _____

How many tablets are in this container? _____

This medication is distributed by whom? _____

What is the trade name of this medication? _____

What is the generic name for this medication? _____

What type of container is necessary for storing this medication? _____

4.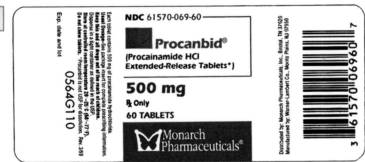

What type of container does this medication need to be dispensed in?

_____

How many tablets are in this container? _____

Who manufactures this medication? _____

What are the storage directions for this medication? _____

What is the generic name for this medication? _____

What is the NDC number for this medication? _____

The label contains the abbreviation "USP." What does this indicate? _____

What is the form of this medication? _____

5.

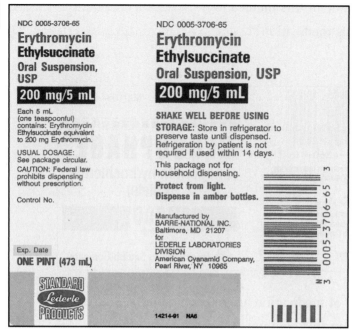

Who is the manufacturer of this medication? _____

What is the NDC number? _____

Storage of this medication is an important factor for palatability. What directions
need to be given to the patient? _____

What directions need to be followed in preparing the medication for dispensing?

_____

What are the storage directions and why are these necessary? _____

What is the trade name for this medication? _____

What is the generic name for this medication? _____

What is the form of this medication? _____

What is the total volume of medication available in this container? _____

What is the dosage strength of this medication? _____

This medication has a time limit for storage at room temperature prior to a decrease
in effectiveness. What is this time limit? _____

6.

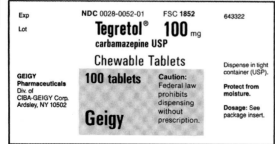

What is the dosage form of this medication? _____

What are the specific directions for the container for dispensing this medication?

_____

What is the medication and what is the dosage strength? _____

How many tablets are in the container? _____

Who manufactures the medication? _____

What is the trade name? _____

What is the generic name? _____

Storage of this medication has a precaution. What is the precaution?

7.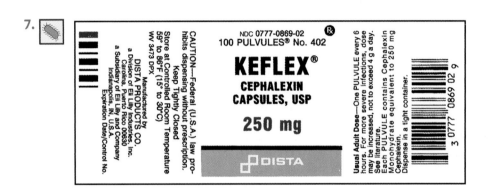

What is the NDC number of this medication? _____

What is the dosage form of this medication? _____

What is the dosage strength found in each unit? _____

Who manufactures the medication? _____

The medication stock bottle contains how many pulvules? _____

8.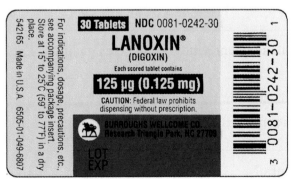

What is the trade name of this medication? _____

What is the generic name of this medication? _____

How many tablets are in this container? _____

What is the NDC number of this medication? _____

What are the storage requirements? _____

The manufacturer of this medication is who? _____

Where is this manufacturer located? _____

9.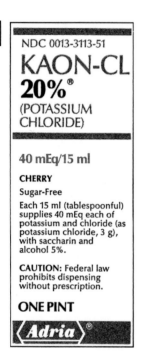

NDC 0013-3113-51

KAON-CL
20%®
(POTASSIUM CHLORIDE)

40 mEq/15 ml

CHERRY

Sugar-Free

Each 15 ml (tablespoonful) supplies 40 mEq each of potassium and chloride (as potassium chloride, 3 g), with saccharin and alcohol 5%.

CAUTION: Federal law prohibits dispensing without prescription.

ONE PINT

⟨*Adria*⟩®

What is the form of this medication? _____

Who manufactures the medication? _____

This medication may be given in household utensils. What is the household equivalent of 40 mEq? _____

What does mEq mean? _____

Can this medication be used with someone who has diabetes mellitus? Explain your answer _____

What is the total volume of medication in the container? _____

What are the two supplements found in this medication? _____

The symbol ® means what? _____

What is the metric dose for 40 mEq? _____

10.

NDC 0031-7890-95

Twenty-Five **2 ml** Single Dose Vials

Robinul®Injectable

Brand of

Glycopyrrolate Injection, USP

0.4 mg/2 ml

(0.2 mg/ml)

Water for Injection, USP q.s./Benzyl Alcohol, NF (preservative) 0.9%.
pH adjusted, when necessary, with hydrochloric acid and/or sodium hydroxide.
For I.M. or I.V. administration.

To open—Cut seal along dotted line

Exp.

Lot

For dosage and other directions for use, consult accompanying product literature.
Store at Controlled Room Temperature, Between 15°C and 30°C (59°F and 86°F).
CAUTION: Federal law prohibits dispensing without prescription.

MANUFACTURED FOR   PHARMACEUTICAL DIVISION
A. H. ROBINS COMPANY, RICHMOND, VA. 23220
by ELKINS-SINN, INC., CHERRY HILL, N.J. 08034
a subsidiary of A. H. Robins Company   10.81

A·H·ROBINS

What is the trade name of this medication? _____

What is the generic name of this medication? _____

What is the form of this medication? _____

What is the dosage strength of this medication? _____

Who is the manufacturer of the medication? _____

How will this medication be administered? _____

How is the medication supplied? _____

What are the storage requirements? _____

USING UNITS AND MILLIEQUIVALENTS AS MEASUREMENTS FOR DOSAGE

Some medications, such as penicillin, heparin, and insulin, as well as others used less often, such as hormones, vitamins, and antitoxins, are measured in units. A unit is a standard of measurement that is set according to a laboratory standard when a biologically based medication contains some product of either plant or animal origin. These may be either USP units or international units. No universal value to a unit is applicable because the value of a unit is measured by the physiological effect a drug has on the body. The effect of a drug varies from medication to medication, so the equivalent given on the label is the guide to the amount of medication that is to be administered to a person. The strength may vary from a few units (less than 100) per milliliter, such as vasopressin and Acthar Gel, to a moderate number of units per milliliter (from 250 to 5000), as is found with heparin and tetanus antitoxin, to 100,000 to 1,000,000 units per milliliter, as is found in the penicillins. Therefore, when working with units, you must be careful interpreting the orders to be sure the correct number of units is indicated on the order or prescription. For example, orders may read as penicillin G 500,000 units, heparin 10,000 units, or NPH insulin 54 units.

TECH NOTE

The amount of medication per unit is not consistent among medications.

As a pharmacy technician, you must be sure to carefully read the label of medications using units as a dosage strength. This is important for obtaining the exact number of units per milliliter, tablet, capsule, or other drug form, because this can vary not only between medications but with the number of units per dosage form found with the same medication. Medications found in vials must be read completely because the potency of the drugs must be stated on the vial, and this is where the differences in potency are seen. Some of the medications that are in injectable form must be given to a hundredth of a milliliter because of potency. Insulin, which also is in units, requires an insulin syringe that matches the potency of the insulin, such as U-100 insulin must be administered with a U-100 syringe.

Milliequivalents (mEq) are used to measure electrolytes that are used as medications, such as potassium (K) and chloride (Cl). A milliequivalent strength represents the amount of electrolyte that is dissolved in a given unit of medication, such as mEq per tablet, milliliter, liter, teaspoon, or tablespoon. In actuality, when using milliequivalents, the amount of medication is a thousandth (1/1000) of an equivalent weight of a chemical.

When using units or milliequivalents, conversions are not necessary because the order will be written in the dosage amount that matches the label strength of the medication to be administered (e.g., insulin is ordered in units, potassium chloride is ordered in milliequivalents). If a prescription is written for KCl 20 mEq and the stock medication is KCl 20 mEq/tablet, a single tablet per dose would be delivered to the patient.

Practice Problems D

Using the labels provided, answer the questions about units and milliequivalents.

1.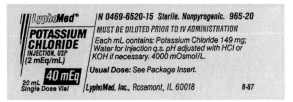

What is the total dosage of the medication in the vial? _____

Who manufactures the medication? _____

What is the metric amount of the medication? _____

What is the dosage form of the medication? _____

2.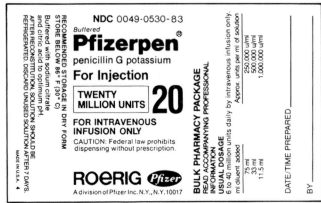

What is the dosage of the medication in units? _____

This medication is to be administered by what route? _____

What is the trade name? _____

What is the generic name? _____

The usual daily dose of the medication is what? _____

How many milliliters of diluent should be added for the medication to have approximately 1,000,000 units/mL? _____

3.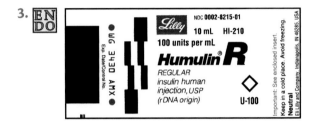

Who manufactures this medication? _____

What does "U-100" mean? _____

What is the total volume of medication in the container? _____

What does "R" mean on the label? _____

4.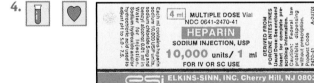

The dosage strength of this medication is what? _____

The container has what total volume of medication? _____

Who manufactures this medication? _____

This medication is administered by what route? _____

What is the generic name of this medication? _____

If there is a trade name for this medication, what is it? _____

From what source is this product manufactured? _____

5.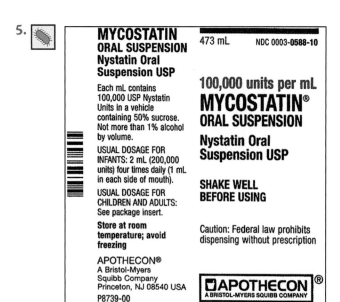

What is the generic name of this medication? _____

What is the trade name of this medication? _____

What is the usual dosage for infants of this medication? _____

The total volume of medication found in this container is what? _____

How much medication is found in 2 mL of suspension? _____

What is the form of this medication? _____

Describe how this medication should be stored. _____

What specific instructions must be given the patient about this medication to be sure
the correct amount of medication is taken? _____

6.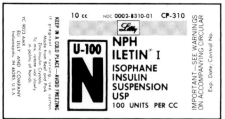

What is the generic name of this medication? _____

What is the trade name of this medication? _____

How many units of insulin are contained in 1 mL of this medication?

_____

The route of administration for this medication is what? _____

Who is the manufacturer of this medication? _____

What is the total volume of medication in milliliters in the container?

_____

7.

The dosage of this medication is what? _____

What are the routes of administration? _____

Who manufactures this medication? _____

Is this the same medication as found in question 4? _____

If so, what is the difference in the dosage strength as found on the two labels?

_____

What is the total volume of medication in the container? _____

8.

The total medication strength found in the container is what? _____

What amount of diluent must be added for the medication to have 500,000 units/mL

after **reconstruction**? _____

The usual adult dosage of this medication for patient safety is what?

_____

What is the generic name of this medication? _____

After reconstitution, how should this medication be stored? _____

9.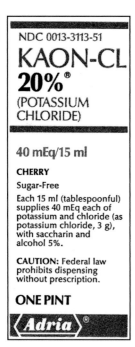

NDC 0002-7185-01
10 ml   VIAL No. 554
Ⓡ   *Lilly*
STERILE PENICILLIN G
PROCAINE
SUSPENSION, USP
300,000 Units per ml
Multiple Dose
DURACILLIN® A.S.

REFRIGERATE   AVOID FREEZING

CAUTION—Federal (U.S.A.) law pro-
hibits dispensing without prescription.
For Intramuscular Use Only
Usual Adult Dose—1 ml intramuscularly
once or twice a day. See literature. Each
ml contains 300,000 units. Crystalline
Penicillin G Procaine, sodium citrate 4%,
lecithin 1%, povidone 0.1% with methyl-
paraben 0.15%, propylparaben 0.02%,
benzyl alcohol 1% as preservatives,
Water for Injection, q.s. .1 ml
SHAKE WELL
TO 1000 AM
Eli Lilly & Co.
Indianapolis, IN 46285, U.S.A

Exp. Date/Control No.

The total volume of medication in the container in metric measurements is what?

_____

What is the total medication strength in the container in units? _____

What strength of medication is found in 1 mL of the suspension?

_____

What specific storage requirements must be followed? _____

What is the generic name of the medication? _____

10.

NDC 0013-3113-51

KAON-CL
20%®
(POTASSIUM
CHLORIDE)

40 mEq/15 ml

CHERRY
Sugar-Free
Each 15 ml (tablespoonful)
supplies 40 mEq each of
potassium and chloride (as
potassium chloride, 3 g),
with saccharin and
alcohol 5%.

CAUTION: Federal law
prohibits dispensing
without prescription.

ONE PINT

⟨*Adria*⟩®

What is the dosage strength of the medication? _____

How much medication will be taken if a tablespoon of medication is administered?

_____

How is the medication administered? _____

REVIEW

It is absolutely necessary that you read medication orders and prescriptions and correctly interpret orders as written by health care professionals to keep patients safe when they take the medications. There must be checks and balances among the prescriber, the pharmacist, and the person responsible for obtaining the medications for dispensing, such as the pharmacy technician. Any break in this cross-check might result in the patient getting the wrong medication, and, more importantly, the mistake could be lethal.

TECH NOTE

As a pharmacy technician, you have the responsibility to be sure you understand any order or prescription and ask for verification if there is even a slight question. Never assume that you understand the prescription or order. As part of the medical team providing medicines, you must assist in continuous quality control for patient safety.

Posttest

Before taking the Posttest, retake the Pretest to check your understanding of the materials presented in this chapter.

Interpret the following prescriptions or medication orders and show the Sig as it would appear on a prescription label. If the prescription calls for liquid form of a medication, be sure your prescription label instructions are ones that can be administered in household measurements.

1.

> Lawrence Merry, M.D.
> 4th Street and Jones Ave.
> Holly, GA 00111
> phone# - 001-555-2176
>
> Patient Name_____ Date _____
> Address_____ Age _____
>
> Rx   Xanax 500 mcg
>   #30
>   Sig: i tab po at bedtime
>
> _____   Refill _____
> DEA#_____

Prescription interpretation: _____

Label instruction: _____

Continued

Posttest, cont.

2.

> Lawrence Merry, M.D.
> 4th Street and Jones Ave.
> Holly, GA 00111
> phone# - 001-555-2176
>
> Patient Name_____ Date _____
> Address_____ Age _____
>
> Rx   K-Clor 20 mEq ℥ xvi
>   Sig: ℥ s̄s̄ po qam p̄ breakfast
>
> _____ Refill _____
> DEA#_____

Prescription interpretation: _____

Label instruction: _____

3.

> Lawrence Merry, M.D.
> 4th Street and Jones Ave.
> Holly, GA 00111
> phone# - 001-555-2176
>
> Patient Name_____ Date _____
> Address_____ Age _____
>
> Rx   Mycostatin Oral Suspension
>   60 mL
>   Sig: Agit then swish and swallow 5 mL
>   q4-6h
>
> _____ Refill _____
> DEA#_____

Prescription interpretation: _____

Label instruction: _____

Posttest, cont.

4.

Lawrence Merry, M.D.
4th Street and Jones Ave.
Holly, GA 00111
phone# - 001-555-2176

Patient Name_____ Date _____
Address_____ Age _____

℞ Dilantin 100 mg caps
   #120
   Sig: cap iv po stat then cap ī po qid

_____ Refill _____

DEA#_____

Prescription interpretation: _____

Label instruction: _____

5.

Lawrence Merry, M.D.
4th Street and Jones Ave.
Holly, GA 00111
phone# - 001-555-2176

Patient Name_____ Date _____
Address_____ Age _____

℞ Zyrtec 1 mg/1 mL
   $\bar{3}$ iii
   Sig: 3 s̄s̄ po qam; rep po at bedtime prn

_____ Refill _____

DEA#_____

Prescription interpretation: _____

Label instruction: _____

Continued

Posttest, cont.

6.

Lawrence Merry, M.D.
4th Street and Jones Ave.
Holly, GA 00111
phone# - 001-555-2176

Patient Name_____ Date _____
Address_____ Age _____

℞   amlodipine 5 mg
              #30
              Sig: tab ī po daily @ 10 am

_____   Refill _____
DEA#_____

Prescription interpretation: _____

Label instruction: _____

7.

Lawrence Merry, M.D.
4th Street and Jones Ave.
Holly, GA 00111
phone# - 001-555-2176

Patient Name_____ Date _____
Address_____ Age _____

℞   Vasotec 10 mg
              #30
              Sig: tab s̄s̄ po x 1 wk then ī tab po daily.
              Check B/p and record daily.

_____   Refill _____
DEA#_____

Prescription interpretation: _____

Label instruction: _____

Posttest, cont.

8.

> Lawrence Merry, M.D.
> 4th Street and Jones Ave.
> Holly, GA 00111
> phone# - 001-555-2176
>
> Patient Name_____ Date _____
> Address_____ Age _____
>
> ℞   Antivert 12.5 mg
>   #60
>   Sig: tab ī po q4-6h prn
>
> _____ Refill _____
> DEA#_____

Prescription interpretation: _____

Label instruction: _____

9.

> Lawrence Merry, M.D.
> 4th Street and Jones Ave.
> Holly, GA 00111
> phone# - 001-555-2176
>
> Patient Name_____ Date _____
> Address_____ Age _____
>
> ℞   Ocuflox Ophthalmic Solution
>   5 mL
>   Sig: i gtt each eye qid x 5 d
>
> _____ Refill _____
> DEA#_____

Prescription interpretation: _____

Label instruction: _____

Continued

Posttest, cont.

ENDO **10.**

Lawrence Merry, M.D.
4th Street and Jones Ave.
Holly, GA 00111
phone# - 001-555-2176

Patient Name_____ Date _____
Address_____ Age _____

℞   Actos 30 mg
       #30
       Sig: i tab po qam ac breakfast

_____ Refill _____
DEA#_____

Prescription interpretation: _____

Label instruction: _____

Interpret the following medication orders using medical terms, and use lay terms where marked with an asterisk.

PAIN **11.** meperidine 75 mg and Phenergan 25 mg IM q4-6h prn extreme pain

_____

12. Septra 3 ii po q4h until all medication is taken*

_____

13. Nafcillin i g q4-6h added to IV fluids

_____

ENDO **14.** Humulin 70/30 25 units subcutaneously qam ac breakfast and ac supper

_____

15. Tagamet 300 mg IM stat

_____

Posttest, cont.

16. ampicillin 250 mg i cap po qid c̄ meals and hs c̄ snack

_____

17. warfarin sodium 5 mg po daily on even days and 2.5 mg po daily on odd days

_____

18. digoxin 250 mcg po qam c̄ pulse ↑60

_____

19. Sudafed 60 mg tab ī po q4-6h prn nasal congestion

_____

20. Celebrex 100 mg cap ī po bid

_____

Interpret these labels by answering the following questions.

21.

NDC 0039-0060-13
3 0039-0060-13
Lasix®
(furosemide)
40 mg
Caution: Federal law prohibits dispensing without prescription. Do not use if bottle closure seal is broken.
100 Tablets

Lot:
Exp:
NSN 6505-00-117-5982
Lasix REG TM HOECHST AG
Lasix®
(furosemide)
100 Tablets
40 mg

Usual Dosage: 20 to 80 mg. See insert for full prescribing information. Dispense in well-closed, light resistant container with safety closure. Store at room temperature. Keep this and all medication out of the reach of children.
HOECHST-ROUSSEL
Pharmaceuticals Incorporated
Somerville, NJ 08876-1258
REG TM HOECHST AG
6601 30-7/92

What is the generic name of this medication? _____

Who manufactures this medication? _____

What is the NDC number of this medication? _____

How many tablets are in a full stock container? _____

What is the dose in each tablet? _____

What is the average adult dose for this medication? _____

Continued

Posttest, cont.

22.

NDC 0028-0051-10   FSC 3602
6505-01-071-6557

Lopressor® 50 mg

metoprolol tartrate USP

EXP
LOT

1000 tablets

Keep this and all drugs out
of the reach of children.

Dispense in tight, light-resistant
container (USP).

Caution: Federal law prohibits
dispensing without prescription.

Geigy

PHARMACIST: Container closure is not child-resistant.
Dosage: See package insert.
Store between 59°- 86°F (15°- 30°C).
Protect from moisture.

Ciba-Geigy Corporation
Pharmaceuticals Division
Summit, NJ 07901

645120

N 3   0028-0051-10   6

What is the warning on the label for patient safety? _____

What is the trade name for this medication? _____

What is the generic name for this medication? _____

What is the NDC number for this medication container? _____

What is the total number of tablets in the container? _____

23.

©Abbott

0074336860

Exp.
Lot
03-2185-3/R5

Store tablets at 15° to 30°C (59° to 86°F).

SPECIMEN

NDC 0074-3368-60
60 Tablets

BIAXIN®
FILMTAB®
clarithromycin tablets
250 mg

Caution: Federal (U.S.A.) law
prohibits dispensing without
prescription.

6505-01-354-8582

Do not accept if seal over bottle
opening is broken or missing.

Dispense in a USP tight,
light-resistant container.

Each tablet contains:
250 mg clarithromycin.

Usual Adult Dose: One or two
tablets every twelve hours.

See enclosure for full prescribing
information.

Filmtab – Film-sealed tablets,
Abbott.
Abbott Laboratories
North Chicago, IL60064, U.S.A.

What is the strength of each tablet? _____

Who manufactures this medication? _____

What is the NDC number? _____

What is the lot number? _____

What is the usual adult dosage of this medication? _____

What is the generic name? _____

What is the trade name? _____

Posttest, cont.

24.

NDC 0002-0313-02
100   TABLETS No. 1571

Lilly

**FERROUS
SULFATE
TABLETS
USP**

5 grs (324 mg)

For Iron Deficiency in
Hypochromic Anemias.

Each Tablet equivalent to 65 mg elemental iron. Also contains cellulose, F D & C Blue No. 1, F D & C Red No. 40, F D & C Yellow No. 6, lactose, magnesium stearate, silicon dioxide, sodium lauryl sulfate, talc, titanium dioxide and other inactive ingredients.

Keep Tightly Closed
YA 8009 AMX
Store at 59° to 86°F
Eli Lilly & Co., Indianapolis, IN 46285, U.S.A.
Expiration Date/Control No.

Do not purchase if Lilly band around cap is missing or broken. After purchasing, do not use initially if red Lilly seal under cap is missing or broken. Tampering may have occurred.

Usual Adult Dose—One or two tablets 3 times a day after meals, or as directed by the physician.

WARNINGS: Keep all medications out of the reach of children. As with any drug, if you are pregnant or nursing a baby, seek the advice of a health professional before using this product. Infants and children only as directed by the physician since indiscriminate use or large doses may be harmful to them.

What is the metric dosage of this medication? _____

What is the apothecary dosage of this medication? _____

What is the use of this medication? _____

What is the dosage form of this medication? _____

What is the average adult dose of this medication? _____

What is the warning for children? _____

What is the quantity in the container when it is full? _____

25.

USUAL ADULT DOSAGE:
See accompanying circular.

Dispense in a well-closed container.

CAUTION: Federal (USA) law prohibits dispensing without prescription.

100 | No. 3297   7603212

NDC 0006-0021-68

100 TABLETS
COGENTIN® 0.5 mg
(BENZTROPINE MESYLATE)

COGENTIN

Dist. by:
MERCK & CO., INC.
West Point, PA 19486, USA

This is a bulk package and not intended for dispensing.

Lot   Exp.

What is the usual adult dose of this medication? _____

What is the strength of each tablet? _____

What is the trade name of this medication? _____

What is the shape of this medication? _____

What is the form of this medication? _____

What is the total number of tablets in the container? _____

Who manufactures this medicine? _____

What is the location of the manufacturer? _____

Continued

Posttest, cont.

26.

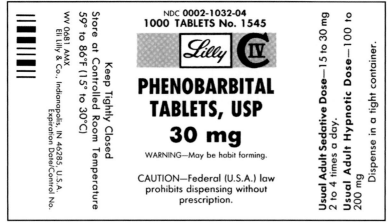

Is this a scheduled medication? _____ If yes, what schedule?

_____

What is the strength of this medication? _____

What is the usual dosage of the medication needed to produce a sedative effect?

_____

What is the usual dosage of the medication necessary to produce a hypnotic effect?

_____

Who manufactures this medication? _____

What is the NDC number? _____

What is the location of the manufacturer? _____

What is the generic name of this medication? _____

What is the trade name of this medication? _____

27.

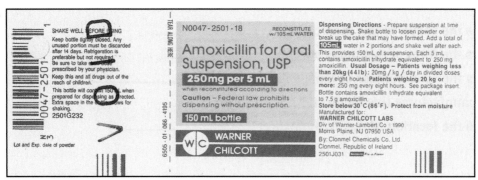

Posttest, cont.

How much water must be added to this medication for reconstitution?

_____

What is the total (volume) of this medication after reconstitution?

_____

What is the dosage strength of this medication after reconstitution?

_____

What is the usual dosage for persons weighing less than 44 pounds?

_____

What is the usual dosage for persons weighing more than 44 pounds?

_____

What is the generic name of this medication? _____

How long can this medication be used after reconstituting? _____

Is refrigeration required? If not, what is suggested? _____

 28.

NDC 0002-2438-05
16 fl oz (1 pt) (473 mL)

Lilly C IV

ELIXIR No. 227
**PHENOBARBITAL
ELIXIR, USP**

Contains 20 mg Phenobarbital
per 5 mL
WARNING—May be habit forming.
Contains Alcohol 14 Percent
CAUTION—Federal (U.S.A.) law
prohibits dispensing without
prescription.

Store at Controlled Room Temperature 59° to 86° F
(15° to 30° C)
Keep Tightly Closed
WV 5931 AMX
Eli Lilly & Company, Indianapolis, IN 46285, U.S.A.
Expiration Date/Control No.

VOID

Usual Adult Sedative Dose—60 mg (1 gr) (3 tea-
spoonfuls) two to four times a day.
Indiscriminate use may be harmful.
Dispense in a tight, light-resistant container.

3 0002 2438 05 9

What is the dosage strength of this medication? _____

What is the form of this medication? _____

What is the adult dose of this medication? _____

What is the NDC number for this medication? _____

Who manufactures this medication? _____

What is the total volume of medication in the container? _____

What would be the household measurement for 20 mg of this medication?

_____

Continued

Posttest, cont.

 29.

N 0047-0606-32

Aspirin
Tablets, USP

Analgesic (Pain Reliever)/
Antipyretic (Fever Reducer)

Directions—Adults: Oral dosage is 1 tablet every three hours; or 1 to 2 tablets every four hours; or 2 to 3 tablets every six hours, while symptoms persist, not to exceed 12 tablets in any 24-hour period, or as directed by a doctor. Drink a full glass of water with each dose. **Children under 12 years of age:** Consult a doctor.

Indications—For the temporary relief of minor aches and pains and to reduce fever.

[**Quality Sealed for your protection***]

*Do not use if the innerseal over the opening of the bottle printed "SEALED for YOUR PROTECTION" is broken or missing.

1000 Tablets
325 mg (5 grains) each

(WC) WARNER CHILCOTT

6505-00-153-8750 .... 325 mg.

Active Ingredient—Each tablet contains Aspirin, USP. Also contains corn starch and microcrystalline cellulose.

Warnings—Children and teenagers should not use this medicine for chicken pox or flu symptoms before a doctor is consulted about Reye syndrome, a rare but serious illness reported to be associated with aspirin.

Keep this and all drugs out of the reach of children. In case of accidental overdose, seek professional assistance or contact a poison control center immediately.

As with any drug, if you are pregnant or nursing a baby, seek the advice of a health professional before using this product. IT IS ESPECIALLY IMPORTANT NOT TO USE ASPIRIN DURING THE LAST 3 MONTHS OF PREGNANCY UNLESS SPECIFICALLY DIRECTED TO DO SO BY A DOCTOR BECAUSE IT MAY CAUSE PROBLEMS IN THE UNBORN CHILD OR COMPLICATIONS DURING DELIVERY.

Do not take this product for pain for more than 10 days or for fever for more than 3 days unless directed by a doctor. If pain or fever persists or gets worse, if new symptoms occur, or if redness or swelling is present, consult a doctor because these could be signs of a serious condition.

Do not take this product if you are allergic to aspirin or if you have asthma, or if you have stomach problems (such as heartburn, upset stomach, or stomach pain) that persist or recur, or if you have ulcers or bleeding problems, unless directed by a doctor. If ringing in the ears or a loss of hearing occurs, consult a doctor before taking any more of this product.

Drug Interaction Precaution: Do not take this product if you are taking a prescription drug for anticoagulation (thinning the blood), diabetes, gout, or arthritis unless directed by a doctor.

Store below 30°C (86°F). Protect from moisture.

Exp date and lot

WARNER CHILCOTT LABS ©1991
Div of Warner-Lambert Co   0606G022
Morris Plains, NJ 07950 USA

N 3   0047-0606-32   1

SPECIMEN

What is the trade name of this medication? _____

What is the apothecary strength measurement for each tablet? _____

What is the metric strength measurement for each tablet? _____

What is the adult dosage of this medication? _____

What are the indications for this medication? _____

What is the maximum amount of time that a person should take this medication as an analgesic? _____ For fever? _____

What precautions are on the label about this medication being taken by pregnant women? _____

REVIEW OF RULES

Interpreting Medication Labels and Orders

● Always read the entire label or prescription/order before making decisions concerning the medication to be administered.

● If you are unfamiliar with the medication, read information concerning the medicine before dispensing.

- The drug label will give the total amount of medication in the package, whether this is in solid doses such as tablets or capsules or in liquid medication such as the total volume in the container.

- Solid medications are usually ordered in the weight of medication per tablet. The label will read in milligrams, grams, grains, or other solid measurements per drug form.

- Liquid medications will be found in the strength (weight) in a volume (or the amount of solvent) of medication such as mg/mL.

- The generic name for the medication will be written in lower case letters, whereas the trade or proprietary name will begin with a capital letter and may be followed by ®.

- If there is a question about the medication ordered, always ask the pharmacist to verify the medication before beginning the process of preparing the medication for dispensing.

- Always read medication labels three times to ensure correctness of the dispensed medication to the medication order/prescription: (1) when removing stock medication from the storage shelf; (2) before preparing medication; and (3) before returning stock medication back to the shelf, if applicable.

CHAPTER 7

Calculation of Solid Oral Doses and Dosages

OBJECTIVES

- Calculate solid oral doses using metric and apothecary measurement systems
- Accomplish conversion of equivalent measurements of oral solid doses between the metric and apothecary systems
- Interpret medical orders and accurately calculate the solid oral dose to be administered using either ratio and proportion, the formula system, or dimensional analysis
- Calculate total dosages of solid oral medication necessary for dispensing a physician's order
- Accomplish patient safety when dispensing medications

KEY WORDS

Buccal Between gum and cheek

Dosage Size, amount, and number of doses of medication for therapeutic care

Dosage form (DF) Physical/structural character of a dose

Dosage strength available (DA) Strength or weight of medication available for doses

Dose Amount of a medication to be administered at one time

Dose ordered (DO) Amount of medication ordered for a single dose

Dose to be given (DG) Amount of medication such as number of tablets or amount of liquid volume to be administered as a dose

Enteric-coated Coating on tablet that allows medication to pass through stomach unchanged and prevents absorption before reaching intestines

Oral medications Medications taken by mouth

Sublingual Under the tongue

Pretest

Calculate the following problems, determining how many capsules or tablets must be given per dose, and provide the answers in the system given for the dosage available and the dosage form. When labels for medication appear, the label is to indicate the dosage available. Show all of your calculations.

1. Dose ordered: phenobarbital 30 mg

Dosage available: phenobarbital 60 mg tablet _____

2. Dose ordered: Tagamet 800 mg

Dosage available: Tagamet 400 mg tab _____

3. Dose ordered: digitoxin 0.25 mg

Dosage available: digitoxin 250 mcg tablet _____

Pretest, cont.

4. Dose ordered: Clinoril 400 mg

Dosage available: Clinoril 200 mg tablet _____

5. Dose ordered: Theophylline 0.4 g

Dosage available: Theophylline 200 mg cap _____

6. Dose ordered: K-Clor 0.6 gm

Dosage available: K-Clor 300 mg tablet _____

7. Dose ordered: aspirin gr x

Dosage available: aspirin gr v tab _____

8. Dose ordered: Pepcid 40 mg

Dosage available: Pepcid 20 mg tablet _____

9. Dose ordered: amoxicillin 1000 mg

Dosage available: amoxicillin 500 mg cap _____

10. Dose ordered: Haldol 2 mg

Dosage available: Haldol 1 mg tablet _____

11. Dose ordered: Synthroid 350 mcg daily _____

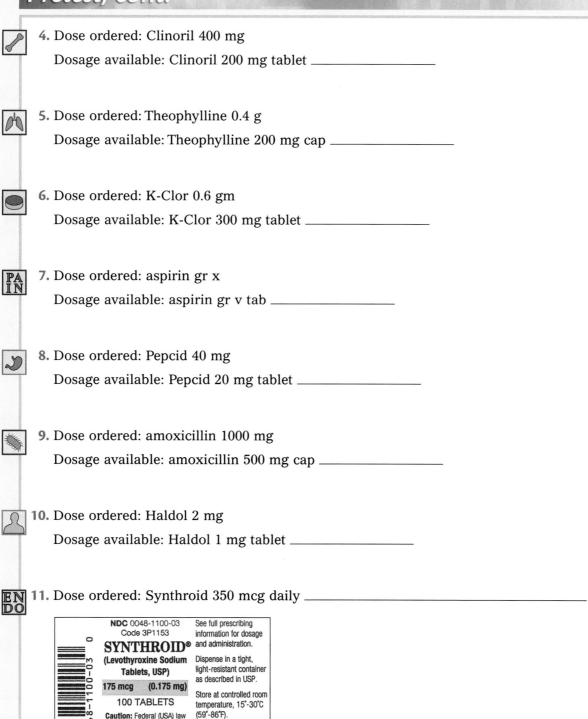

NDC 0048-1100-03
Code 3P1153

SYNTHROID®
(Levothyroxine Sodium Tablets, USP)

175 mcg   (0.175 mg)

100 TABLETS

Caution: Federal (USA) law prohibits dispensing without prescription.

BASF Pharma   knoll®

See full prescribing information for dosage and administration.

Dispense in a tight, light-resistant container as described in USP.

Store at controlled room temperature, 15°-30°C (59°-86°F).

Knoll Pharmaceutical Company
Mount Olive, NJ 07828
USA
7893-02

0048-1100-03

Continued

Pretest, cont.

12. Dose ordered: ferrous sulfate 325 mg _____

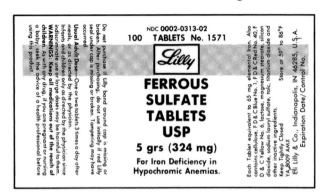

13. Dose ordered: Glyset 50 mg _____

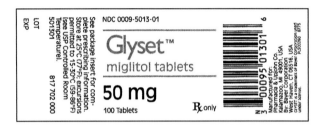

14. Dose ordered: Cogentin 1.5 mg _____

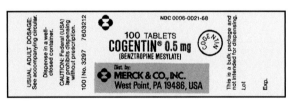

15. Dose ordered: Zyvox 0.6 g _____

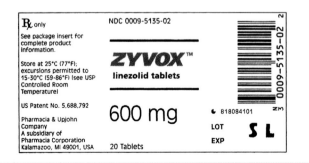

Pretest, cont.

16. Dose ordered: Sinequan 20 mg _____

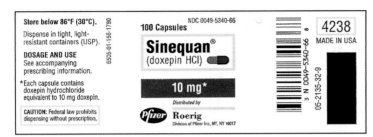

Store below 86°F (30°C).

Dispense in tight, light-resistant containers (USP).

DOSAGE AND USE
See accompanying prescribing information.

*Each capsule contains doxepin hydrochloride equivalent to 10 mg doxepin.

CAUTION: Federal law prohibits dispensing without prescription.

6505-01-156-1790

NDC 0049-5340-66
100 Capsules

Sinequan®
(doxepin HCl)

10 mg*

Distributed by
Pfizer   Roerig
Division of Pfizer Inc, NY, NY 10017

3 N 0049-5340-66 8
05-2135-32-9

4238
MADE IN USA

EN DO

17. Dose ordered: Synthroid 50 mcg _____

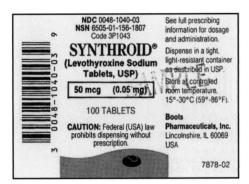

NDC 0048-1040-03
NSN 6505-01-156-1807
Code 3P1043

SYNTHROID®
(Levothyroxine Sodium Tablets, USP)

50 mcg   (0.05 mg)

100 TABLETS

CAUTION: Federal (USA) law prohibits dispensing without prescription.

3 0048-1040-03 9

See full prescribing information for dosage and administration.

Dispense in a tight, light-resistant container as described in USP.

Store at controlled room temperature. 15°-30°C (59°-86°F).

Boots Pharmaceuticals, Inc.
Lincolnshire, IL 60069 USA

7878-02

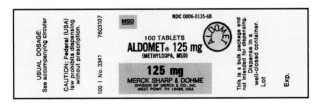

18. Dose ordered: Aldomet 0.25 g _____

USUAL DOSAGE:
See accompanying circular.

CAUTION: Federal (USA) law prohibits dispensing without prescription.

7603107

100 I No. 3341

MSD

NDC 0006-0135-68

100 TABLETS
ALDOMET® 125 mg
(METHYLDOPA, MSD)

125 mg
MERCK SHARP & DOHME
DIVISION OF MERCK & CO., INC.
WEST POINT PA 19486, USA

ALDOMET

This is a bulk package and not intended for dispensing. Dispense in a well-closed container.

Lot   Exp.

Continued

Pretest, cont.

19. Dose ordered: Cardizem 60 mg _____

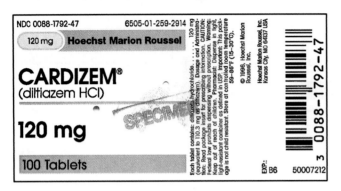

20. Dose ordered: cimetidine 400 mg _____

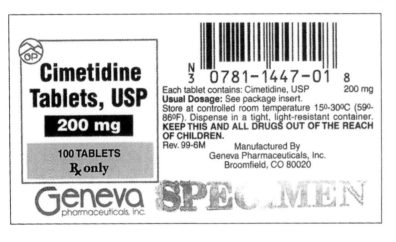

INTRODUCTION

Using the oral route for medication administration is the safest and most frequently used means of administering medicines. **Oral medications** come in solid forms (such as tablets and capsules) and liquid forms. Variations of these solid forms, such as powders and granules, are dissolved in liquids for administration (see Chapters 8 and 9). Other advantages of administering medications orally include convenience for the patient, absence of damage to skin, and reduced cost of manufacturing the medication because the drug does not require the use of sterile technique, allowing the drug to be more economical.

Oral medications are absorbed in the gastrointestinal tract, primarily in the small intestine. Because of the differences in absorption rates due to age, gastric motility, gastric contents, and illnesses, the amount of medication that each patient receives may not be the same amount as the usually prescribed **dose**, therefore, a prescription or medical order is written to accommodate individual differences. These differences must be considered by the physician and are further checked and verified by the pharmacy professional as a means of checks and balances. Therefore, drug manufacturers often provide drugs in different strengths to meet the needs of each patient and to allow dispensing of the therapeutic dose necessary for each person. When the dose ordered is available in the needed **dosage** strength and form, fewer errors will occur with administration of the medication. The pharmacy technician must be aware of the various strengths of medications and take care in choosing the correct drug strength when preparing medications for dispensing.

Some medications may be irritating to the intestinal tract and may require eating a meal or snack to aid in absorption or to prevent irritation in the stomach. Others must have special instructions for taking the medicine, such as iron elixir, which can stain teeth and should be administered through a straw, or Fosamax, which requires the person receiving the drug remain in an upright position for at least 30 minutes after administration. Some tablets may be divided or crushed for ease in swallowing; the ability to divide the tablets is usually indicated by the tablet being scored. Remember, capsules should not be crushed or divided, although some may be opened and sprinkled on food for ease of administration after obtaining special permission from the physician.

Because solid oral medications are dispensed according to specific instructions for safety and for providing the correct doses, the pharmacy technician must be aware that calculation of exact dosages is an important factor in administering medications. Many drug dosages will be in the exact amounts that are found on medication labels, whereas others must be calculated to be sure the correct amount of medication is provided for administration. This chapter is designed to ensure that you can calculate doses and dosages from prescriptions and medication orders, using physician's orders and drug labels.

CALCULATING SOLID ORAL MEDICATION DOSES

To provide the necessary medication for the administration of a solid oral dose, the label must be read carefully and the correct medication must be used in dispensing the drug. After choosing the appropriate medication, the pharmacy technician must be sure to calculate the amount of medicine to be given to the patient both in the individual dose and the entire amount of medication, or dosage. Care is necessary to supply the treatment prescribed for patient safety. The calculation of a dose depends on the amount of medicine that has been ordered at a given time, whereas dosage indicates the total amount of medicine that is necessary for the complete order or prescription. This chapter covers calculating both doses and dosages. Just as a reminder, the label on the medication provided and the prescribed medication must be either in the same measurement system or a form that can be converted to provide the prescribed medicine dose and dosage. Another important rule of thumb is that when converting among measurement systems, be sure the final conversion is in the same measurement system as that found on the label of the medication. In other words, if you are converting between milligrams and grams and the label on the medication is in grams per tablet, the final answer should be in grams per tablet or the number of tablets. Finally, be sure that the medication names are exactly the same, because many medications have sound-alike or look-alike names that are similar. If there is ever a doubt about the medicine to be used or if the calculation does not seem to be what you expected it to be, obtain clarification from the pharmacist before preparing the medicine, a practice that is always safe, important, and acceptable. The pharmacist—the person ultimately responsible for dispensing the medication—would prefer to answer questions before medication preparation rather than make a medication error by dispensing incorrect doses or medications.

Remember that dose refers to the amount of medication given at a single time; dosage refers to the amount of medication for the physician's entire order.

More rules that should be considered when calculating medication dosage follow:

- Capsules are not made to be opened or divided, although in some special circumstances this may occur with permission from the physician.
- Scored tablets may be divided, but tablets not scored are not intended to be divided or broken.
- **Enteric-coated, buccal,** and **sublingual** tablets are not intended for crushing.
- Buccal and sublingual tablets should not be swallowed whole but should be dissolved within the oral cavity in the designated location.
- If a part of a tablet is the answer to the dose problem, be sure that altering the tablet by breaking or crushing will not alter the pharmaceutical action or purpose of the medication and that the calculations have been correctly made and the correct medication strength has been chosen.

! TECH ALERT

If your calculation provides an answer that seems incorrect, check your formula and calculations. Recalculate as necessary. If the answer still does not seem correct, ALWAYS ask for help from a co-worker or the pharmacist. Never fill an order or prescription if you still have a question regarding the correctness of your calculation.

Drug calculations may be obtained by using one of three methods. The method that you feel the most comfortable using is the correct method for you to use. One method is using ratio and proportion (discussed in Chapter 2). Dimensional analysis is an extended form of ratio and proportion and may also be used for calculating a dose of medication. Finally, the following formula may be used for calculations:

$$\frac{DD \text{ (Dose desired)}}{DH \text{ (Dose on hand)}} \times Qty \text{ (Quantity or form)} = Dose \text{ to be given (DG)}$$

! TECH ALERT

Always check to be sure the measurement system of the medication available with the drug order before performing calculations.

In the next section, each problem will be calculated using each of the three methods. Again, find the method with which you feel the most comfortable and use it for all your calculations. Always using the same methodology for calculations will assist in avoiding possible confusion during calculations.

Calculating Medications Using Ratio and Proportion

When using the proportional method of calculating doses, the **dosage strength available** (DA) and the **dosage form** (DF) must be one ratio, and the **dose ordered** (DO) and the **dose to be given** (DG) must be the second ratio in the proportion. Remember that in using a mathematical equation for ratio and proportion, the ratio shows the relationship between two numbers, and proportion shows the relationship between two ratios. When setting up a problem for calculation by ratio and proportion, the formula then appears as follows:

DA (Dosage available) : DF (Dosage form) :: DO (Dose ordered) : DG (Dose to be given)

Remember that these relationships may also be written as fractional units if this is easier for your calculations. A fractional formula is as follows:

$$\frac{DA}{DF} = \frac{DO}{DG}$$

TECH NOTE

Note that the **known** dosage and the dosage form are on the left side of the proportion.

Also remember that when part of the ratio is missing, the unknown number is represented by "x". If a calculation is necessary and one of the components of the proportion is missing, the missing part or x can be found by filling in the known parts of the proportion and then completing the problem as with any proportional problem. To use proportion, the dosage available (DA) and the dose ordered (DO) must be in the same measurement system. If the systems differ, conversion must be done to bring these components into the same system. (See Chapter 4 for help in remembering the measurement systems and Chapter 5 for help in converting among systems.) Later in this chapter you will calculate problems requiring conversion. Now you can begin performing calculations with medications in the same system.

EXAMPLE 7-1

An order is written for 500 mg of medication, and the available medication strength is 250 mg/capsule.

In this proportion, if you know that 250 mg (DA) of a medication is found in 1 capsule (DF) and the order reads for the patient to be given 500 mg (DO), the ratio would look like this:

250 mg (DA) : 1 cap (DF) :: 500 mg (DO) : x (DG)

OR

$$\frac{250 \text{ mg (DA)}}{1 \text{ cap (DF)}} = \frac{500 \text{ mg (DO)}}{x \text{ (DG)}}$$

TECH NOTE

DA and DO in this example are both in milligrams in the metric system so conversion to the same weight is not necessary.

Now multiply the means versus extremes or cross-multiply if in fractional components.

$$250 \text{ mg} : 1 \text{ cap} :: 500 \text{ mg} : x \text{ cap} \quad \text{or} \quad \frac{250 \text{ mg}}{1 \text{ cap}} \;\times\; \frac{500 \text{ mg}}{x \text{ cap}}$$

Drop the "mg" because this appears in both parts of the equation, and the equation now looks like this:

$$250x = 500 \times 1 \text{ cap}$$

$$x = \frac{500 \text{ cap}}{250}$$

x = 2 cap, or the prescribed amount of medication to be given is 2 capsules

Let's try another medication order as an example, but this time we will use measurements in the apothecary system.

EXAMPLE 7-2

A medication order is written for gr ¾ (DO) to be given, and dose available is gr ¼ (DA) in each tablet (DF). What is the dose to be given to the patient?

$$gr \frac{1}{4} (DA) : 1 \ tab \ (DF) :: gr \frac{3}{4} (DO) : x \ (DG)$$

OR

$$\frac{gr \ \frac{1}{4} \ (DA)}{1 \ tab \ (DF)} = \frac{gr \ \frac{3}{4} \ (DO)}{x \ (DG)}$$

As previously, drop the "gr" because this appears on both sides of the equation. Again, either multiply means and extremes or cross-multiply the fractional components. The resultant formula is as follows:

$$\frac{1}{4}x = \frac{3}{4} \times 1$$

$$x = \frac{3}{4} \times \frac{4}{1}$$

$$x = \frac{3}{\cancel{4}} \times \frac{\cancel{4}}{1}$$

$$x = \frac{3}{1} \quad or \quad 3 \ tablets$$

Calculating Medications Using Dimensional Analysis

Dimensional analysis is actually just an elongated form of ratio and proportion using multiple fractional units. To use dimensional analysis, ratios must allow for the cancellation of measurements from one ratio into the next. (See Chapter 5 for a review of dimensional analysis basics.)

If the previous problems were calculated in dimensional analysis, the first problem would read as follows:

EXAMPLE 7-3

An order is written for 500 mg of medication, and the available strength is 250 mg/capsule.

$$x \text{ caps} = \frac{1 \text{ cap}}{250 \text{ mg}} \times \frac{500 \text{ mg}}{1}$$

Reduce the equations to lowest terms: $x \text{ caps} = \frac{1 \text{ cap}}{\cancel{250} \text{ mg}_1} \times \frac{\cancel{500}^{2} \text{ mg}}{1}$

$$x \text{ caps} = \frac{1 \times 2}{1 \times 1} \quad \text{or} \quad x \text{ caps} = \frac{2}{1}$$

$$x \text{ caps} = 2 \text{ capsules}$$

EXAMPLE 7-4

A medication order is written for gr ¾ (DO) to be given, and the dose available is gr ¼ (DA) in each tablet (DF). What is the dose to be given (DG) to the patient?

$$x \text{ tabs} = \frac{1 \text{ tab}}{\text{gr } \frac{1}{4}} = \frac{\text{gr } \frac{3}{4}}{1}$$

$$x \text{ tabs} = \frac{1 \text{ tab}}{\text{gr } 1} = \frac{\text{gr } 3}{1} \quad \text{or} \quad x \text{ tabs} = \frac{1 \times 3 \text{ tab}}{1 \times 1}$$

$$x \text{ tabs} = \frac{3}{1} \text{ or } 3 \text{ tablets}$$

Dose to be given will be 3 tablets.

Calculating Medications Using the Formula Method

Many professionals use the formula method to calculate doses. Using the formula, replace each component of the formula with the correct information and then calculate the problem. This is the same means of replacement as is used with ratio and proportion, but the formula is used for placing the given amounts. The formula follows:

$$\frac{\text{DD (Dose desired)}}{\text{DH (Dose on hand [DA])}} \times \text{Qty (Quantity [DF])} = \text{Dose to be given (DG)}$$

Quantity in solid medications will appear as capsules or tablets, whereas in liquid form the quantity may be found in the number of mg, g, or other weight measurement in the volume of medication, or may be given mL, drops, or other liquid volume measurements.

EXAMPLE 7-5

An order is written for 500 mg of medication, and the available strength is a 250 mg capsule.

$$\frac{500 \text{ mg (DD)}}{250 \text{ mg (DA)}} \times 1 \text{ cap (Qty [DF])} = \text{Dose to be given (DG)}$$

$$\frac{500 \text{ mg}}{250 \text{ mg}} \times 1 \text{ cap} = DG$$

TECH NOTE

Because "mg" is found in both the numerator and denominator, it may be canceled. Also notice the dosage form (a capsule in this example) has remained in place as the quantity in this formula.

$$\frac{500}{250} \times 1 \text{ cap} = DG$$

$$500 \div 250 = 2$$

$$2 \times 1 = 2 \text{ capsules to be given}$$

EXAMPLE 7-6

A medication order is written for gr ¾ (DO) to be given and the dose on hand is gr ¼ (DH or DA) in each tablet (Qty or DF). What is the dose to be given (DG) to the patient?

$$\frac{\text{gr } ¾}{\text{gr } ¼} \times 1 \text{ tab} = \text{Dose to be given (DG)}$$

$$\frac{\text{gr } ¾}{\text{gr } ¼} \times 1 \text{ tab} = \text{Dose to be given} \quad \text{or} \quad x = \frac{3}{4} \times \frac{4}{1} \times 1 \text{ tab} = \text{Dose to be given}$$

Again, remember that "=" has been crossed and the fraction has been inverted

$$\frac{3}{4} \times \frac{4}{1} \times 1 \text{ tab} = \text{Dose to be given} \quad \text{or} \quad \frac{3}{1} \times 1 \text{ tab} = \text{Dose to be given}$$

Dose to be given = 3 tabs

Please notice that both of these problems are done within the same measurement system. After the practice problems, you will begin working between measurement systems for calculating doses and dosages.

Practice Problems A

Calculate the practice problems below. Show all your calculations. Remember to use the method of conversion that is most comfortable for you. Indicate how the medication order would be shown on a prescription label.

TECH NOTE

Medications in tablets, capsules, syrups, elixirs, suspensions, and the like may or may not have "po" within the medication order or prescription; however it is assumed professionally that these forms of medications are to be taken by mouth.

NOTE: This chapter concerns oral medications so when interpreting orders for labels be sure to include that the medications are to be taken by mouth.

1. **EN DO** Order: Synthroid 175 mcg po daily in am

NDC 0048-1100-03 Code 3P1153 **SYNTHROID®** (Levothyroxine Sodium Tablets, USP) **175 mcg (0.175 mg)** 100 TABLETS **Caution:** Federal (USA) law prohibits dispensing without prescription. **BASF** Pharma **knoll®**	See full prescribing information for dosage and administration. Dispense in a tight, light-resistant container as described in USP. Store at controlled room temperature, 15°-30°C (59°-86°F). **Knoll Pharmaceutical** **Company** Mount Olive, NJ 07828 USA 7893-02

Interpret the order. _____

Dose to be given: _____

Prescription label: _____

2. Order: ferrous sulfate gr x̄ po qam

Do not purchase if Lilly band around cap is missing or broken. After purchasing, do not use initially if red Lilly seal under cap is missing or broken. Tampering may have occurred. **Usual Adult Dose—**One or two tablets 3 times a day other meals, or as directed by the physician. Infants and children only as directed by the physician since indiscriminate use or large doses may be harmful to them. **WARNINGS: Keep all medications out of the reach of children.** As with any drug, if you are pregnant or nursing a baby, seek the advice of a health professional before using this product.	**NDC** 0002-0313-02 **100 TABLETS No. 1571** *Lilly* **FERROUS** **SULFATE** **TABLETS** **USP** **5 grs (324 mg)** For Iron Deficiency in Hypochromic Anemias.	Each Tablet equivalent to 65 mg elemental Iron. Also contains cellulose, F.D.& C.Blue No. 1, F.D.& C.Red No. 40, F.D. & C.Yellow No. 6, lactose, magnesium stearate, silicon dioxide, sodium lauryl sulfate, talc, titanium dioxide and other inactive ingredients. Keep Tightly Closed Store at 59° to 86°F YA.B009 AMX Eli Lilly & Co., Indianapolis, IN 46285, U.S.A. Expiration Date/Control No.

Interpret the order. _____

Dose to be given: _____

Prescription label: _____

3. Order: ciprofloxacin 1.5 gm po qam

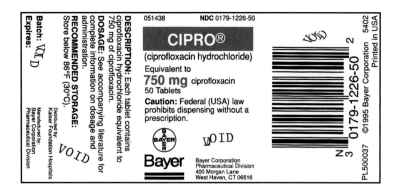

Interpret the order. _____

Dose to be given: _____

Prescription label: _____

4. Order: digoxin cap 0.1 mg po qam $\bar{c}$ P ↑ 60 until changed by MD

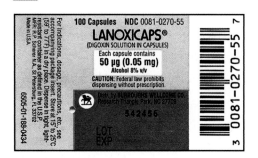

Interpret the order. _____

Dose to be given: _____

Prescription label: _____

5. Order: Lopid 1.2 gm qam c̄ am meal

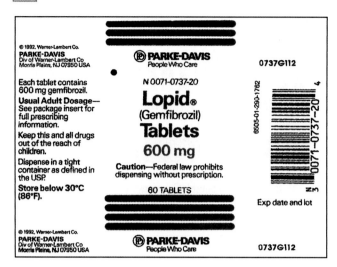

Interpret the order. _____

Dose to be given: _____

Prescription label: _____

6. Order: Dilantin 0.5 gm bid c̄ breakfast and evening meal

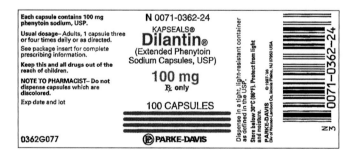

Interpret the order. _____

Dose to be given: _____

Prescription label: _____

7. ENDO   Order: metformin HCl 1 gm po bid c̄ meals. Ck BS before taking medication

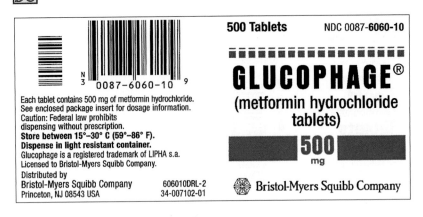

Interpret the order. _____

Dose to be given: _____

Prescription label: _____

8. Order: Biaxin 500 mg po bid c̄ food

NDC 0074-3368-60
60 Tablets

BIAXIN®
FILMTAB®
clarithromycin tablets
250 mg

Caution: Federal (U.S.A.) law
prohibits dispensing without
prescription.

6505-01-354-8582

Do not accept if seal over bottle
opening is broken or missing.
Dispense in a USP tight,
light-resistant container.
Each tablet contains:
250 mg clarithromycin.
Usual Adult Dose: One or two
tablets every twelve hours.
See enclosure for full prescribing
information.
Filmtab – Film-sealed tablets,
Abbott.
Abbott Laboratories
North Chicago, IL60064, U.S.A.

©Abbott   0074336860   SPECIMEN   Store tablets at 15° to 30°C (59° to 86°F).

Exp.   Lot 03-2185-3/R5

Interpret the order. _____

Dose to be given: _____

Prescription label: _____

9. Order: pravastatin 20 mg po daily hs*

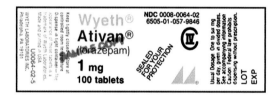

Interpret the order. _____

Dose to be given: _____

Prescription label: _____

10. Order: Ativan 0.5 mg po q6-8h or hs prn anxiety*

Interpret the order. _____

Dose to be given: _____

Prescription label: _____

*These abbreviations are found on the TJC Do Not Use List and ISMP's List of Error-Prone Abbreviations, Symbols, and Dose Designations due to medication safety issues. They should not be used. You are being tested on them here because these abbreviations may still appear in the pharmacy setting.

11. Order: Retrovir 200 mg po qhs*

```
Rev. 2/96                                    100 Capsules        NDC 0173-0108-55
U.S. Patent Nos. 4818538 and 4828838 (Product Patents);
4724232, 4833130, and 4837208 (Use Patents)
For indications, dosage, precautions, etc., see accom-
panying package insert.
Store at 15° to 25°C (59° to 77°F) and protect from
moisture. Dispense in a tight container as defined in
the U.S.P.
Made in U.S.A.
                                            RETROVIR® (zidovudine)
                                            Capsules
                                            Each capsule contains
                                            100 mg
                                            CAUTION: Federal law prohibits
                                            dispensing without prescription.
                                            Glaxo Wellcome Inc.
                                            Research Triangle Park, NC 27709
                                                587019
                                            LOT
                                            EXP              6505-01-253-2515
                                                        0173-0108-55   5
```

Interpret the order. _____

Dose to be given: _____

Prescription label: _____

12. PA IN   Order: ASA gr x × po q4-6h prn aching; do not exceed 8 tab q24h

```
N 0047-0606-32

Aspirin
Tablets, USP
Analgesic (Pain Reliever)/
Antipyretic (Fever Reducer)

Directions—Adults: Oral dosage is 1 tablet
every three hours; or 1 to 2 tablets every four
hours; or 2 to 3 tablets every six hours, while
symptoms persist, not to exceed 12 tablets in
any 24-hour period, or as directed by a doctor.
Drink a full glass of water with each dose.
Children under 12 years of age: Consult a
doctor.
Indications—For the temporary relief of minor
aches and pains and to reduce fever.

Quality Sealed for your protection*

*Do not use if the innerseal over the opening
of the bottle printed "SEALED for YOUR
PROTECTION" is broken or missing.

1000 Tablets
325 mg (5 grains) each

WC WARNER
CHILCOTT

6505-00-153-8750        325 mg.

Active Ingredient—Each tablet contains Aspirin, USP
Also contains corn starch and microcrystalline cellulose.
Warnings—Children and teenagers should not use this medicine for chicken pox or flu
symptoms before a doctor is consulted about Reye syndrome, a rare but serious illness
reported to be associated with aspirin.
Keep this and all drugs out of the reach of children. In case of accidental overdose,
seek professional assistance or contact a poison control center immediately.
As with any drug, if you are pregnant or nursing a baby, seek the advice of a health
professional before using this product. IT IS ESPECIALLY IMPORTANT NOT TO USE ASPIRIN
DURING THE LAST 3 MONTHS OF PREGNANCY UNLESS SPECIFICALLY DIRECTED TO DO SO BY
A DOCTOR BECAUSE IT MAY CAUSE PROBLEMS IN THE UNBORN CHILD OR COMPLICATIONS
DURING DELIVERY.
Do not take this product for pain for more than 10 days or for fever for more than 3 days
unless directed by a doctor. If pain or fever persists or gets worse, if new symptoms occur,
or if redness or swelling is present, consult a doctor because these could be signs of a
serious condition.
Do not take this product if you are allergic to aspirin or if you have asthma, or if you have
stomach problems (such as heartburn, upset stomach, or stomach pain) that persist or
recur, or if you have ulcers or bleeding
problems, unless directed by a doctor. If
ringing in the ears or a loss of hearing
occurs, consult a doctor before taking any
more of this product.
Drug Interaction Precaution: Do not take this
product if you are taking a prescription drug
for anticoagulation (thinning the blood),
diabetes, gout, or arthritis unless directed by
a doctor.
Store below 30°C (86°F). Protect from
moisture.
Exp date and lot

                        0047-0606-32   1
                        WARNER CHILCOTT LABS
                        Div of Warner-Lambert Co
                        Morris Plains, NJ 07950 USA
                        ©1991
                        0606G022

SPECIMEN
```

Interpret the order. _____

Dose to be given: _____

Prescription label: _____

*These abbreviations are found on the TJC Do Not Use List and ISMP's List of Error-Prone Abbreviations, Symbols, and Dose Designations due to medication safety issues. They should not be used. You are being tested on them here because these abbreviations may still appear in the pharmacy setting.

13. Order: cephalexin 0.75 gm po bid c̄ breakfast and hs

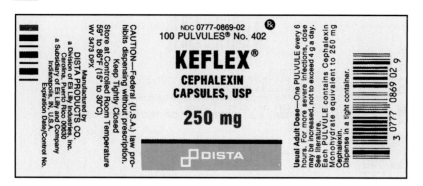

Interpret the order. _____

Dose to be given: _____

Prescription label: _____

14. Order: Decadron 0.75 mg daily @ same time

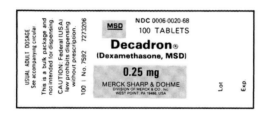

Interpret the order. _____

Dose to be given: _____

Prescription label: _____

15. Order: promethazine 0.0375 gm q4-6h prn N&V

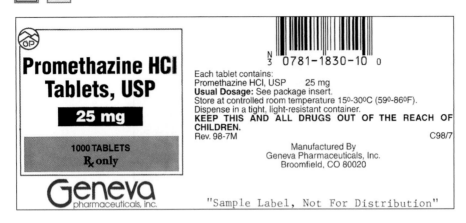

Interpret the order. _____

Dose to be given: _____

Prescription label: _____

16. Order: Lotrel 5/20 daily in am

NDC 0078-0404-05

Lotrel® 2.5/10

amlodipine besylate
(equivalent to amlodipine 2.5 mg)
benazepril HCl 10 mg

100 capsules

Rx only

Ů NOVARTIS

Dosage: See package insert.
Store at 25°C (77°F); excursions
permitted to 15-30°C (59-86°F).
See USP controlled room temperature.
Protect from moisture.
Dispense in tight container (USP).
Keep this and all drugs out of the
reach of children.
Mfd. by: Novartis Pharmaceuticals Corp.
Suffern, New York 10901
Dist. by: Novartis Pharmaceuticals Corp.
East Hanover, New Jersey 07936
©Novartis
5000183

Interpret the order. _____

Dose to be given: _____

Prescription label: _____

17. Order: isoniazid 250 mg tid c̄ meals

BARR LABORATORIES, INC.   **NDC** 0555-0066-05

Isoniazid Tablets, USP

100 mg

Caution: Federal law prohibits dispensing without prescription.

0555-0066-05

Interpret the order. _____

Dose to be given: _____

Prescription label: _____

18. Order: Evista 0.12 gm po daily

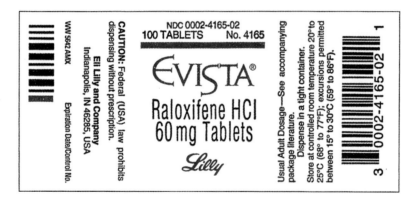

WW 5642 AMX

Expiration Date/Control No.

CAUTION: Federal (USA) law prohibits dispensing without prescription.

Eli Lilly and Company Indianapolis, IN 46285, USA

NDC 0002-4165-02
100 TABLETS   No. 4165

EVISTA®

Raloxifene HCl 60 mg Tablets

Lilly

Usual Adult Dosage—See accompanying package literature.
Dispense in a tight container.
Store at controlled room temperature 20° to 25°C (68° to 77°F); excursions permitted between 15° to 30°C (59° to 86°F).

0002-4165-02

Interpret the order. _____

Dose to be given: _____

Prescription label: _____

19. Order: Voltaren 0.05 gm bid c̄ meals

```
EXP                 NDC 0028-0262-01    FSC 8820
LOT                 6505-01-296-3174
Do not store above 86°F    Voltaren® 50 mg
(30°C).                    diclofenac sodium
Protect from moisture.
Dosage: See package
insert.

Mfd. by:                   100 enteric-coated tablets
CiBA-GEIGY Caribe, Inc.    Dispense in tight container (USP).
Caguas, PR  00726
                           Caution: Federal law prohibits
Dist. by:                  dispensing without prescription.
GEIGY Pharmaceuticals
Division of CIBA-GEIGY     Geigy              NEW
Corporation                                  EASY-GRASP
Ardsley, NY 10502                            TABLET

PHARMACIST: Container closure is
not child resistant.

0028-0262-01

N 3
                                             644910
```

Interpret the order. _____

Dose to be given: _____

Prescription label: _____

20. Order: carbamazepine 0.2 gm qid with meals and hs*

```
Exp           NDC 0028-0052-01    FSC 1852       643322
Lot
              Tegretol®  100 mg
              carbamazepine USP

              Chewable Tablets
                                                 Dispense in tight
GEIGY         100 tablets    Caution:            container (USP).
Pharmaceuticals             Federal law
Div. of                     prohibits            Protect from
CIBA-GEIGY Corp.            dispensing           moisture.
Ardsley, NY 10502          without
              Geigy        prescription.         Dosage: See
                                                 package insert.
```

Interpret the order. _____

Dose to be given: _____

Prescription label: _____

CALCULATING SOLID MEDICATIONS AMONG DIFFERENT MEASUREMENT SYSTEMS

Remember from Chapter 5 that conversions among measurement systems are approximates, and amounts are often not exact but as close as possible with the medications ordered and medications available. To figure the dose to be given, you must first convert so that the medication ordered (DO) and the medication on hand (DA) are in the same measurement system. (Solid medications taken orally do not require the use of conversions to the household system, so this is covered in Chapter 8.)

*These abbreviations are found on the TJC Do Not Use List and ISMP's List of Error-Prone Abbreviations, Symbols, and Dose Designations due to medication safety issues. They should not be used. You are being tested on them here because these abbreviations may still appear in the pharmacy setting.

TECH NOTE

The general rule for converting the medication order to the measurement system of the medication on hand should be followed. That is, if the medication is ordered in the apothecary system and the medication is in the metric system, you should use the metric system for the calculation or vice versa, being sure the drug on hand is the system used in the final answer.

TECH NOTE

Round answers to the nearest whole number unless tablets are scored; in that case, round to the nearest half tablet.

EXAMPLE 7-7

The physician orders ASA gr $\overline{\text{iiss}}$ daily for a patient with coronary disease. The medication on hand is labeled ASA 81 mg tab.

First, the order as written by the physician must be interpreted, and then the calculation of the dose must be completed. In this order, the physician wants the patient to take aspirin (ASA) 2½ grains daily. Now you know that the dose will be 2½ grains of medication, but you do not know the number of tablets that are to be administered or (DG). The order is written in the apothecary system, whereas the medication available is in the metric system. So, you must now make a conversion for this order to be filled. Under the general rule to convert to the available medications, in this case the conversion should be from apothecary to metric. In Chapter 5 you learned that one grain is equal to 60 mg, or the conversion necessary for this order. Also remember that the known equivalency should be placed on the left of the ratio and proportion formula with the unknown on the right of the equation.

$$\textit{Known} \qquad \textit{Unknown}$$

$$\text{gr i} : 60 \text{ mg} :: \text{gr } \overline{\text{iiss}} : x$$

$$\text{gr 1} : 60 \text{ mg} :: \text{gr } 2\tfrac{1}{2} : x$$

$$x = 60 \times 2\frac{1}{2}$$

$$x = 60 \times \frac{5}{2} \quad \text{or} \quad \frac{60 \times 5}{2} \quad \text{or} \quad \frac{300}{2}$$

$$x = 150 \text{ mg}$$

Following the conversion, the amount necessary is 150 mg of ASA, so now the formula, ratio and proportion, or dimensional analysis calculation may be used to figure the number of tablets necessary for the dose ordered.

Ratio and Proportion Method

81 mg (DA) : 1 tab (DF) :: 150 mg (DO) : x (Dose to be given)

81 mg : 1 tab :: 150 mg : x

$$81x = 150 \times 1 \text{ tab (150)}$$

$$x = 150 \div 81$$

$$x = 1.85, \text{ rounded to 1.9 or 2 tablets (then round to the nearest whole number)}$$

Dose to be given = 2 tablets.

Dimensional Analysis Method

Dimensional analysis will allow you to make the entire conversion in one proportional equation. Using dimensional analysis, the step of changing from apothecary to metric may be done as part of the equation in the following:

$$x \text{ tabs} = \frac{\text{gr } \overset{..}{\text{ii}}\ \overline{\text{ss}}\ (DO)}{1} \times \overset{\text{conversion factor}}{\frac{60 \text{ mg}}{\text{gr } 1}} \times \frac{1 \text{ tab (DF)}}{81 \text{ mg (DH)}}$$

$$x \text{ tabs} = \frac{\text{gr } 2\frac{1}{2}}{1} \times \frac{60 \text{ mg}}{\text{gr } i} \times \frac{1 \text{ tab}}{81 \text{ mg}}$$

$$x \text{ tabs} = \left(2\frac{1}{2} \times 60 \times 1 \right) \div (1 \times 1 \times 81) \text{ or } 150 \div 81$$

$$x \text{ tablets} = 1.85 \text{ round to } 1.9 \quad \text{or} \quad 2 \text{ tabs}$$

> **TECH NOTE**
>
> Remember that when converting, the answer may be approximate rather than exact. The exact answer is 1.85 or 1.9, which will be rounded to 2 tablets.

If you prefer, you can make your conversion from apothecary to metric before figuring the dose. Then calculate the dose by dimensional analysis as follows:

$$x \text{ tabs} = \frac{1 \text{ tab}}{81 \text{ mg}} \times \frac{150 \text{ mg}}{1}$$

$$x \text{ tabs} = 150 \div 81$$

$$x \text{ tabs} = 1.85 \text{ round to } 1.9 \quad \text{or} \quad 2 \text{ tablets (see Tech Note above)}$$

Formula Method

$$\frac{150 \text{ mg (DD)}}{81 \text{ mg (DA)}} \times 1 \text{ tabs (DF)} = \text{Dose to be given (DG)}$$

$$\frac{150 \text{ mg}}{81 \text{ mg}} \times 1 \text{ tab (DF)} = \text{Dose to be given (DG)}$$

$$(150 \div 81) \times 1 = \text{Dose to be given (DG)}$$

$$\text{Dose to be given} = 1.85 \text{ round to } 1.9 \quad \text{or} \quad 2 \text{ tablets (see Tech Note above.)}$$

In some cases you must convert within a system such as micrograms to milligrams or milligrams to grams or vice versa. If so, make the conversion within the system before converting between systems.

> **TECH NOTE**
>
> All the methods of conversion between systems are included, choose the method that is most comfortable for you to use and use it consistently.

Practice Problems B

Calculate the following problems, using the method that is most comfortable for you. Show all calculations. Indicate how the medication order would appear on the prescription label.

1. A physician orders ferrous sulfate gr v po bid. The available medication is labeled ferrous sulfate 325 mg tabs.

   Interpret the order. _____

   Dose to be given: _____ tablet(s)

   Prescription label: _____

2. A physician orders phenobarbital grss̄ tab po hs.* The medication available is labeled phenobarbital 60 mg tabs.

   Interpret the order. _____

   Dose to be given: _____ tablet(s)

   Prescription label: _____

3. A physician orders codeine sulfate 60 mg q4-6h prn pain. The medication available is labeled codeine sulfate gr ¼ tab.

   Interpret the order. _____

   Dose to be given: _____ tablet(s)

   Prescription label: _____

4. A physician orders Nitrostat gr 1/150 SL q5min up to 3 doses prn angina. The medication available is labeled Nitrostat 0.4 mg tab.

   Interpret the order. _____

   Dose to be given: _____ tablet(s)

   Prescription label: _____

*These abbreviations are found on the TJC Do Not Use List and ISMP's List of Error-Prone Abbreviations, Symbols, and Dose Designations due to medication safety issues. They should not be used. You are being tested on them here because these abbreviations may still appear in the pharmacy setting.

5. [PA IN] The physician orders aspirin gr x po q4-6h prn high fever or aching for a patient with influenza. The medication available is labeled aspirin-DS 650 mg tab.

Interpret the order. _____

Dose to be given: _____ tablet(s)

Prescription label: _____

6. [pill] A physician orders ferrous sulfate 650 mg bid c̄ breakfast and evening meal. The medication available is labeled ferrous sulfate gr v tab.

Interpret the order. _____

How many tablets will be given with each dose? _____

Prescription label: _____.

7. [PA IN] A physician orders codeine sulfate gr s̄s̄ po q4h prn pain or cough. The medication available is labeled codeine sulfate 15 mg tab.

Interpret the order. _____

How many tablets will be given with each dose? _____

Prescription label: _____

8. [brain] A physician orders phenobarbital 30 mg po tid and hs* for epilepsy. The medication available is labeled gr ¼ tab.

Interpret the order. _____

How many tablets will be given with each dose? _____

Prescription label: _____

*These abbreviations are found on the TJC Do Not Use List and ISMP's List of Error-Prone Abbreviations, Symbols, and Dose Designations due to medication safety issues. They should not be used. You are being tested on them here because these abbreviations may still appear in the pharmacy setting.

9. ♥ A physician orders Nitrostat 0.6 mg SL q5min × 3 doses prn angina; call 911 if no relief. The medication available is labeled Nitrostat gr 1/100 tab.

Interpret the order. _____

How many tablets will be given with each dose? _____

Prescription label: _____

10. PA IN   A physician orders codeine sulfate 90 mg po q4-6h prn pain in left hip. The medication available is codeine sulfate gr 3/4 tab.

Interpret the order. _____

How many tablets will be given with each dose? _____

Prescription label: _____

CALCULATE TOTAL DOSAGES OF MEDICATION FROM PHYSICIAN'S ORDERS

Physicians may state an order for a medication to be given so many times a day over a desired length of time. To be able to complete this order in an inpatient setting, the order will be dispensed on a daily basis for the desired time. If this same prescription is provided in a retail environment, the pharmacy technician will be required to calculate the number of doses that will be necessary for dispensing the complete prescription to the patient. This will require the pharmacy technician to find the number of doses in a specific day and then multiply this by the days that the medication is necessary.

EXAMPLE 7-8

Dr. Ho orders amoxicillin 500 mg tid × 10 days.

This order reads to dispense amoxicillin 500 mg capsules to be taken 3 times a day for 10 days. Amoxicillin is available in 500 mg capsules. 3 capsules per day × 10 days = 30 capsules.

The pharmacy technician in a retail pharmacy would prepare 30 capsules for the pharmacist to check for dispensing. In the inpatient setting, such as a nursing home, the date of the order would be noted and the ending date would be noted, so the medication would be discontinued 10 days later.

Practice Problems C

Interpret the orders and calculate the number of tablets or capsules necessary for each order. Show all calculations. Indicate how the prescription label would read.

1. Dr. Jones orders naproxen 500 mg bid × 30 d. The available dose is Naprosyn 500 mg tablets.

   Interpret the order. _____

   How many tablets need to be dispensed for the entire prescription? _____

   Prescription label: _____

2. Dr. Ho orders KCl 20 mEq to be given daily with furosemide for 30 days. The available medication is KCl 10 mEq tablets.

   Interpret the order. _____

   How many tablets need to be dispensed for this prescription? _____

   Prescription label: _____

3. Dr. Assad orders Flagyl 250 mg po bid × 7 days. Available are Flagyl 500 mg tabs.

   Interpret the order. _____

   How many tablets should be dispensed for this prescription? _____

   Prescription label: _____

4. **EN DO** Dr. Mills orders Decadron 0.75 mg on a declining scale of 0.75 mg tid × 3 d, 0.75 mg bid × 3 d, 0.75 mg daily × 3 d. Available medication is Decadron 0.75 mg tablets.

Interpret the order. _____

How many Decadron tablets need to be dispensed for the entire prescription?

_____

How many tablets would be dispensed on the first day in the inpatient setting?

_____

How many tablets would be dispensed for the fourth day for the inpatient?

_____

Prescription label: _____

5. A physician orders Coumadin 5 mg on even days and Coumadin $7\frac{1}{2}$ mg on odd days. The dose available is Coumadin 5 mg tablets.

Interpret the order. _____

How many tablets would you dispense for the month of June? _____

Prescription label: _____

6. Mrs. Jones is having difficulty sleeping. In the past she has taken Valium 5 mg for anxiety. Dr. Santo wants her to take 5 mg daily qam for anxiety and $7\frac{1}{2}$ mg hs* for sleep. The medication available is Valium 5 mg scored tablets.

Interpret the order. _____

How many tablets would you prepare for dispensing for a 4-day supply to see if this

helps Mrs. Jones? _____

Prescription label: _____

*These abbreviations are found on the TJC Do Not Use List and ISMP's List of Error-Prone Abbreviations, Symbols, and Dose Designations due to medication safety issues. They should not be used. You are being tested on them here because these abbreviations may still appear in the pharmacy setting.

7. Mr. Casto has lower back pain. Dr. Gero prescribes Skelaxin 400 mg tid × 10 days. Available dosage is Skelaxin 800 mg scored tablets.

Interpret the order. _____

How many tablets should be prepared for dispensing for Mr. Casto for the entire

prescription? _____

Prescription label: _____

8. Dr. Burke wants Johnny to take prednisone 5 mg in descending doses beginning with 7 tabs on the first day, 6 tabs on the second day, and decreasing one tablet daily until only one tablet is taken for 2 days.

Interpret the order. _____

How many total tablets should be dispensed? _____

Prescription label: _____

9. Dr. Shu, a urologist, orders Septra DS for Mr. King for a urinary tract infection. Dr. Shu wants Mr. King to take Septra DS bid × 7 days and then daily × 21 days.

Interpret the order. _____

How many tablets should be prepared for dispensing? _____

Prescription label: _____

10. Dr. Green orders metformin for Mrs. Forrester to be taken 1000 mg qam and 500 mg hs.* Metformin is available in 500 mg tablets or 750 mg tablets.

Interpret the order. _____

Which dosage on hand (DH) would you use? _____

How many tablets would you prepare for dispensing for 30 days?

_____

Prescription label: _____

*These abbreviations are found on the TJC Do Not Use List and ISMP's List of Error-Prone Abbreviations, Symbols, and Dose Designations due to medication safety issues. They should not be used. You are being tested on them here because these abbreviations may still appear in the pharmacy setting.

PATIENT SAFETY WHEN CALCULATING DOSES AND DOSAGES

As a pharmacy technician, you must always be aware that patient safety and accurate calculations are a necessity when preparing medications for dispensing. Medication orders or prescriptions are the physician's determination of the medication and the amount that should be safe for the patient. The triangulation among the physician, pharmacist, and pharmacy technician or other health care team member is necessary to ensure this safety. In the center of the triangle is the patient, who is dependent on health care professionals to provide medications that are as risk-free as possible.

To be certain that the medication is correct and in the correct dosage, you should follow certain safety rules.

- Always check calculations after the dose has been figured. To do this, the procedure necessary for accurate calculations should be learned to confidence level so that you do not have to depend on any of your co-workers to do the calculation for you; ultimately, you are responsible for the medication you prepared for dispensing.
- If you have any question about the dosage or your calculations, check with the pharmacist. Remember that he or she is responsible for the medication that is dispensed.
- As you work from either a medication order or a prescription, verify that what you have on hand is the medication ordered and that it is in a dosage form that can be used.
- Check labels three times before providing the prescription for dispensing—before taking the medication from the shelf, before preparing the medication, and before returning the medication to the stock area or passing to the pharmacist after preparation.
- Compare the labels on the medication with the order from the physician. Be sure these are the same, being careful of sound-alike and spell-alike medications. Do not allow yourself to be distracted when examining the labels; keep your full attention on the task at hand.
- If you are working with unit dose medications, be sure that you are preparing the medication for dispensing in the unit dose, not the multidose amount.
- Know your medications and the approximate dose that is usually given to a patient of the age, gender, and size of the person for whom the prescription or medication order is made. If in doubt of the usual dose, read the drug insert or other reference materials related to the medications before preparing the medicine so that you are aware of the usual dose for the specific medication.
- Finally, remember that the pharmacist would rather have you ask a question than have the incorrect medication dispensed for the patient.

REVIEW

When calculating solid oral medication doses, the amount of medication should be calculated to that of the physician's order. Remember that the DA and the DO must be in the same system before calculating doses. When the medication label contains an amount of medication within one measurement system and the order does not agree with the measurement within the system for the available amount, you calculate the amount of medication necessary for the order by making conversions within the system. However, if the medication order and the available medications are in different measurement systems, you must use conversions as found in Chapter 5 to be sure the medications are converted to the same system. (See Chapter 4 for the measurement in the metric, household, and apothecary systems.) If a conversion must be made, it should be made to the measurement system found on the medication label.

Medication doses can be calculated using ratio and proportion (using the equation below):

DA (Dosage available) : DF (Dosage form) :: DO (Dose ordered) : DG (Dose to be given)

OR

Medication doses can also be calculated using dimensional analysis in which the available medication should begin the ratios found in the proportional equation with the necessary conversions following your initial entry.

OR

The formula method, using the formula shown below may be used:

$$\frac{DD\ (Dose\ desired)}{DH\ (Dose\ on\ hand)} \times Qty\ (Quantity\ or\ form) = Dose\ to\ be\ given$$

As a pharmacy technician, you should find the method that is most comfortable for you and use it for all calculations.

A physician may give an order that requires the calculation of the total amount of medication necessary for dispensing a medication. To make this calculation, find the number of doses necessary in a day and then multiply this total amount by the total number of days that the prescription is to be taken.

Posttest

Before taking the Posttest, retake the Pretest to check your understanding of the materials presented in this chapter.

For the following problems, pick the correct label from the set below and put the label letter in the space indicated. Then, using the label, interpret the order and calculate the ordered medications. On the fourth line, indicate how the order would look on the prescription label. Figure the dose to be given in the dose form (i.e., tabs or caps) and indicate the form in the answer. Months are 30 days unless otherwise stated. Show all calculations.

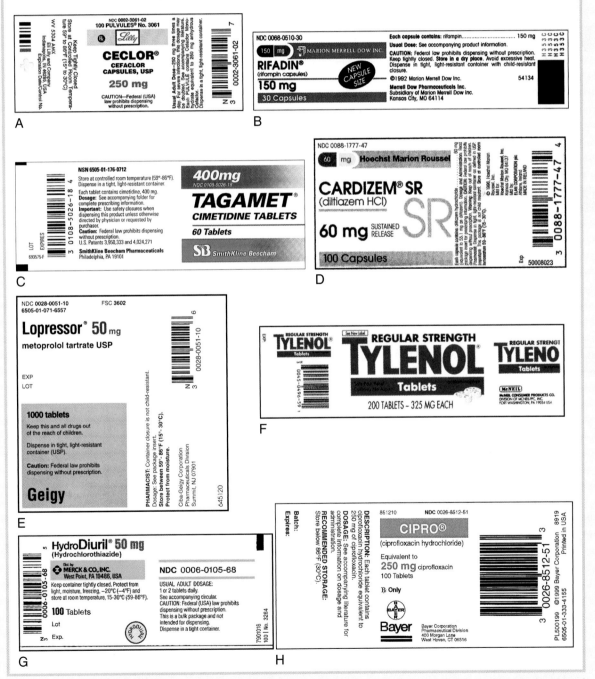

A

B

C

D

E

F

G

H

Continued

Posttest, cont.

1. Order: Tagamet 0.8 g bid

Correct label: _____

Interpret the order. _____

Dose to be given: _____

Prescription label: _____

2. Order: HydroDIURIL 100 mg qam pc am meal

Correct label: _____

Interpret the order. _____

Dose to be given: _____

Prescription label: _____

3. Order: Tylenol gr x q4-6h prn fever

Correct label: _____

Interpret the order. _____

Dose to be given: _____

Prescription label: _____

4. Order: ciprofloxacin HCl 0.5 g tid c̄ meals

Correct label: _____

Interpret the order. _____

Dose to be given: _____

Prescription label: _____

5. Order: cefaclor 0.75 g daily in 3 divided doses

Correct label: _____

Interpret the order. _____

Dose to be given: _____

Prescription label: _____

Posttest, cont.

6. Order: diltiazem-SR 120 mg po stat then 60 mg po daily

   Correct label: _____

   Interpret the order. _____

   Total number of tablets needed for a 30-day supply: _____

   Dose to be given stat: _____

   Dose to be given daily: _____

   Prescription label: _____

7. Order: rifampin 300 mg po daily in 2 divided doses

   Correct label: _____

   Interpret the order. _____

   .

   Dose to be given: _____

   Dosage for a month's supply in September: _____

   Prescription label: _____

8. Order: Lopressor 100 mg po bid today and then 50 mg po bid × 15 days then 50 mg po qam for the remainder of December. (Today is December 1.)

   Correct label: _____

   Interpret the order. _____

   Total dosage to be given today: _____

   How many capsules are in each dose today? _____

   Total daily dosage to be given starting tomorrow: _____

   Number of capsules for each dose starting tomorrow: _____

   Total capsules that should be dispensed to fill the order: _____

   Prescription label: _____

Continued

Posttest, cont.

Using the following labels, interpret the order and calculate the ordered medications. Figure the dose to be given in the dose form (i.e., tabs or caps) and indicate the form in the answer. Months are 30 days unless otherwise stated. Show your calculations.

9. Order: tetracycline 500 mg qid × 5 d; then 500 mg bid × 5 d; then 500 mg daily × 5 d for acne

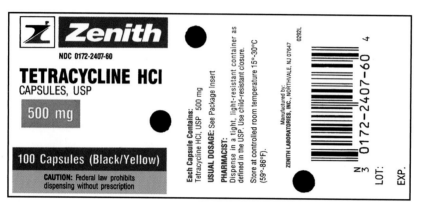

Interpret the order. _____

Dose to be given with each administration: _____

Total number of capsules that will be given in the first 5 days: _____

Total number of capsules in days 6-10: _____

Total number of capsules necessary to fill the prescription: _____

What is the total dosage per day in the first 5 days? _____

What is the total dosage per day for days 6-10? _____

What is the total dosage per day for the last 5 days? _____

Prescription label: _____

10. Order: codeine phosphate gr $\overline{ss}$ po stat and q4-6h prn pain

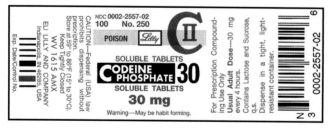

Interpret the order. _____

Dose to be given: _____

Prescription label: _____

Posttest, cont.

11. Order: nitroglycerin gr 1/150 subl q5min × 3 doses as a maximum dose for chest pain or until ↓ pain

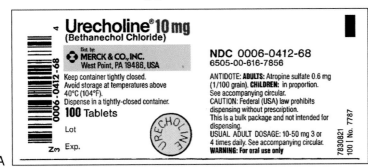

N 0071-0570-24

Nitrostat®
(Nitroglycerin
Tablets, USP)
0.4 mg (1/150 gr)
℞ only
100 SUBLINGUAL TABLETS

Ⓟ **PARKE-DAVIS**

Warning—To prevent loss of potency, keep these tablets in the original container. Close tightly immediately after each use.

Usual Dosage—0.3 to 0.6 mg sublingually as needed.
See package insert for full prescribing information.
Keep this and all drugs out of the reach of children.
Dispense in original, unopened container.
Store up to 25°C (77°F).
Protect from moisture.

6505-00-687-3663

0570G038

PARKE-DAVIS
Div of Warner-Lambert Co   © 1997-'98
Morris Plains, NJ 07950 USA

Interpret the order. _____

Dose to be given: _____

Prescription label: _____

12. Order: Urecholine 20 mg po bid c̄ meals × 10 d

A

Urecholine® 10 mg
(Bethanechol Chloride)

Dist. by:
MERCK & CO., INC.
West Point, PA 19486, USA

Keep container tightly closed.
Avoid storage at temperatures above
40°C (104°F).
Dispense in a tightly-closed container.

100 Tablets

Lot

Exp.

0006-0412-68

NDC 0006-0412-68
6505-00-616-7856

ANTIDOTE: **ADULTS:** Atropine sulfate 0.6 mg
(1/100 grain). **CHILDREN:** in proportion.
See accompanying circular.
CAUTION: Federal (USA) law prohibits
dispensing without prescription.
This is a bulk package and not intended for
dispensing.
USUAL ADULT DOSAGE: 10-50 mg 3 or
4 times daily. See accompanying circular.
WARNING: For oral use only

7830821
100 | No. 7787

B

Urecholine® 25 mg
(Bethanechol Chloride)

Dist. by:
MERCK & CO., INC.
West Point, PA 19486, USA

Keep container tightly closed.
Avoid storage at temperatures above
40°C (104°F).
Dispense in a tightly-closed container.

100 Tablets

Lot

Exp.

0006-0457-68

NDC 0006-0457-68
6505-00-912-7440

ANTIDOTE: **ADULTS:** Atropine sulfate 0.6 mg
(1/100 grain). **CHILDREN:** in proportion.
See accompanying circular.
CAUTION: Federal (USA) law prohibits
dispensing without prescription.
This is a bulk package and not intended for
dispensing.
USUAL ADULT DOSAGE: 10-50 mg 3 or
4 times daily. See accompanying circular.
WARNING: For oral use only

7830514
100 | No. 7788

Interpret the order. _____

Choose the correct container of medication. _____

Dose to be given: _____

Dosage to be dispensed for the order: _____

Prescription label: _____

Continued

Posttest, cont.

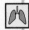

13. Order: Benadryl 50 mg po tid prn itching

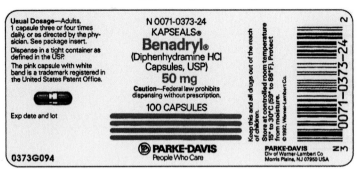

Interpret the order. _____

Dose to be given: _____

Prescription label: _____

14. Order: Cipro 0.75 g po bid × 10 days

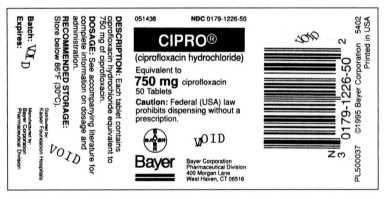

Interpret the order. _____

Dose to be given: _____

Dosage to be dispensed to fill the prescription: _____

Prescription label: _____

Posttest, cont.

15. Order: ampicillin 1 gm po stat, then 500 mg po qid × 12 d

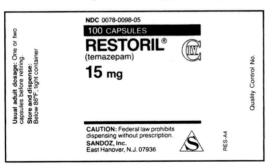

Manufactured for
WARNER CHILCOTT LABORATORIES
Div of Warner-Lambert Co ©1991
Morris Plains, NJ 07950 USA.
By: Clonmel Chemicals Co. Ltd.
Clonmel, Republic of Ireland

0404G161
6505-00-931-0702

Lot

Expiration date

N 0047-0404-24

**Ampicillin
Capsules, USP**

500mg

Caution — Federal law prohibits
dispensing without prescription.

100 Capsules

WC WARNER
CHILCOTT

Each capsule contains
ampicillin trihydrate
equivalent to 500 mg
ampicillin.
Usual Adult Dosage —
250 or 500 mg every
6 hours. See package
insert.
**PHARMACY STOCK
PACKAGE**
Dispense in a tight, light
resistant container as
defined in the USP.
**Store below 30°C (86°F).
Protect from moisture.**
0404J030

Interpret the order. _____

Dose to be given stat: _____

Dose to be given qid: _____

Dosage necessary to correctly dispense the medication: _____

Prescription label: _____

16. Order: temazepam 0.015 g po hs* prn sleep

NDC 0078-0098-05
100 CAPSULES
RESTORIL® Ⓒ IV
(temazepam)
15 mg

Usual adult dosage: One or two
capsules before retiring.
Store and dispense:
Below 86°F; tight container

Quality Control No.

CAUTION: Federal law prohibits
dispensing without prescription.
SANDOZ, Inc.
East Hanover, N.J. 07936

RES A4

Ⓢ

Interpret the order. _____

Dose to be given prn: _____

Prescription label: _____

*These abbreviations are found on the TJC Do Not Use List and ISMP's List of Error-Prone Abbreviations, Symbols, and Dose Designations due to medication safety issues. They should not be used. You are being tested on them here because these abbreviations may still appear in the pharmacy setting.

Continued

Posttest, cont.

17. Order: Strattera 0.05 g po daily c̄ breakfast

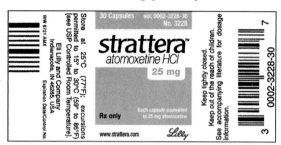

Interpret the order. _____

Dose to be given: _____

How many capsules should be included in the entire prescription for a month?

_____

Prescription label: _____

Dosage of medication to be supplied for a 45-day supply: _____

18. Order: Surfak i or ii cap po qhs* prn

An aid in the treatment of temporary constipation.
Keep this and all medication out of the reach of children.
Warning: As with any drug, if you are pregnant or nursing a baby, seek the advice of a health professional before using this product.
Caution: If cramping pain occurs, discontinue the medication.
Manufactured by R.P. Scherer
Clearwater, Florida 33518
Expressly for:
HOECHST-ROUSSEL Pharmaceuticals Inc.
Somerville, New Jersey 08876
REG. TM HOECHST AG
60210-2/85

NDC 0039-0002-10
Surfak®
docusate calcium USP
STOOL SOFTENER
Seal Under Cap
Printed Hoechst-Roussel
100 CAPSULES
50 MG EACH

Each capsule contains 50 mg docusate calcium USP and the following inactive ingredients: alcohol USP up to 1.3% (w/w), corn oil NF, FD&C Red #3, FD&C Red #40, gelatin NF, glycerin USP, parabens NF, sorbitol NF, soybean oil USP and other ingredients.
Usual Dosage: Adults—two or three capsules daily; children 6 to 12 and adults with minimal needs — one to three capsules daily. Continue for several days or until bowel movements are normal. For children under 6 consult a physician. Preserve in a tight container. Store at controlled room temperature (59°-86°F) in a dry place.

Interpret the order. _____

Dose to be given: _____

Total number of mg taken when ii cap are taken hs: _____

Prescription label: _____

*These abbreviations are found on the TJC Do Not Use List and ISMP's List of Error-Prone Abbreviations, Symbols, and Dose Designations due to medication safety issues. They should not be used. You are being tested on them here because these abbreviations may still appear in the pharmacy setting.

Posttest, cont.

19. Order: Synthroid 0.1 mg qam

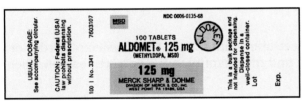

Interpret the order. _____

Dose to be given: _____

Prescription label: _____

20. Order: Aldomet 0.25 g po qam and 0.125 g po @ 5 pm

Interpret the order. _____

Dose to be given in tablets in am: _____

Dose to be given in tablets @ 5 pm: _____

Total dosage to be dispensed for 30 days: _____

Prescription label: _____

REVIEW OF RULES

Calculating Solid Oral Medications

- Calculations for oral solid medications may be accomplished by using ratio and proportion, dimensional analysis, or formula methods.

- Before beginning calculations, unless using dimensional analysis, the medications must be in the same unit of measure within the same measurement system. If the measurement systems are different, convert to the measurement system that is on the available medication label.

- Solid medications usually have a quantity of a single solid form such as per tablet or package of powder. Remember that scored tablets may be broken at scores or on indented marks.

- To solve using the ratio and proportion method, set the known measurements on one side of the equation with the unknowns on the other side of the equation. Remember to label the units in each ratio so that the units are in the same position in each ratio and the proportion is therefore equal.

- Dimensional analysis is an extended means of ratio and proportion placed in fractional units. See the rules at the end of Chapter 5 for a review of this means of solving dosage.

- The formula method requires the use of the following formula:

$$\frac{DD\ (Dose\ desired)}{DH\ (Dose\ on\ hand)} \times Qty\ (Quantity\ or\ DF) = Dose\ to\ be\ given\ (DG)$$

- To use this formula, place the correct information from the physician's order or prescription, the available medication, and the quantity in the correct position. Then calculate the problem.

CHAPTER 8

Calculate Doses of Oral and Parenteral Liquid Medications

OBJECTIVES

- Interpret orders and calculate the volume of oral and parenteral liquid medications necessary to administer ordered doses using either ratio and proportion, formula, or dimensional analysis method
- Accomplish conversion of equivalent measurements among metric, household, and apothecary systems as needed for oral or parenteral liquid medication doses
- Measure parenteral medications in ordered amounts in the appropriate syringe
- Calculate total doses of parenteral medications when two or more medications are ordered to be given together

KEY WORDS

Act-O-Vial System Two-section vial divided by a seal holding a premeasured active ingredient in the lower section and a premeasured diluent in the upper section; mixing occurs when the two sections of the vial are combined either through puncturing the seal or moving the seal through pressure similar to Mix-O-Vial

Ampule Small glass container that is sealed and holds a single dose of medication, usually for injection

Depot Long-acting oil based medications that are gradually released for prolonged drug administration

Elixir Clear, sweetened, flavored medication containing alcohol and water

Intradermal Into or within the dermis of the skin

Intramuscular Into or within the muscle

Intravenous Into or within a vein

Meniscus Curved line that develops on the upper surface of a liquid when poured into a container

Parenteral Medications administered outside the gastrointestinal tract or those applied to the skin such as topically; most are usually considered to be those given by injection or infusion; medications given through the skin by injection

Subcutaneous Beneath the skin; medications injected into the subcutaneous tissue

Suspension Medication consisting of small particles that are not dissolved but are dispersed throughout the liquid

Syrup Aqueous solution sweetened with sugar or a sugar substitute to disguise taste

Tincture Alcohol-based liquid; commonly used as a skin preparation

Vial Glass or plastic container with metal-enclosed rubber seal for injectable medications; may hold single or multiple doses

Pretest

Interpret each medical order that follows. Show all of your mathematical calculations. Round answers to nearest tenth.

1. A physician orders Ceclor 250 mg po tid for a child with otitis media.

   Interpret the order. _____

   If the drug available is Ceclor 125 mg/5 mL, how many teaspoons of medication should be given to the child for each dose? _____

2. A physician orders Atarax Syrup 15 mg po qid.

   Interpret the order. _____

   How many milliliters should be administered if the drug available is Atarax Syrup 10 mg/5 mL? _____

3. A physician orders Tylenol gr v q4h prn fever and aches for a child who has a high fever. The drug available is Tylenol elixir 160 mg/tsp.

   Interpret the order. _____

   How many milliliters of Tylenol should the parent give the child? _____

4. A physician orders Amoxil 62.5 mg po tid for an infant. The drug available is 125 mg/5 mL.

   Interpret the order. _____

   What is the volume of medication for the child in the metric system?

   _____

5. Using the medication order in question No. 4, what amount of medication should be administered in the household measurement? _____

Pretest, cont.

6. A physician orders Zofran 2 mg IM to be given 30 minutes before the treatment for a chemotherapy patient. The drug dosage available is Zofran 2 mg/mL.

Interpret the order. _____

How many milliliters would be administered to the patient? _____

7. A physician orders Ticar 500 mg IM bid. The reconstituted strength of the medication is 1 gm/2.6 mL.

Interpret the order. _____

What is the correct volume of medication to be administered to the patient in a dose? _____

8. The physician orders vitamin B_{12} 1000 mcg IM qwk. The available drug dosage is 1 mg/mL.

Interpret the order. _____

How many milliliters should be given as a weekly dose? _____

9. A physician orders meperidine 75 mg IM stat for a patient who has had cardiac surgery. The drug dosage available is meperidine 50 mg/mL.

Interpret the order. _____

How many milliliters should be administered stat to this patient?

_____

10. A physician orders 50 mg of meperidine and 25 mg of promethazine IM q4-6h prn for a postsurgical patient with pain and nausea. The drug dosage available is meperidine 75 mg/mL and promethazine 25 mg/mL.

Interpret the order. _____

How many mL will be given of the promethazine and how many mL of meperidine?

_____

What is the total amount of medication in mL if this is prepared in one syringe?

_____

Continued

Pretest, cont.

 11. Ordered medication: amoxicillin 375 mg po tid

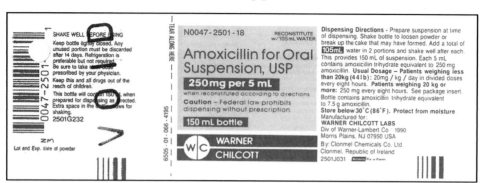

Volume to be administered in household measurements for a dose:

_____

What is the metric volume for each dose? _____

Interpret the order. _____

 12. Ordered medication: streptomycin 750 mg IM

Volume of medication to be administered: _____

Interpret the order. _____

Pretest, cont.

13. Ordered medication: codeine phosphate gr i subcutaneous q4h prn

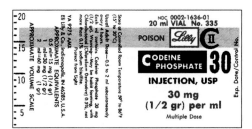

Volume of medication to be administered: _____

Interpret the order. _____

14. Ordered medication: Mycostatin 500,000 units po tid

MYCOSTATIN
ORAL SUSPENSION
Nystatin Oral
Suspension USP

473 mL   NDC 0003-0588-10

Each mL contains
100,000 USP Nystatin
Units in a vehicle
containing 50% sucrose.
Not more than 1% alcohol
by volume.

USUAL DOSAGE FOR
INFANTS: 2 mL (200,000
units) four times daily (1 mL
in each side of mouth).

USUAL DOSAGE FOR
CHILDREN AND ADULTS:
See package insert.

**Store at room
temperature; avoid
freezing**

APOTHECON®
A Bristol-Myers
Squibb Company
Princeton, NJ 08540 USA

P8739-00

100,000 units per mL
MYCOSTATIN®
ORAL SUSPENSION

Nystatin Oral
Suspension USP

SHAKE WELL
BEFORE USING

Caution: Federal law prohibits
dispensing without prescription

APOTHECON ®
A BRISTOL-MYERS SQUIBB COMPANY

Volume of medication to be administered: _____

What volume will be given in household measurements? _____

Interpret the order. _____

Continued

Pretest, cont.

15. Ordered medication: erythromycin 0.3 gm po tid

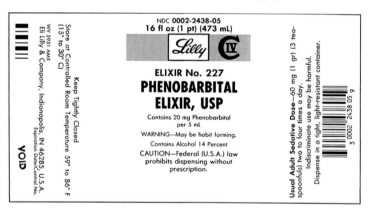

TO PATIENT:
Shake well before using.
Keep tightly closed. Store in refrigerator and discard unused portion after ten days. Oversize bottle provides shake space.
TO THE PHARMACIST:
When prepared as directed, each 5 mL teaspoonful contains erythromycin ethylsuccinate equivalent to 200 mg of erythromycin in a cherry-flavored suspension.
Bottle contains erythromycin ethylsuccinate equivalent to 8 g of erythromycin.
Usual Dose: See package outsert.
Store at room temperature in dry form.
Child-Resistant closure not required; Reference: Federal Register Vol.39 No.29.
DIRECTIONS FOR PREPARATION: Slowly add 140 mL of water and shake vigorously to make 200 mL of suspension.
BARR LABORATORIES, INC.
Pomona, NY 10970
R11-90

BARR LABORATORIES, INC.

NDC 0555-0215-23
NSN 6505-00-080-0653

Erythromycin Ethylsuccinate
for Oral Suspension, USP

200 mg of erythromycin activity per 5 mL reconstituted

Caution: Federal law prohibits dispensing without prescription.

200 mL (when mixed)

0555-0215-23   SAMPLE

Exp. Date: _____ Lot No.: _____

Volume of medication to be administered as a dose: _____

Interpret the order. _____

16. Ordered medication: phenobarbital 30 mg po hs*

Store at Controlled Room Temperature (15° to 30° C)
WV 5931 AMX
Eli Lilly & Company, Indianapolis, IN 46285, U.S.A.
Expiration Date/Control No.
Keep Tightly Closed
Store at Controlled Room Temperature 59° to 86° F
VOID

NDC 0002-2438-05
16 fl oz (1 pt) (473 mL)

Lilly **C IV**

ELIXIR No. 227
PHENOBARBITAL ELIXIR, USP

Contains 20 mg Phenobarbital per 5 mL

WARNING—May be habit forming.
Contains Alcohol 14 Percent
CAUTION—Federal (U.S.A.) law prohibits dispensing without prescription.

Usual Adult Sedative Dose—60 mg (1 gr) (3 tea-spoonfuls) two to four times a day. Indiscriminate use may be harmful. Dispense in a tight, light-resistant container.

3 0002 2438 05 9

Volume of medication to be administered in household measurements:

_____

Interpret the order. _____

*These abbreviations are found on the TJC Do Not Use List and ISMP's List of Error-Prone Abbreviations, Symbols, and Dose Designations due to medication safety issues. They should not be used. You are being tested on them here because these abbreviations may still appear in the pharmacy setting.

Pretest, cont.

17. Ordered medication: Prozac 10 mg po qam

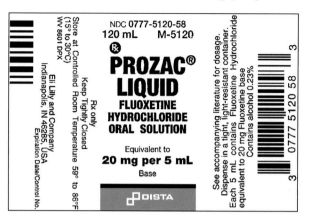

What utensil would you tell the patient to use for household administration when person calls and states that the dose spoon is lost? _____

Volume of medication to be administered in metric system: _____

Volume of medication to be administered in household system: _____

Interpret the order. _____

18. Ordered medication: Benadryl 25 mg po prn

N 0071-2220-17	Elixir P-D 2220 for prescription dispensing only.
ELIXIR	**Contains**—12.5 mg diphenhydramine hydrochloride in each 5 mL. Alcohol, 14%.
Benadryl®	**Dose**—Adults, 2 to 4 teaspoonfuls; children over 20 lb, 1 to 2 teaspoonfuls; three or four times daily.
(Diphenhydramine Hydrochloride Elixir, USP)	See package insert.
	Keep this and all drugs out of the reach of children.
Caution—Federal law prohibits dispensing without prescription.	**Store below 30°C (86°F). Protect from freezing and light.**
4 FLUIDOUNCES	Exp date and lot
PARKE-DAVIS Div of Warner-Lambert Co Morris Plains, NJ 07950 USA	2220G102

Volume of medication to be administered in household measurements:

_____

What metric volume will be given? _____

Interpret the order. _____

Continued

Pretest, cont.

19. Ordered medication: morphine sulfate gr 1/10 IV q4h

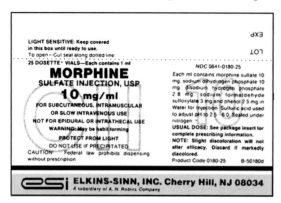

Volume of medication to be administered: _____

Interpret the order. _____

20. Ordered medication: Colace syrup 80 mg po at bedtime

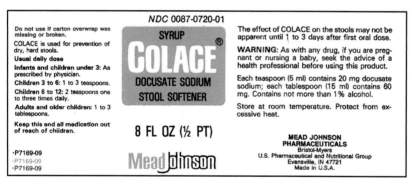

Volume of medication to be administered with each dose in metric system:

_____

Interpret the order. _____

INTRODUCTION

For some patients, solid medications such as tablets and capsules are difficult to swallow, and the physician will order oral liquid preparations. These preparations are usually stated in weight or strength/volume such as milligrams/milliliter. Because liquid medications may be dispensed in either drams from the apothecary system or teaspoons in the household measurement system, conversions among all three measurement systems are often required for dispensing or administering the prescription as written. As with solid medications, these conversions may be accomplished by either ratio and proportion or dimensional analysis. If ratio and proportion is used, then the formula method may be used for preparation of the medication for dispensing. If dimensional analysis is used, the conversion among systems may be accomplished by use of additional ratios for conversion in the equation. Thus the entire conversion and calculation may be completed with one elongated proportional step. (Examples are shown later in this chapter.) Some medications for oral administration are prepared in a powder form for reconstitution to a liquid form before dispensing—the subject of Chapter 9.

! TECH ALERT

When it is necessary to compute medication doses and equivalencies, the equivalent should be no more than 10% above or below the amount of the prescribed dose. Some doses will require rounding to a measureable quantity; however, the dose, once rounded, should be within the 10% margin. Be aware that some medications require that rounding be within a much lower percentage of variation. This is due to the narrow range between effectiveness and toxicity. If you have questions regarding acceptable rounding techniques, ask your pharmacist for assistance.

Injectable medications may be given when a person is unable to swallow solid medications or when a quicker effect is necessary. **Parenteral** medications are given by injection into body tissue and may also be given intravenously or directly into the bloodstream. Because solid medications cannot be injected under the skin except as special **intradermal** forms such as pellets, most injectable medications must be in liquid form. As with oral liquid medications, some parenteral medications come in powders for injection, requiring reconstitution before administration. These medications usually will not be stable in liquid form for an extended period, so they must be handled for stability at the time of administration (reconstitution of parenteral medications is discussed in Chapter 9).

CALCULATION OF ORAL LIQUID MEDICATIONS

Oral medications are available in solid form as discussed in the previous chapter and in liquid form as discussed in this chapter. When oral medications are given in a liquid form, the absorption is usually faster because solids have to dissolve before absorption. The absorption of a medicine is controlled, in part, by the dosage form administered. Most oral medications are absorbed in the small intestine, although some are absorbed beginning in the mouth or stomach. These medications may be administered with oral syringes that are available in 1-mL, 5-mL, and 10-mL sizes (Figure 8-1), a medication cup (Figure 8-2), a dropper that is available in different measurements and is usually tailored by the

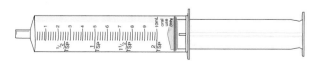

FIGURE 8-1 Typical oral syringe.

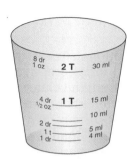

FIGURE 8-2 Typical medication cup.

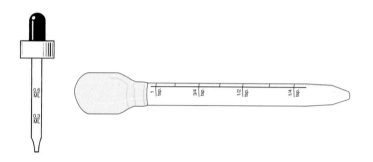

FIGURE 8-3 Typical medicine droppers.

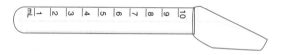

FIGURE 8-4 Typical measuring spoon found with oral liquid pediatric medications.

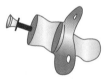

FIGURE 8-5 Pacifier used to administer oral liquid medication to infant.

manufacturer for a specific drug (Figure 8-3), dosage spoons (Figure 8-4), or by using household devices such as teaspoons and tablespoons. The newest form of administration of oral liquid medications is through a nipple or with a pacifier that will hold a measured amount of medication (Figure 8-5). The choice of administration implement for oral liquid medications depends on the volume of medication to be administered and the availability of supplies. Medication cups are found in institutional settings, whereas droppers and oral syringes may be used either in institutions or at home. Teaspoons and tablespoons are the measurements occasionally used for larger doses in the home setting or when the calibrated utensils are not available. The use of kitchen utensils is usually discouraged, because oral syringes and calibrated cups are more accurate.

TECH NOTE

When a medication dropper is provided by the manufacturer, that dropper should be used for administration of the medication.

Liquid medications may be found in **tinctures, elixirs, suspensions**, and **syrups**, some of which may be irritating to the gastric system and must be diluted before administration. Some medications such as cough syrups should not be diluted even after the administration; therefore the information about the medication and its use and proper administration is necessary before administering a dose or providing patient education.

Liquid drug preparations are labeled with the strength of the drug (such as milligrams) in the total volume (such as milliliters) of the liquid. Remember that liquid medications may be expressed in metric (milliliters, cubic centimeters, and liters), apothecary (drams and minims), and household (teaspoons, tablespoons, pints, and the like) measurement systems. Doses of medication are also calculated based on strength/volume. This fact is then used to prepare liquid medications for administration. For example, a physician may order amoxicillin 500 mg to be given to a child who requires a liquid dosage form. The medication on hand is amoxicillin 250 mg (weight or strength) per 5 mL (volume). In this case the known amounts will be placed into the formula, ratio and proportion, or dimensional analysis equations for preparing the correct amount of medication. If you need to review the formulas for any of these ways of ascertaining the correct dose to be given or if you need to review the safety measures necessary for medication preparation and administration, return to Chapter 7.

TECH NOTE

Volume is usually the unknown that needs to be found when calculating oral liquid medications.

As with the previous chapter, you will calculate doses for competency. You must remember that *dose* is the amount of medication to be administered at a specific given time, whereas *dosage* (to be discussed in Chapter 14) is the total amount of medication that will be administered over a particular length of time. Again, as a reminder, the label on the medication must be in the same system of measurement as that found on the prescription or medication order. If these do not agree, conversion should be accomplished to the system found on the label. Also, be sure the medication names are exactly the same, because many drug names look and sound alike.

Calculating Oral Liquid Medications Using Ratio and Proportion

As you learned in Chapter 7, when using the ratio and proportion method of drug calculation, the dose available (DA) and the dosage form (DF) must be one ratio, and the dose ordered (DO) and dose to be given (DG) must be the other ratio in the proportion. With liquids, DF and DG will be in volume, whereas DA and DO will be in strength or weight of drug.

TECH NOTE

When using this formula to calculate a dose of medication for an oral liquid order, the dose to be given will be in a liquid form such as milliliters (mL) or cubic centimeters (cc). Also remember that if the dose desired and the dose available or on hand are not in the same measurement system, a conversion to the system of the dose available should be made. (See Chapter 4 to review the measurement systems and Chapter 5 for help with conversions between systems.)

EXAMPLE 8-1

A physician orders amoxicillin 500 mg oral suspension. The medication available is amoxicillin 250 mg/5 mL. How much medication would be administered to the patient for a single dose?

Remember the formula for using ratio and proportion appears as follows:

DA : DF :: DO : DG

If you prefer using fractional units for the relationships between the ratios in the proportions, the formula to be used is as follows:

$$\frac{DA}{DF} = \frac{DO}{DG}$$

Now that you have reviewed the formula, you can calculate the problem given because all of the given measurements are in the metric system.

The DA is 250 mg in the DF of 5 mL. The DO is 500 mg. The proportion is set up as follows:

250 mg (DA) : 5 mL (DF) :: 500 mg (DO) : x (DG)

OR

$$\frac{250 \text{ mg (DA)}}{5 \text{ ml (DF)}} = \frac{500 \text{ mg (DO)}}{x \text{ (DG)}}$$

Either multiply the means versus the extremes or cross-multiply if using the fractional components.

$$250 \text{ mg} : 5 \text{ mL} :: 500 \text{ mg} : x \quad \text{or} \quad \frac{250 \text{ mg}}{5 \text{ mL}} \bowtie \frac{500 \text{ mg}}{x}$$

As previously learned, drop the mg because it appears in both sides of the equation, so the equation now appears as follows:

$250x = 500 \times 5 \text{ mL}$

$x = 500 \times 5 \text{ mL} \div 250 \quad \text{or} \quad 2500 \text{ mL} \div 250$

$x = 10 \text{ mL}$ or 10 mL is the prescribed amount of amoxicillin to be administered to the patient

Try another medication order as an example. Because most oral liquid medications must be calculated to the metric system, the examples are in the metric system.

EXAMPLE 8-2

A physician orders Ceftin oral suspension 187 mg. The medication on hand is Ceftin 125 mg/5 mL. Because this prescription will be given at home, the medication order for the label should read the amount to be given in household measurements. Again, review Chapters 4 and 5 as needed.

125 mg (DA) : 5 mL (DF) :: 187 mg (DO) : x (DG)

OR

$$\frac{125 \text{ mg (DA)}}{5 \text{ ml (DF)}} \bowtie \frac{187 \text{ mg (DO)}}{x \text{ (DG)}}$$

Again, either multiply means and extremes or cross-multiply the fractional equivalents as previously accomplished. The resultant formula follows:

$$125 \times x = 187 \times 5 \text{ mL} \quad \text{or} \quad 125x = 935 \text{ mL}$$

$$x = 7.48 \text{ or } 7.5 \text{ mL after rounding}$$

TECH NOTE

Round all doses to a measurable quantity for the utensil being used.

Now change this to the household measurement as requested by the physician.

$$5 \text{ mL} : 1 \text{ tsp} :: 7.5 \text{ mL} : x$$

$$5x = 7.5$$

Remember that the "mL" designation may be removed because it appears in both equivalents following cross-multiplication.

$$x \text{ tsp} = 7.5 \div 5 \quad \text{or} \quad 1\frac{1}{2}$$

Therefore the dose to be given in household measures is $1\frac{1}{2}$ tsp. Remember that household measurements are in fractional units rather than decimal units.

Calculating Oral Liquid Medications Using Dimensional Analysis

Remember that dimensional analysis is really just an elongated form of ratio and proportion using fractional components. To review dimensional analysis as a means of calculating doses, please review Chapter 5. The problem in Example 8-1 would appear as follows for calculation with dimensional analysis:

EXAMPLE 8-3

A physician orders amoxicillin 500 mg oral suspension. The dosage available is amoxicillin 250 mg/5 mL. How much medication would be administered to the patient for a single dose?

$$x \text{ mL} = \frac{5 \text{ mL}}{250 \text{ mg}} \times \frac{500 \text{ mg}}{1}$$

$$x \text{ mL} = \frac{5 \text{ mL} \times 500}{250} \quad \text{or} \quad \frac{2500 \text{ mL}}{250}$$

$$x = 10 \text{ mL}$$

EXAMPLE 8-4

A physician orders Ceftin 187 mg oral suspension. The medication on hand is Ceftin 125 mg/5 mL. Because this prescription will be given at home, the medication order for the label should read the amount to be given in household measurements. With dimensional analysis the problem will have an unknown in teaspoons (x = teaspoons). To obtain the answer in teaspoons, one step of fractional components is added to the calculation, thus eliminating the need for two separate calculations as was necessary with the ratio and proportion or formula methods.

$$x \text{ tsp} = \frac{187 \text{ mg}}{1 \text{ dose}} \times \frac{5 \text{ mL}}{125 \text{ mg}} \times \frac{1 \text{ tsp}}{5 \text{ mL}}$$

$$x \text{ tsp} = \frac{187 \text{ mg}}{1 \text{ dose}} \times \frac{5 \text{ mL}}{125 \text{ mg}} \times \frac{1 \text{ tsp}}{5 \text{ mL}}$$

$$x \text{ tsp} = \frac{187 \times 1}{125 \times 1}$$

$x = 1.49$ tsp or 1.5 tsp after rounding to a measurable quantity

The dose to be given is 1½ tsp.

Calculating Oral Liquid Medications Using the Formula Method

Remember that the formula method is another means for calculating doses of medications. As with ratio and proportion methods of dosage calculations, the units in the formula are replaced with the desired and known factors. As a review, the formula is as follows:

$$\frac{\text{DD (Dose desired)}}{\text{DH (Dose on hand)}} \times \text{Qty (Quantity/Volume or DF)} = \text{DG}$$

Although quantity for oral solid measurements is in capsules or tablets, the quantity in oral liquid medications will be in liquid form, usually in milliliters (mL) in the metric system or teaspoons (tsp) or tablespoons (tbsp) in the household system. The use of dram (℥) in the apothecary system may be used to write prescriptions, but this would not be used when providing the instructions on a medication label for home use. Now take the same problems seen before and calculate using the formula method.

TECH NOTE

Remember that a dram (℥) is approximately equal to a teaspoon or approximately 5 mL. When converting among systems, use the conversion factor that gives the closest accurate dose. (For further review of conversions among measurement systems, refer to Chapters 4 and 5.)

EXAMPLE 8-5

A physician orders amoxicillin 500 mg oral suspension. The dosage available is amoxicillin 250 mg/5 mL. How much medication would be administered to the patient for a single dose?

$$\frac{500 \text{ mg (DD)}}{250 \text{ mg (DH)}} \times 5 \text{ mL (Qty)} = \text{Dose to be given (DG)}$$

$$\frac{\overset{2}{\cancel{500}} \text{ mg} \times 5 \text{mL}}{\underset{1}{\cancel{250}} \text{ mg}} = (\text{DG}) \quad \text{OR} \quad \frac{10 \text{ mL}}{1} = (\text{DG})$$

DG = 10 mL as a single dose

Note that because "mg" is found in both the numerator and denominator, "mg" may be canceled. Also notice that the metric volume measurement has remained in place as the quantity in this formula.

EXAMPLE 8-6

A physician orders Ceftin 187 mg oral suspension. The medication on hand is Ceftin 125 mg/5 mL. Because this prescription will be given at home, the medication order on the label should read the amount to be given in household measurements.

$$\frac{187 \text{ mg (DD)}}{125 \text{ mg (DA)}} \times 5 \text{ mL (Qty)} = \text{Dose to be given (DG)}$$

$$\frac{187 \text{ mg} \times \overset{1}{\cancel{5}} \text{ mL}}{\underset{25}{\cancel{125}} \text{ mg}} = \text{(DG)} \quad \text{or} \quad \frac{187 \text{ mL}}{25} = \text{(DG)}$$

$$7.48 \text{ mL or } 7.5 \text{ mL} = \text{DG}$$

Now, by ratio and proportion, complete the desired medication calculation in household measurements.

$$5 \text{ mL} : 1 \text{ tsp} :: 7.5 \text{ mL} : x \text{ tsp}$$

$$5x \text{ tsp} = 7.5$$

Remember that the "mL" designation may be removed because it appears in both equivalents following cross-multiplication.

$$x \text{ tsp} = 7.5 \div 5 \quad \text{or} \quad 1\frac{1}{2}$$

Therefore the dose to be given in household measures is 1½ tsp.

> **TECH NOTE**
>
> Remember that an apothecary dram (ℨ) is approximately 4 to 5 mL and is considered a teaspoon in the household measurement system because it is not possible to measure 4 mL in a household teaspoon. Always use the conversion that is measurable in the utensil to be used for dose administration.

Using a Medication Cup and Oral Syringe to Measure Oral Liquid Medications

When measuring oral liquid medications using a medicine cup, read the line of the medication to the **meniscus** at eye level. The meniscus is the curved line that develops on the cup when a medication is poured into the container (Figure 8-6). For medications that must be more accurately measured, an oral syringe should be used. With the oral syringe, the accurate dose is measured from 0.1 mL dose increments in the 1-mL syringe. In the 5-mL and 10-mL oral syringes the increments are in 0.2 mL.

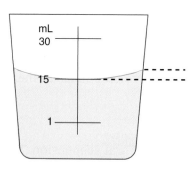

FIGURE 8-6 Reading the meniscus or curved line to 15 mL.

! **TECH ALERT**

Household measurement utensils are sources of potential errors and are not the ideal means of measuring doses. The abbreviations for teaspoon (tsp) and tablespoon (tbsp) can be easily confused, leading to errors in administration. Patient safety is better ensured if calibrated medication administration utensils are used. However, household utensils are used in some necessary instances and understanding these conversions is needed to assist people with proper dosing.

TECH NOTE

Remember that with oral liquid medication the quantity is given in either weight or strength per volume, not in single tablets or capsules as found with solid preparations. Therefore in most cases, the final volume of medication to be given will be in milliliters.

Practice Problems A

Calculate the following medication orders and answer the questions listed. If there is a dispensing device shown, draw the medication to the correct volume. Show your calculations.

Remember to use the method of calculation and conversion that is most comfortable for you. Choose one conversion system and continue to use it when doing drug calculations.

1. Ordered medication: dicloxacillin suspension 100 mg po bid

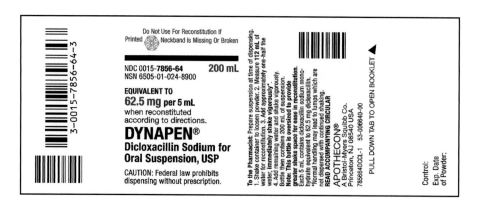

Interpret the order. _____

Volume of medication to be given in a dose: _____

2. Medication order: phenobarbital elixir 60 mg po qid

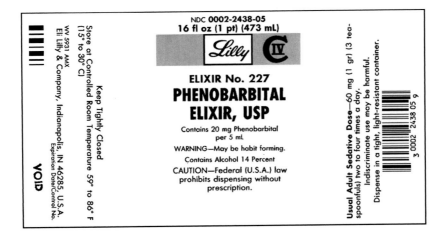

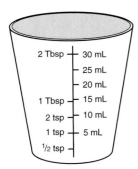

Interpret the order. _____

Volume of medication to be given in a dose: _____

3. 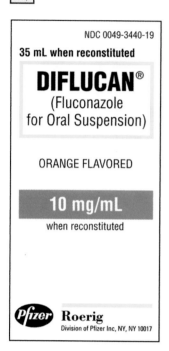   Prescribed: Diflucan suspension 35 mg po daily

NDC 0049-3440-19

35 mL when reconstituted

DIFLUCAN®
(Fluconazole
for Oral Suspension)

ORANGE FLAVORED

10 mg/mL

when reconstituted

Pfizer **Roerig**
Division of Pfizer Inc, NY, NY 10017

Interpret the order. _____

Volume of medication to be given in a dose: _____

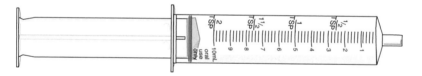

4.   Prescribed: cephalexin oral suspension 62.5 mg po tid $\bar{c}$ food

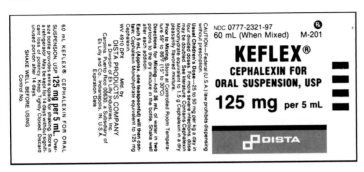

Interpret the order. _____

Volume of medication to be given in a dose: _____

How would this be administered using household measurements?

_____

5. 🫃   Prescribed: docusate sodium syrup 100 mg hs prn dry hard stools

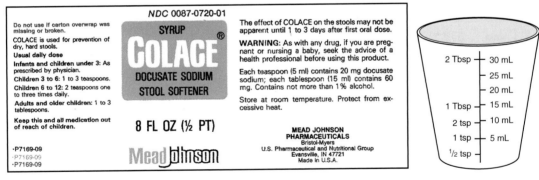

Interpret the order. _____

Volume of medication to be given with each dose in metric system:

_____

Volume of medication to be given with each dose in household measurements:

_____

6. 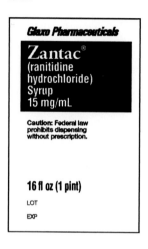 Prescribed: ranitidine syrup 150 mg bid q12h

Glaxo Pharmaceuticals

Zantac®
(ranitidine
hydrochloride)
Syrup
15 mg/mL

Caution: Federal law
prohibits dispensing
without prescription.

16 fl oz (1 pint)

LOT

EXP

2 Tbsp — 30 mL
— 25 mL
— 20 mL
1 Tbsp — 15 mL
2 tsp — 10 mL
1 tsp — 5 mL
1/2 tsp —

Interpret the order. _____

Volume of medication to be given with each dose: _____

7. 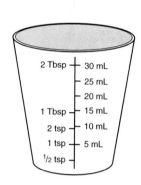 Prescribed: fluoxetine oral solution 10 mg po bid

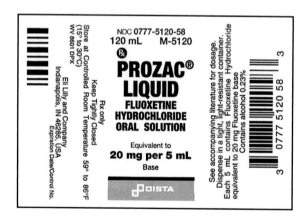

NDC 0777-5120-58
120 mL   M-5120

®
**PROZAC®
LIQUID**
FLUOXETINE
HYDROCHLORIDE
ORAL SOLUTION

Equivalent to
20 mg per 5 mL
Base

DISTA

Store at Controlled Room Temperature 59° to 86°F
(15° to 30°C)
WW 8601 DPX
Rx only
Keep Tightly Closed
Eli Lilly and Company
Indianapolis, IN 46285, USA
Expiration Date/Control No.

See accompanying literature for dosage.
Dispense in a tight, light-resistant container.
Each 5 mL contains Fluoxetine Hydrochloride
equivalent to 20 mg Fluoxetine base
Contains alcohol 0.23%

3 0777 5120 58 3

Interpret the order. _____

Volume of medication to be given in metric measurements with each dose:

_____

Volume of medication to be given in household measurements: _____

What type of medication administration unit should be given for administration of
this dose? _____

8. 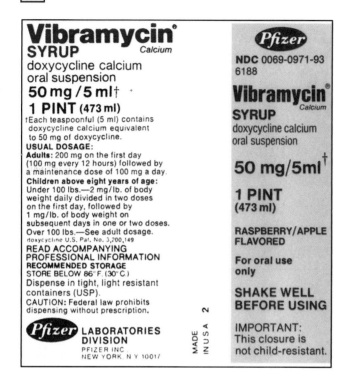 Prescribed: Vibramycin oral suspension 150 mg stat and then 75 mg q12h

Interpret the order. _____

Initial volume of medication to be given with each initial dose in metric system:

_____

Initial volume of medication to be given with each initial dose in household measurements: _____

Subsequent volume with each subsequent dose to be given in metric system:

_____

Subsequent volume with each subsequent dose to be given in household measurements: _____

9. 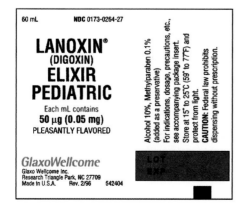 Prescribed: Lanoxin elixir 75 mcg bid if P ↑ 60

Interpret the order. _____

_____

Volume of medication to be given:

_____

Should this medication be administered with household utensils?

_____

10. Prescribed: Mellaril oral solution 45 mg bid q12h

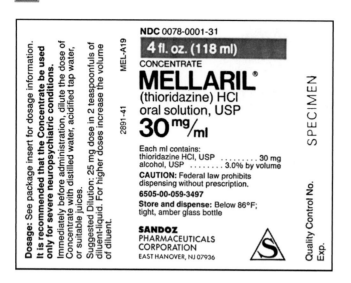

Interpret the order. _____

Volume of medication to be given as a dose: _____

11. Prescribed: amoxicillin oral suspension 375 mg tid q8h

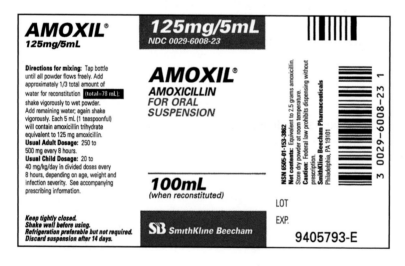 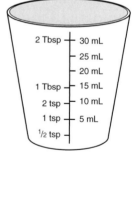

Interpret the order. _____

Volume of medication to be given as a dose: _____

12. 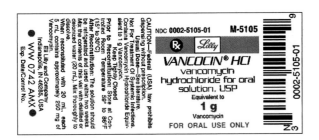   Prescribed: Vancocin HCl oral solution 250 mg bid for bacterial infection

Interpret the order. _____

Volume of medication to be given as a dose: _____

13. 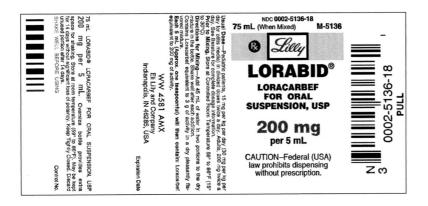   Prescribed: loracarbef oral suspension 160 mg bid for acute bronchitis

Interpret the order. _____

Volume of medication to be given as a dose: _____

14. Prescribed: cefaclor oral suspension 250 mg tid c̄ food

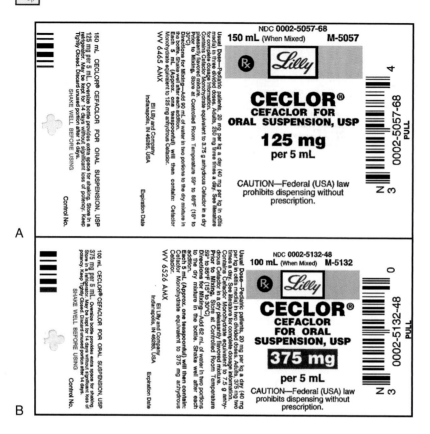

A

B

Interpret the order. _____

Of the labels provided, which container of cefaclor should be selected for ease of accurate administration for this prescription? _____

What is the volume of the medication from the selected medication bottle? _____

15. Prescribed: Duricef oral suspension 0.5 g q6h c̄ food

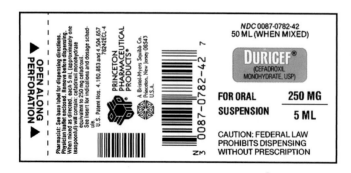

Interpret the order. _____

Volume of medication to be given as a dose: _____

16. Prescribed: amoxicillin/clavulanate potassium oral suspension 0.75 g daily in three divided doses

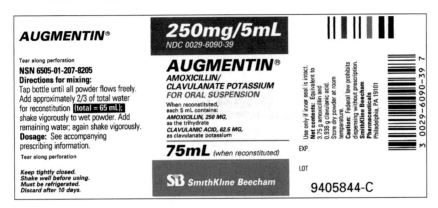

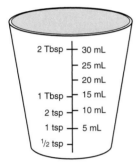

Interpret the order. _____

Volume of medication to be given as a dose: _____

17. Prescribed: cephalexin oral suspension 0.375 g tid

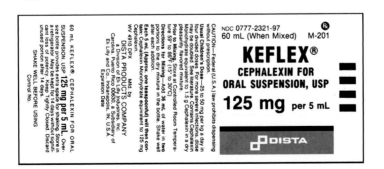

Interpret the order. _____

Volume of medication to be given as a dose: _____

18. PA IN   Prescribed: acetaminophen 60 mg q4h prn fever and aching

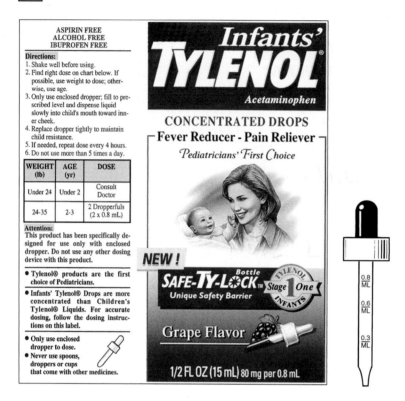

Interpret the order. _____

Volume of medication to be given as a dose: _____

What would the dose be if the physician ordered the medication using the label for a child weighing 33 lb? _____

19.   Prescribed: V-Cillin K oral suspension 100,000 Units qid c̄ food

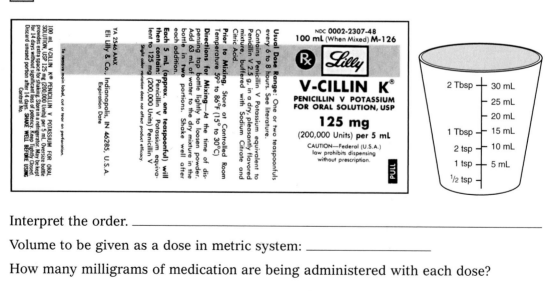

Interpret the order. _____

Volume to be given as a dose in metric system: _____

How many milligrams of medication are being administered with each dose?

_____

20. Prescribed: Lorabid oral suspension 50 mg bid

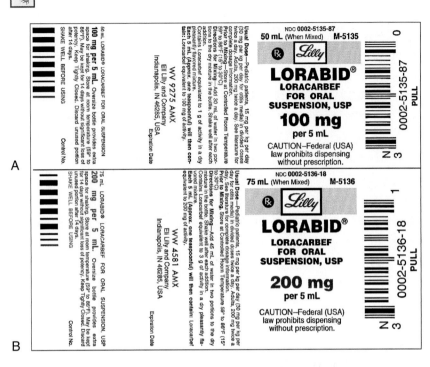

Interpret the label. _____

Which bottle of medication would be used to prepare this medication for a more accurate administration? _____

Volume of medication per dose from the bottle selected in metric system:

_____

Volume of medication for the above dose from the bottle selected in household measurement: _____

Volume of medication for the above dose as found on the label not selected:

_____

CALCULATING PARENTERAL MEDICATIONS IN VIALS AND AMPULES

Parenteral medications are those administered outside the gastrointestinal tract and are usually considered to be those given by injection. These medications may be given directly into the bloodstream (**intravenous**), into the muscle (**intramuscular**), beneath the skin (**subcutaneous** or **intradermal**) through appropriate parenteral routes. When medications are administered by these means, absorption is typically faster than with most oral medications, with the exception of some slow-release or **depot** injectables. For the person who cannot swallow medications taken orally or for medications that cannot be administered

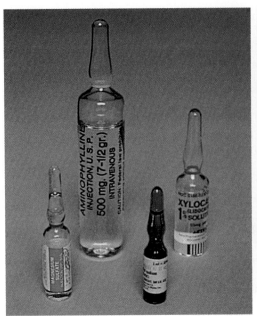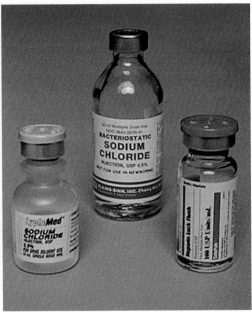

FIGURE 8-7 Typical ampule and vial containers.

orally because of absorption incompatibilities, the parenteral route of administration may be used.

Parenteral medications are available in **ampules** and **vials** (Figure 8-7) and are most often prepared as a liquid either in an aqueous or oil base by the drug manufacturer. Other medications that are not stable in the liquid form come in powders and crystals that must be reconstituted to a liquid form before being given parenterally. (Chapter 9 discusses the reconstitution of medications.)

! TECH ALERT

All medications administered parenterally (by injection) must be in a sterile liquid form. Once these medications have been injected, the medication cannot be retrieved, so special care is needed to ensure the medication and its dose are correct prior to administration.

As with oral liquid medications, parenteral medications are identified on the container as the strength of the medication in a specific volume of liquid. The strength is usually provided in the metric system—milligrams, grams, and micrograms—and usually in milliliters for volume. The apothecary system's units of grains per milliliter may also be used, although this is not as common today as previously. (International units are found with some medications, and this unit of measurement is discussed in Chapter 11.)

TECH NOTE

The label will read as the strength per volume, such as mg/mL or g/mL.

Some parenterals will also be expressed in percentage strength, but they will usually also have the drug strength per volume in metric measures included on the label. Large doses of parenteral medications may be drawn into syringes holding larger volumes such as 5 mL, 10 mL, 20 mL, and 50 mL per syringe. Tuberculin syringes are calibrated in 0.01-mL increments. Three-milliliter syringes have increments of 0.1 mL. Five-milliliter syringes may have indications for 0.1 or 0.2 mL, whereas the larger syringe volumes are usually marked with 0.2-mL increments except in syringes holding more than 20 ML and depending on the total volume that can be measured in the specific syringe. The choice of syringe size is based on the amount of medication that is to be administered.

TECH NOTE

Large syringes are seldom used for medication administration because large doses of medications (more than 10 mL) are usually given using intravenous fluids.

! TECH ALERT

Some syringes still may have minim (m̥) markings. If these syringes are used, care must be taken to read the correct measurement such as mL in the metric system and dram (ʒ) in the apothecary system. This is extremely important for patient safety because the dosage will be affected greatly by reading the incorrect markings.

! TECH ALERT

If the answer to a dose calculation does not agree with an anticipated answer based on the amount of medication prescribed and the dose of medication on hand, ALWAYS recalculate and ask for assistance as necessary. A dose that seems too large or too small should always have calculations checked.

TECH NOTE

The calibrations between markings on the syringe are usually found as four spaces as in increments of 0.1 ml on the 3-mL syringe or 0.2 ml on the 5-mL syringe. Always be sure to understand the markings prior to using the syringe for preparing medications to ensure that the correct amount of medication is being prepared.

Once the parenteral medication has been calculated, the correct syringe must be chosen according to the volume of medication to be administered. If the volume of medication has a dose of less than 0.1 mL or is in increments of tenths of a mL, such as 0.25 mL, it should be measured with a tuberculin syringe (Figure 8-8). Syringes for larger volumes are chosen by the amount of medication to be either administered or added to intravenous fluids. A 3-mL syringe is the usual choice for medication volumes between 1 mL and 3 mL or when medications can be measured in tenths of milliliter above 0.1 mL, such as 0.3 mL or 1.9 mL (Figure 8-9). As seen in this figure, on some syringes that are manufactured with the needle attached, the needle has a safety cap as required by Occupational Safety and Health Administration regulations. The measurement of medications in larger syringes is not as accurate and is shown in 0.2 mL (Figure 8-10). The selection of the correct syringe depends on the volume of medication dose and the precision of the accurate dose. Note that medication volumes are measured with the bottom of the rubber stopper of the plunger placed at the calibration mark of the syringe for the correct fluid level of the medication. For example, in Figure 8-11 the volume would be 1.7 mL and in Figure 8-12 the volume would be 2.3 mL.

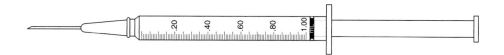

FIGURE 8-8   Typical tuberculin syringe measured in 0.01 mL.

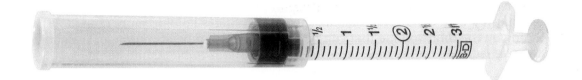

FIGURE 8-9   BD Safety-LOK 3-mL syringe.

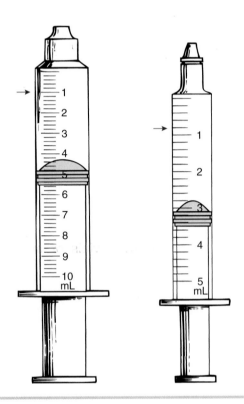

FIGURE 8-10   Measurement of liquids in larger syringes in 0.2 mL increments.

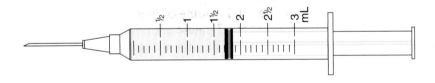

FIGURE 8-11   Syringe containing volume of 1.7 mL.

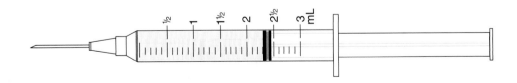

FIGURE 8-12   Syringe containing volume of 2.3 mL.

3. 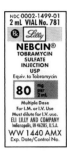 Prescribed: tobramycin 60 mg IM q8h

NDC 0002-1499-01
2 mL VIAL No. 781
Ⓡ *Lilly*
NEBCIN®
TOBRAMYCIN
SULFATE
INJECTION
USP
Equiv. to Tobramycin
80 mg per 2 mL
Multiple Dose
For I.M. or I.V. Use
Must dilute for I.V. use.
ELI LILLY AND COMPANY
Indianapolis, IN 46285, U.S.A.
WW 1440 AMX
Exp. Date/Control No.

Interpret the order. _____

Volume of medication to be given in a dose: ___1.5 ML___

Choose the correct syringe and show the amount of medication on that syringe.

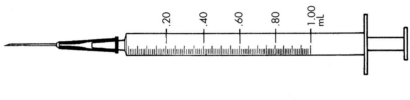

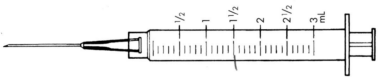

4. 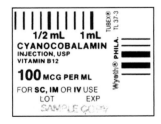 Prescribed: vitamin B$_{12}$ 0.2 mg IM qwk

| | | | | | | | | | TUBEX® TL 37-3
1/2 mL   1 mL
CYANOCOBALAMIN
INJECTION, USP
VITAMIN B12
100 MCG PER ML
FOR **SC, IM** OR **IV** USE
LOT   EXP
SAMPLE COPY

Interpret the order. _____

Volume of medication to be given in a dose: _____

Can the medication vial shown be used to fulfill the order? _____

Explain your answer: _____

5. [PA IN] Prescribed: meperidine 75 mg IM q4-6h prn pain

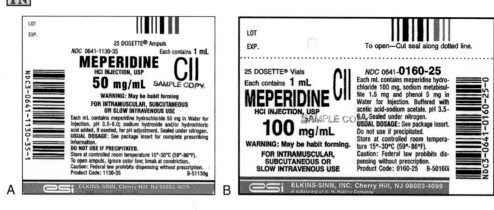

Interpret the order. _____

Which vial of meperidine is the best choice to be used? _____

Why did you choose the vial that is to be used? _____

Volume of medication to be given with the dose of the medication chosen:

_____

Choose the correct syringe and show the amount of medication on that syringe.

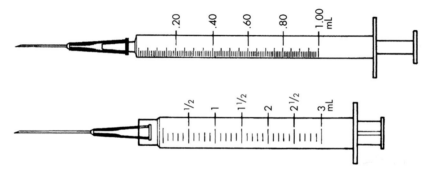

6. [image] Prescribed: benztropine mesylate 1 mg IM daily

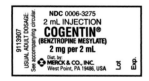

Interpret the order. _____

Volume of medication to be given in a dose: _____

Show the amount of medication on the syringe supplied.

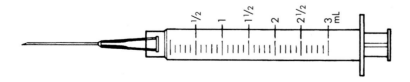

7. 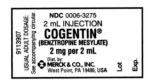 Prescribed: Cogentin 1.5 mg IM daily

NDC 0006-3275
2 mL INJECTION
COGENTIN®
(BENZTROPINE MESYLATE)
2 mg per 2 mL
Dist. by:
MERCK & CO., INC.
West Point, PA 19486, USA

9113907
USUAL ADULT DOSAGE:
See accompanying circular

Lot
Exp.

Interpret the order. _____

Volume of medication to be given in a dose: _____

Choose the correct syringe and show the amount of medication on that syringe.

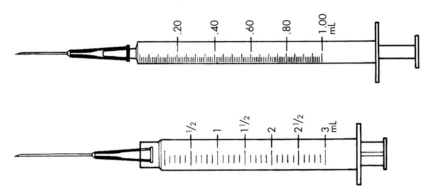

8. 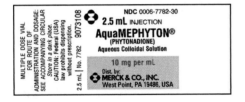 Dose ordered: AquaMEPHYTON 2 mg stat

NDC 0006-7782-30
2.5 mL INJECTION
AquaMEPHYTON®
(PHYTONADIONE)
Aqueous Colloidal Solution

10 mg per mL
Dist. by:
MERCK & CO., INC.
West Point, PA 19486, USA

MULTIPLE DOSE VIAL
FOR ROUTE OF
ADMINISTRATION AND DOSAGE:
SEE ACCOMPANYING CIRCULAR
Store in a dark place.
CAUTION: Federal (USA)
law prohibits dispensing
without prescription.
2.5 mL | No. 7782   9073108

Interpret the order. _____

Volume of medication to be given in a dose: _____

Choose the correct syringe and show the amount of medication on that syringe.

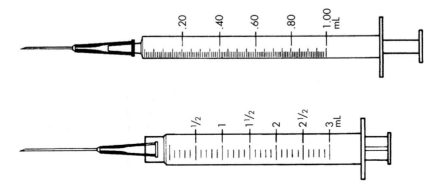

9. 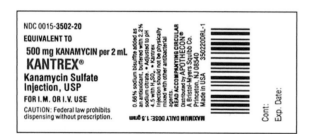 Prescribed: Amikin 250 mg IM q8h

NDC 0015-3020-20

Amikin®
AMIKACIN SULFATE
INJECTION For I.M. or I.V. Use
EQUIVALENT TO

500 mg AMIKACIN Per 2 mL

CAUTION: Federal law prohibits
dispensing without prescription.
©Bristol-Myers Company

BRISTOL LABORATORIES
Bristol-Myers
U.S. Pharmaceutical and
Nutritional Group
Evansville, Indiana 47721

0.66% sodium bisulfite added as an
antioxidant; buffered with 2.5% sodium
citrate, adjusted to pH 4.5 with H₂SO₄.
U.S. 3,781,268 / 4,424,343
READ CIRCULAR   3020200RL-06

Lot
Exp. Date

Interpret the order. _____

Volume of medication to be given in a dose: _____

Choose the correct syringe and show the amount of medication on that syringe.

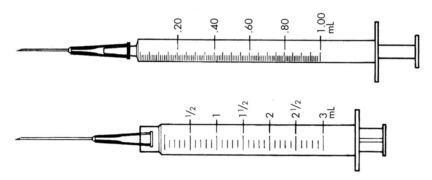

10. 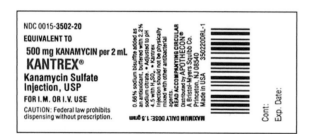 Prescribed: Kantrex 125 mg IM q12h until discontinued

NDC 0015-3502-20

EQUIVALENT TO

500 mg KANAMYCIN per 2 mL

KANTREX®

Kanamycin Sulfate
Injection, USP

FOR I.M. OR I.V. USE

CAUTION: Federal law prohibits
dispensing without prescription.

MAXIMUM DAILY DOSE: 1.5 gram

0.66% sodium bisulfite added as
an antioxidant, buffered with 2.2%
sodium citrate. • Adjusted to pH
4.5 with H₂SO₄. • Kantrex
Injection should not be physically
mixed with other antibacterial
agents.
READ ACCOMPANYING CIRCULAR
Distributed by APOTHECON®
A Bristol-Myers Squibb Co.
Princeton, NJ 08540
Made in USA   3502200RL-1

Cont:
Exp. Date:

Interpret the order. _____

Volume of medication to be given in a dose: _____

Choose the correct syringe and show the amount of medication on that syringe.

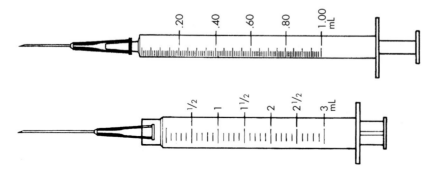

11. 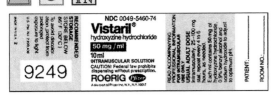 Prescribed: Vistaril 75 mg and meperidine 50 mg IM q6h prn pain

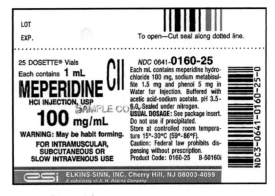

Interpret the order. _____

Volume of Vistaril that will be given in a dose: _____

Volume of meperidine to be given in a dose: _____

Show the amount of combined medication on the syringe supplied:

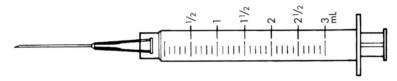

12. 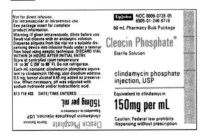 Prescribed: Cleocin phosphate 0.25 g IM stat then q8h

Interpret the order. _____

Volume of medication to be given in a dose: _____

Choose the correct syringe and show the amount of medication on that syringe.

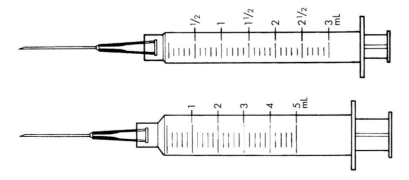

13. Prescribed: lincomycin 0.45 g IM stat

Caution: Federal law prohibits dispensing
without prescription.
For intramuscular or intravenous use.
See package insert for complete product
information.
Warning: If given intravenously, must be
diluted before use.
Store at controlled room temperature
15° to 30° C (59° to 86° F).
Each mL contains lincomycin hydrochloride equivalent to lincomycin, 300 mg.
Also benzyl alcohol, 9.45 mg added
as preservative.

The Upjohn Company
Kalamazoo, MI 49001, USA

811 218 303

Upjohn NDC 0009-0555-02
10 mL

Lincocin®

Sterile Solution

lincomycin
hydrochloride
injection, USP

Equivalent to
300mg per mL
lincomycin
3 grams per 10 mL

Interpret the order. _____

Volume of medication needed for the order: _____

14. Prescribed: Solu-Cortef 125 mg IM stat

Single-Dose Vial   For IV or IM use
Contains Benzyl Alcohol as a Preservative
See package insert for complete
product information.
Per 2 mL (when mixed):
* hydrocortisone sodium succinate equiv.
to hydrocortisone, 250 mg. Protect
solution from light. Discard after 3 days.

814 070 205   Reconstituted ....

The Upjohn Company
Kalamazoo, MI 49001, USA

2 mL Act-O-Vial®   NDC 0009-0909-08

Solu-Cortef® Sterile Powder
hydrocortisone sodium succinate
for injection, USP
250 mg*

Interpret the order. _____

Volume of medication needed for a dose: _____

Choose the correct syringe and show the amount of medication on that syringe.

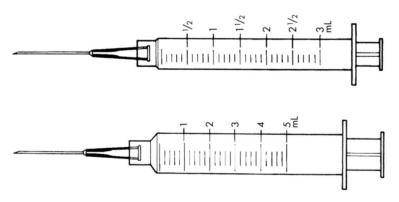

15. 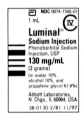 Prescribed: Depo-Provera 0.3 g IM qmo

For IM use only
See package insert for
complete product information
Shake vigorously immediately
before each use
812 224 302

The Upjohn Company
Kalamazoo, MI 49001 USA

NDC 0009-0626-01
2.5 mL Vial
Depo-Provera®
Sterile Aqueous Suspension
sterile medroxyprogesterone
acetate suspension, USP
400mg per mL

Interpret the order. _____

Volume of medication to be given as a dose: _____

16.   Prescribed: Luminal gr ¾ IM prn rest

NDC 0074-1540-01
1 mL
Luminal®
Sodium Injection
Phenobarbital Sodium
Injection, USP
130 mg/mL
(2 grains)
(in water 10%,
alcohol 10%, and
propylene glycol 67.8%)
Abbott Laboratories,
N. Chgo., IL 60064, USA
58-0130-2/R1-11/97

Interpret the order. _____

Volume of medication to be given as a dose: _____

Strength of medication to be given in the metric system: _____

Choose the correct syringe and show the amount of medication on that syringe.

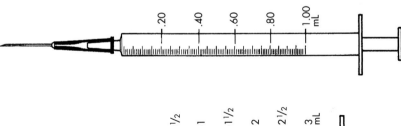

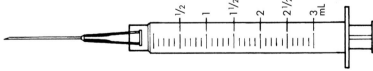

17. PA IN   Prescribed: codeine phosphate gr ¾ IM prn pain

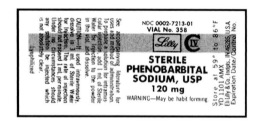

Interpret the order. _____

Volume of medication to be given in a dose: _____

Strength of medication to be given in the metric system: _____

18. 🧠   Prescribed: phenobarbital sodium gr i̇ss IM q4h prn agitation

Interpret the order. _____

Volume of medication to be given in a dose: _____

Strength of medication in metric system: _____

Choose the correct syringe and show the amount of medication on that syringe.

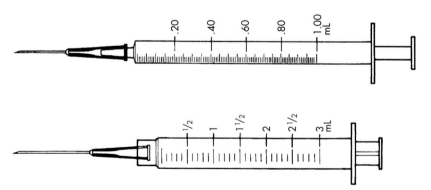

19. 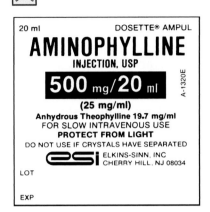 Prescribed: aminophylline 125 mg IV q6h

20 ml   DOSETTE® AMPUL

AMINOPHYLLINE
INJECTION, USP

500 mg/20 ml

(25 mg/ml)
Anhydrous Theophylline 19.7 mg/ml
FOR SLOW INTRAVENOUS USE
PROTECT FROM LIGHT
DO NOT USE IF CRYSTALS HAVE SEPARATED

ELKINS-SINN, INC
CHERRY HILL, NJ 08034

LOT

EXP

A-1320E

Interpret the order. _____

Volume of medication to be given with a single dose: _____

20. 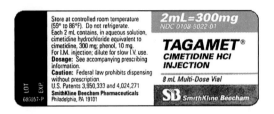 Prescribed: Tagamet 75 mg IM q6h

Store at controlled room temperature
(59° to 86°F). Do not refrigerate.
Each 2 mL contains, in aqueous solution,
cimetidine hydrochloride equivalent to
cimetidine, 300 mg; phenol, 10 mg.
For I.M. injection; dilute for slow I.V. use.
Dosage: See accompanying prescribing
information.
Caution: Federal law prohibits dispensing
without prescription.
U.S. Patents 3,950,333 and 4,024,271
SmithKline Beecham Pharmaceuticals
Philadelphia, PA 19101

LOT EXP
693957-P

2mL=300mg
NDC 0108-5022-01

TAGAMET®
CIMETIDINE HCl
INJECTION

8 mL Multi-Dose Vial

SB SmithKline Beecham

Interpret the order. _____

Volume of medication to be given with a single dose: _____

Choose the correct syringe(s) and show the amount of medication on the syringe(s).

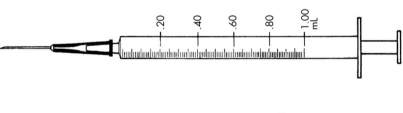

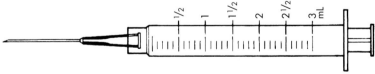

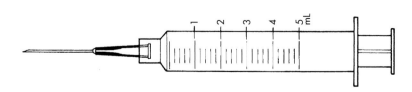

REVIEW

As with the previous chapter, on the calculation of oral solid medications, this chapter shows how to calculate the dose desired for parenteral and oral liquid medications. The same methods for calculation—ratio and proportion, dimensional analysis, and formula methods—are used for these calculations. These medications are then dispensed in the measurements for liquids in the three systems—metric, household, and apothecary. Conversions for the correct volume of medication depend on the measurement system to be used for administration. The household system is often used for home delivery of oral medications: when a more accurate utensil for administration is not provided. The metric and apothecary systems are most often used with inpatient settings, especially with parenteral medications. If the medication is to be given parenterally, the correct syringe and needle must be chosen. Liquid oral medications may be administered from a medicine cup, dose spoon, dose syringe, medicine dropper, or medication pacifier depending on the volume of medication and the age and ability to take medication of the patients. In some instances, liquid medications may be combined with oral or with parenteral administration. In those instances the correct dose amount for each medication must be properly calculated and prepared in the appropriate administration container. As with all medications, the proper calculation and appropriate containers for parenteral and oral liquid medications are important for patient safety. Patient safety should always be the utmost concern when preparing and delivering medications.

Posttest

Before taking the Posttest, retake the Pretest to check your understanding of the materials presented in this chapter.

Using the following labels, interpret the orders and calculate the ordered medications. Figure the dose to be given in the dose form and indicate the form in the answer. Show all calculations. Round to the nearest tenth after completing all calculations, unless marked with an asterisk, and then round to the nearest hundredths. Always be sure the answer is a measurable volume.

1. Prescribed: Stadol 1 mg stat then q4h

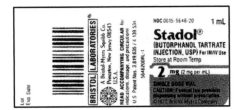

Interpret the order. _____

Volume of medication to be given as a single dose: _____

Choose the correct syringe and show the amount of medication on that syringe.

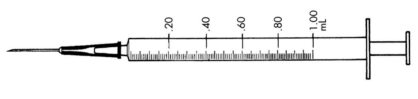

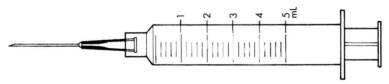

Continued

Posttest, cont.

2. Prescribed: phenobarbital elixir gr $\overline{ss}$ q4h for epilepsy

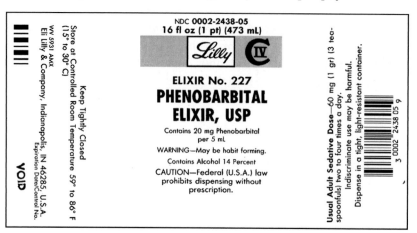

Interpret the order. _____

Volume of medication to be given as a dose in metric system: _____

Volume of medication to be given in apothecary system: _____

Posttest, cont.

3. Prescribed: penicillin V potassium oral solution 0.25 g po qid

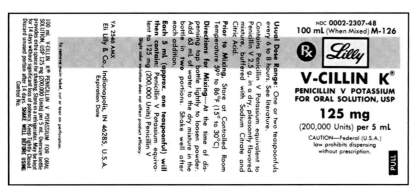

NDC 0002-2307-48
100 mL (When Mixed) M-126

℞ *Lilly*

V-CILLIN K®
PENICILLIN V POTASSIUM
FOR ORAL SOLUTION, USP

125 mg
(200,000 Units) per 5 mL

CAUTION—Federal (U.S.A.)
law prohibits dispensing
without prescription.

PULL

Usual Dose Range: One or two teaspoonfuls every 6 to 8 hours. See literature.

Contains Penicillin V Potassium equivalent to Penicillin V 2.5 g, in a dry, pleasantly flavored mixture, buffered with Sodium Citrate and Citric Acid.

Prior to Mixing. Store at Controlled Room Temperature 59° to 86°F (15° to 30°C).

Directions for Mixing—At the time of dispensing tap bottle lightly to loosen powder. Add 63 ml of water to the dry mixture in the bottle in **two** portions. Shake well after each addition.

Each 5 mL (approx. one teaspoonful) will then contain: Penicillin V Potassium equivalent to 125 mg (200,000 Units) Penicillin V

Slight color variation does not affect product efficacy.

YA 2546 AMX
Eli Lilly & Co.,
Indianapolis, IN 46285, U.S.A.
Expiration Date

100 mL V-CILLIN K® PENICILLIN V POTASSIUM FOR ORAL SOLUTION, USP 125 mg (200,000 Units) per 5 mL. Oversize bottle provides extra space for shaking. Store in a refrigerator. May be kept for 14 days without significant loss of potency. Keep Tightly Closed. Discard unused portion after 14 days. SHAKE WELL BEFORE USING.
Control No.

To remove main label, cut or tear on perforation.

Interpret the order. _____

Volume of medication to be given with a dose in metric system: _____

Volume of medication to be given in household measurements with each dose:

_____

Indicate the amount of medication in the medication cup.

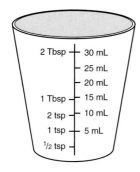

2 Tbsp — 30 mL
— 25 mL
— 20 mL
1 Tbsp — 15 mL
2 tsp — 10 mL
1 tsp — 5 mL
½ tsp —

Continued

Posttest, cont.

4. Prescribed: Keflex oral suspension 32 mg q6h

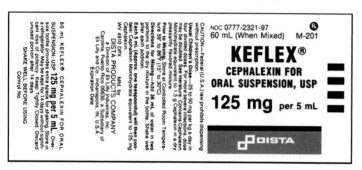

NDC 0777-2321-97
60 mL (When Mixed)   M-201

KEFLEX®
CEPHALEXIN FOR
ORAL SUSPENSION, USP

125 mg per 5 mL

DISTA

Interpret the order. _____

Volume of medication to be given in metric units for each dose: _____

Indicate the amount of medication in the correct utensil for administration.

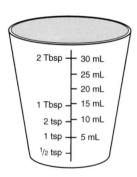

2 Tbsp —— 30 mL
        —— 25 mL
        —— 20 mL
1 Tbsp —— 15 mL
2 tsp —— 10 mL
1 tsp —— 5 mL
½ tsp

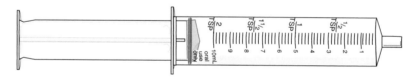

Posttest, cont.

5. Prescribed: Garamycin 0.06 g IM q8h

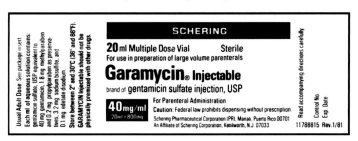

Interpret the order. _____

Volume of medication to be given in metric system for each dose:

_____

Indicate the correct amount of medication on the appropriate syringe.

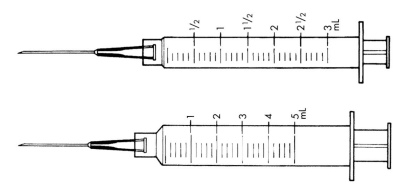

6. Prescribed: scopolamine gr 1/150 subcutaneously 30 min before surgery

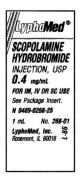

Interpret the order. _____

Volume of medication to be given in metric system: _____

Continued

Posttest, cont.

7. Prescribed: Solu-Medrol 37.5 mg IM stat

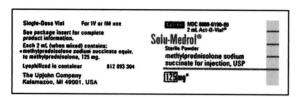

Single-Dose Vial   For IV or IM use

See package insert for complete
product information.

Each 2 mL (when mixed) contains:
• methylprednisolone sodium succinate equiv.
to methylprednisolone, 125 mg.

Lyophilized in container   812 893 304

The Upjohn Company
Kalamazoo, MI 49001, USA

NDC 0009-0190-09
2 mL Act-O-Vial®

Solu-Medrol®
Sterile Powder
methylprednisolone sodium
succinate for injection, USP

125 mg*

Interpret the order. _____

Volume of medication to be given: _____

Indicate the correct amount of medication on the appropriate syringe.

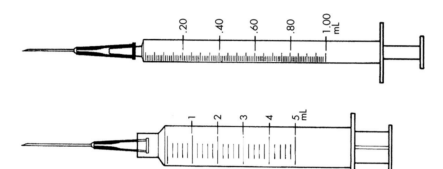

Posttest, cont.

8. Prescribed: Mellaril oral solution 45 mg bid

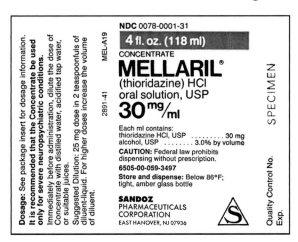

Interpret the order. _____

Volume of medication to be given with each dose: _____

Indicate the amount of medication in the correct utensil for administration.

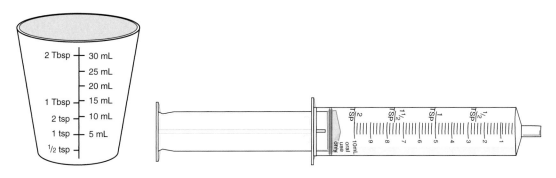

9. Prescribed: diazepam 2 mg IM stat and then q6h prn for anxiety

Interpret the order. _____

Volume of medication to be given as a single dose: _____

Continued

Posttest, cont.

10. Prescribed: amoxicillin oral suspension 125 mg q8h

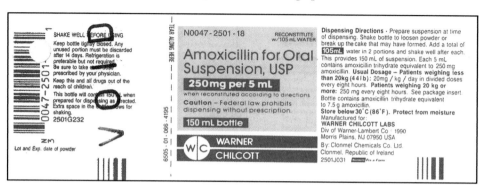

Interpret the order. _____

Volume of medication to be given as a dose in metric system: _____

Volume of medication in household measurements: _____

Indicate the amount of medication in the most accurate utensil for administration.

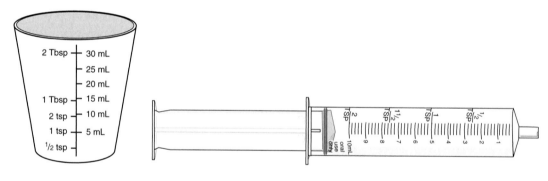

Posttest, cont.

11. Prescribed: Zantac syrup 75 mg bid 30 min ac meals

Glaxo Pharmaceuticals

Zantac®
(ranitidine
hydrochloride)
Syrup
15 mg/mL

Caution: Federal law
prohibits dispensing
without prescription.

16 fl oz (1 pint)

LOT

EXP

Interpret the order. _____

Volume of medication to be given with a dose in the metric system: _____

Volume of medication to be given with each dose in household measurements: _____

Indicate the volume of medication on the utensils to be used for administration.

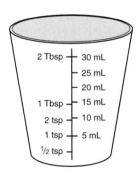

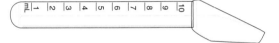

12. Prescribed: Cipro 0.4 g IV q12h

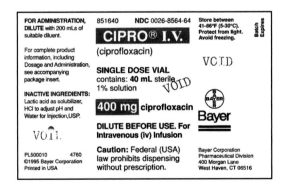

Interpret the order. _____

Metric volume of medication for each dose that will be added to an IV bag for administration: _____

Continued

Posttest, cont.

13. Prescribed: Dilaudid 500 mcg IM q4h prn severe pain

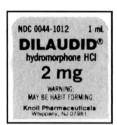

NDC 0044-1012   1 mL
DILAUDID®
hydromorphone HCl
2 mg
WARNING:
MAY BE HABIT FORMING.
Knoll Pharmaceuticals
Whippany, NJ 07981

Interpret the order. _____

*Volume of medication to be given with each dose in metric system:

_____

Indicate the amount of medication on the correct syringe for administration.

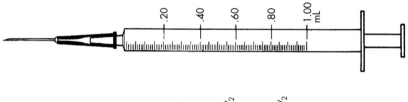

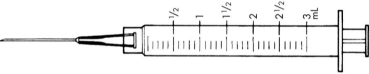

14. Prescribed: digoxin 0.1 mg IM stat then daily

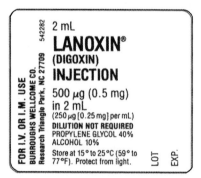

2 mL
LANOXIN®
(DIGOXIN)
INJECTION
500 μg (0.5 mg)
in 2 mL
(250 μg [0.25 mg] per mL)
DILUTION NOT REQUIRED
PROPYLENE GLYCOL 40%
ALCOHOL 10%
Store at 15° to 25°C (59° to
77°F). Protect from light.
FOR I.V. OR I.M. USE
BURROUGHS WELLCOME CO.
Research Triangle Park, NC 27709   542282
LOT
EXP.

Interpret the order. _____

Volume of medication to be given in a dose in metric system: _____

Posttest, cont.

15. Prescribed: Duricef 750 mg po stat then 0.5 g q12h

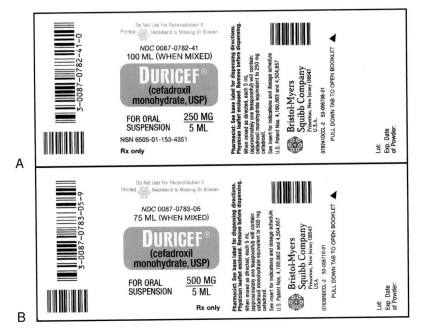

Do Not Use For Reconstitution If
Printed ❄ Neckband Is Missing Or Broken

NDC 0087-0782-41
100 ML (WHEN MIXED)

DURICEF®
(cefadroxil
monohydrate, USP)

FOR ORAL   250 MG
SUSPENSION   5 ML

NSN 6505-01-153-4351
Rx only

Pharmacist: See base label for dispensing directions.
Physician leaflet enclosed. Remove before dispensing.
When mixed as directed, each 5 mL
(approximately one teaspoonful) will contain:
cefadroxil monohydrate equivalent to 250 mg
cefadroxil.
See insert for indications and dosage schedule.
U.S. Patent Nos. 4,160,863 and 4,504,657

Bristol-Myers
Squibb Company
Princeton, New Jersey 08543
U.S.A.
0782410CL-2 53-006708-01   PULL DOWN TAB TO OPEN BOOKLET

Lot:
Exp. Date
of Powder:

A

Do Not Use For Reconstitution If
Printed ❄ Neckband Is Missing Or Broken

NDC 0087-0783-05
75 ML (WHEN MIXED)

DURICEF®
(cefadroxil
monohydrate, USP)

FOR ORAL   500 MG
SUSPENSION   5 ML

Rx only

Pharmacist: See base label for dispensing directions.
Physician leaflet enclosed. Remove before dispensing.
When mixed as directed, each 5 mL
(approximately one teaspoonful) will contain:
cefadroxil monohydrate equivalent to 500 mg
cefadroxil.
See insert for indications and dosage schedule.
U.S. Patent Nos. 4,160,863 and 4,504,657

Bristol-Myers
Squibb Company
Princeton, New Jersey 08543
U.S.A.
0783060CL-2 53-006710-01   PULL DOWN TAB TO OPEN BOOKLET

Lot:
Exp. Date
of Powder:

B

Interpret the order. _____

Which drug bottle should be used? _____

Volume of medication to be given in stat dose in metric system: _____

Volume of medication to be given in stat dose in household system:

_____

Volume of medication to be given q12h in metric system: _____

Volume of medication to be given q12h in household measurements:

_____

Indicate the correct amount of medication on the appropriate utensil for each administration.

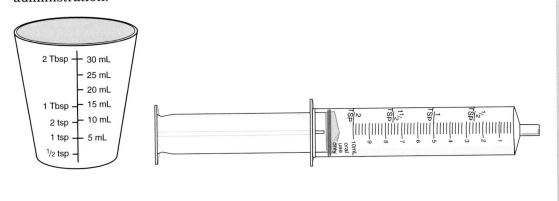

Continued

Posttest, cont.

16. Prescribed: dicloxacillin suspension 100 mg po q6h for acute bronchitis

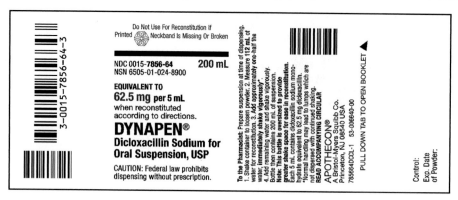

Interpret the order. _____

Metric volume of medication to be given as a dose: _____

What is the volume of medication in household measurements? _____

17. Prescribed: secobarbital sodium gr $\overline{\text{iss}}$ IM prn sleep

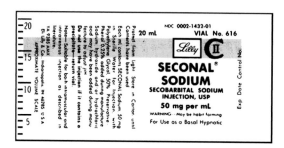

Interpret the order. _____

Volume of medication to be given as a single dose: _____

Indicate the amount of medication on the correct syringe for administration.

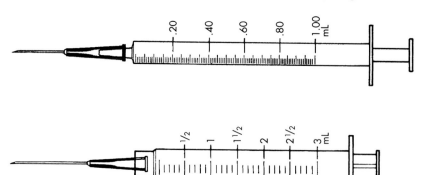

Posttest, cont.

18. Prescribed: Garamycin 30 mg IM q8h

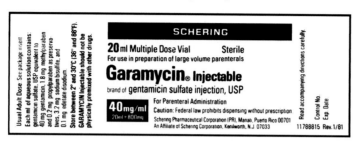

SCHERING

20 ml Multiple Dose Vial   Sterile
For use in preparation of large volume parenterals

Garamycin® Injectable
brand of gentamicin sulfate injection, USP

For Parenteral Administration
40 mg/ml Caution: Federal law prohibits dispensing without prescription.
20ml = 800mg Schering Pharmaceutical Corporation (PR), Manati, Puerto Rico 00701
An Affiliate of Schering Corporation, Kenilworth, N.J. 07033   11788815 Rev. 1/81

Usual Adult Dose See package insert
Each ml of aqueous solution contains:
gentamicin sulfate, USP equivalent to
40 mg gentamicin, 1.8 mg methylparaben
and 0.2 mg propylparaben as preservatives, 3.2 mg sodium bisulfite, and
0.1 mg edetate disodium.
Store between 2° and 30°C (36° and 86°F).
GARAMYCIN Injectable should not be
physically premixed with other drugs.

Read accompanying directions carefully.
Control No.
Exp. Date

Interpret the order. _____

*Volume of medication to be given as a dose: _____

19. Lasix 20 mg IM q4h

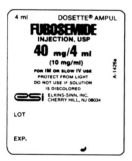

4 ml   DOSETTE® AMPUL

FUROSEMIDE
INJECTION, USP

40 mg/4 ml
(10 mg/ml)

FOR IM OR SLOW IV use
PROTECT FROM LIGHT
DO NOT USE IF SOLUTION
IS DISCOLORED

ESI ELKINS-SINN, INC.
CHERRY HILL, NJ 08034

LOT

EXP.

Interpret the order. _____

Volume of medication to be given as a single dose: _____

Indicate the amount of medication on the correct syringe for administration.

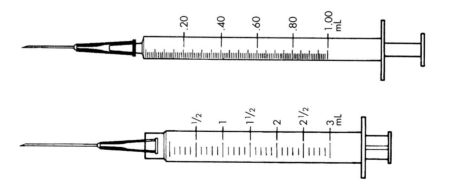

Continued

Posttest, cont.

20. meperidine 50 mg IM q4h prn pain

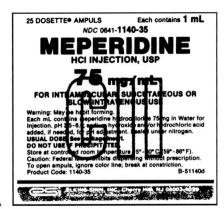

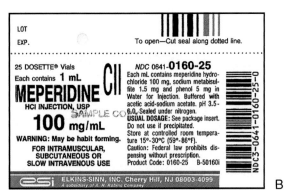

A

B

Interpret the order. _____

Which container of meperidine would you choose to use? _____

Volume of medication to be given from the vial of medication selected:

_____

*Volume of medication to be given from the other vial of medication:

_____

REVIEW OF RULES

Calculating Parenteral Medications

- Calculations for parenteral medications may be accomplished using ratio and proportion, dimensional analysis, or formula methods.

- Before beginning calculations of liquid medications, be sure the dose desired and the dose available are in the same measurement system. If the measurement systems are different, convert to the measurement system that is on the label of available medication.

- Liquid medication quantities are usually given in the strength of medication in the volume of solvent or the liquid amount. This proportion will vary with each liquid medication depending on how it is manufactured. You must carefully read the quantity of medication on each label.

- Liquid medications found on prescriptions for household administration are often converted to household measurements for dispensing unless a specific dispensing utensil is provided by the manufacturer or pharmacy.

- Medication orders and prescriptions for oral liquid medications can be calculated using the ratio and proportion, dimensional analysis, or formula method.

- To solve using the ratio and proportion method, set the known measurements in the equation with the unknown correctly placed in the equation. The following change in the ratio and proportion is necessary for liquid medications:

DA : DF :: DO : DG

- Dimensional analysis is an extended method of ratio and proportion placed in fractional units. See the rules at the end of Chapter 5 for a review of this means of solving dosage.

- The formula method uses the same formula as found in Chapter 7. In the case of liquid preparations, the quantity will vary with each medication. Manufacturers provide the strength of medication in a volume (qty). Be sure that the measurement system for the dose desired and the dose on hand are the same, but remember that the quantity may vary in measurement system (e.g., the medication strength may be in milligrams, but the quantity may be in either teaspoons, milliliters, or drams).

- Calculate the problem with the method that is most comfortable for you, but be consistent in the calculation technique.

CHAPTER 9

Reconstitution of Powders or Crystals into Liquid Medications

OBJECTIVES

- Read labels of powders or crystals (lyophilized) medications to determine correct diluent and correct volume necessary to reconstitute powders
- Check labels for expiration dates and storage conditions before and after reconstitution of solid medication to a liquid form
- Understand the importance of labeling reconstituted medications with date, time, and initials of person performing the medication reconstitution
- Determine the appropriate amount of diluent necessary when using a single-dose container of a powder or crystals
- Determine the appropriate amount of diluent necessary when preparing a multidose container of a powder or crystals
- Determine the appropriate dilution concentration when more than one dosage strength in the multidose container is possible, and then determine amount of diluent necessary to meet desired concentration
- Calculate the amount of medication of a reconstituted medication to be dispensed to meet the physician's order

KEY WORDS

Diluent Agent that dilutes a substance; in pharmacology, the liquid added to a powder to change the powder to a liquid or the liquid used to dilute another liquid

Graduates Containers marked with progressive series of lines or markers, usually in the metric system, for measuring liquids or solids

Lyophilized Freeze dried

Powder displacement Amount of solute that causes displacement in the total volume of medication

Powder volume Space occupied by dry powder or freeze-dried (lyophilized or crystalline)

active ingredient related to total volume of medication following reconstitution with indicated diluent volume

Reconstitution Process of adding fluid, such as distilled water, sterile water for injection, or sterile saline, to a powdered or crystalline form of medication, making a specific liquid dosage strength

Vehicle Inert substance in which a medication is mixed for administration

Pretest

Complete the following reconstitution of the medications to supply the dosage necessary for a physician's order. Show your calculations. Be sure all calculations are made to a measurable amount.

 1. A physician orders penicillin G 200,000 units to be given IM q12h × 5 d for a child. As the pharmacy technician in the hospital pharmacy, you are to prepare the powdered medication for administration by injection. It is desirable for the intramuscular (IM) injection dose not to exceed 1 mL in volume for this child. You have the label for a multidose vial from which to prepare the medication. Determine the correct reconstituted concentration for use with this patient.

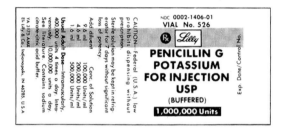

What is the volume of diluent necessary to meet the requirements for this dosage?

_____

After reconstitution, what volume of medication is given for each dose? _____

How long is the medication potent after reconstitution? _____

 2. A physician orders penicillin G 250,000 units q6h IM. The medication is available in a 1,000,000-unit multidose vial. The label reads to reconstitute the medication with either sterile water for injection or isotonic sodium chloride for injection using the following instructions:

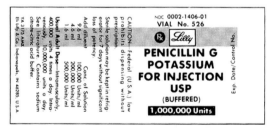

Which reconstituted concentration would you choose for the medication ordered?

_____

What volume of diluent would you add to the powder for this order?

_____

Continued

Pretest, cont.

3. A physician orders Mefoxin 1.2 g IM q8h. The medication available is a 2-g vial for reconstitution. The label reads as follows:

MEFOXIN CONCENTRATION	AMOUNT OF DILUENT TO BE ADDED	AMOUNT THAT CAN BE DRAWN
400 mg/mL	4 mL for IM use	5 mL
180 mg/mL	10 mL for IV use	10.5 mL

What is the total strength of medication in the vial? _____

What volume of diluent would you add to reconstitute the medication for the order?

_____

What volume of medication is needed for a dose? _____

What is the powder volume of this medication for IM use? _____

What is the powder volume for this medication for intravenous (IV) use?

_____

4. A physician orders ampicillin 500 mg IM q6h. The available medication is a 1-g vial. The following label is on the vial:

AMPICILLIN CONCENTRATION	AMOUNT OF DILUENT
250 mg/mL	3.4 mL

What is the volume of diluent to be added to the vial? _____

What is the concentration following reconstitution? _____

What is the total strength of medication in the vial? _____

What volume of medication is prepared for a dose as ordered? _____

What is the powder volume? _____

Pretest, cont.

 5. A bottle of ampicillin is marked 125 mg/5 mL for a child. The 200-mL bottle instructs that 158 mL of water be added for an oral suspension. The physician wants the child to receive ampicillin 250 mg qid.

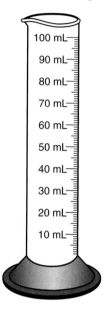 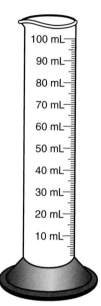

What is the total strength of medication in milligrams in the bottle? _____

Hint: Use ratio and proportion to complete this answer.

What volume of water is added for the bottle to have the correct concentration? _____ Show on the graduates the volume of water needed for reconstitution.

What is the volume per dose that the child should receive? _____

What dose volume would you tell the parent to give in household measurements?

_____

Is the volume in the one container sufficient for 10 days? _____

Show your work. Explain your answer. _____

If necessary, how many mL of medication are needed to complete the prescription as designated? _____

What is the total volume of liquid in milliliters in the container after reconstitution?

_____

What is the powder volume of this medication? _____

Continued

Pretest, cont.

6. A bottle of Veetids after reconstitution will contain 125 mg/5 mL. The bottle states that the total volume in the bottle will be 100 mL after reconstitution.

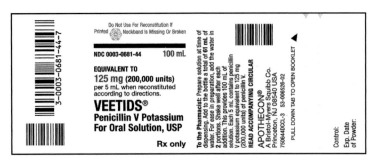

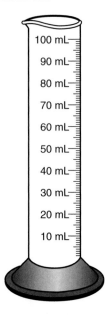

What volume of water is added to the bottle to provide the required concentration?

_____

What is the powder volume of the medication before reconstitution? _____

Show on the graduate the volume of water to be added.

What is the final concentration of the medication? _____

How long would this bottle last if the person takes 1 tsp 3 times a day? _____

7. A label for ticarcillin for injection for IV and IM use shows that the vial contains 1 g of medication in 2.6 mL of reconstituted medication for IM use. The instructions state to use at least 4 mL of sterile water for injection for IV use. To prepare an IM solution, add 2 mL of sterile diluent. Use the solution promptly after reconstitution.

What is the dosage strength found in this vial once prepared for IM use?

_____

What is the diluent volume for IM use? _____

Pretest, cont.

If 5 mL of sterile water has been added to the medication for IV use, what volume of medication would be added to the IV fluids to provide the medication for an order of 750 mg? Base your answer on the fact that the entire vial will contain 6 mL of medication. _____

What volume of medication is prepared for injection if the physician orders 500 mg IM stat? _____

The physician then orders 250 mg IM every 8 hours. What volume of medication would be given with each dose? _____

Can the remainder of the vial be used for the subsequent injections?

_____ Explain your answer. _____

ENDO

8. A vial of Solu-Medrol is being reconstituted for a patient with severe allergies. The label reads to reconstitute the medication with 8 mL of bacteriostatic water for injection with benzyl alcohol. When reconstituted, each 8 mL will contain 500 mg. The solution will remain stable between 15° and 30° C for 48 hours after mixing.

What diluent volume is added to the vial for the indicated dosage of the medication?

_____

What diluent is used for this reconstitution? _____

How long would the Solu-Medrol remain potent at room temperature? _____

If the reconstitution occurs at 10:00 AM on October 15, at what time should the medication be discarded if it has not been used? _____

What is the dosage strength per milliliter of medication? _____

Hint: Use ratio and proportion to obtain this answer.

What volume of medication is given for 125 mg dose? _____

What volume of medication is given for a 275 mg dose? _____

What is the storage temperature in Fahrenheit? _____

Continued

Pretest, cont.

9.

EXP.	equivalent to **1gram** cefazolin NDC 0007-3130-16 **ANCEF®** STERILE CEFAZOLIN SODIUM (LYOPHILIZED) LOT **25 Vials for Intramuscular or Intravenous Use**	NSN 6505-01-262-9508 **Before reconstitution protect from light and store at controlled room temperature (15° to 30°C; 59° to 86°F).** **Usual Adult Dosage:** 250 mg to 1 gram every 6 to 8 hours. See accompanying prescribing information. For I.M. administration add 2.5 mL of Sterile Water for Injection. SHAKE WELL. Withdraw entire contents. Provides an approximate volume of 3.0 mL (330 mg/mL). For I.V. administration see accompanying prescribing information. Reconstituted *Ancef* is stable for 24 hours at room temperature or for 10 days if refrigerated (5°C or 41°F). **SmithKline Beecham Pharmaceuticals** Philadelphia, PA 19101 694115-N **K3130-16**

What is the total strength of medication in a vial? _____

What is the diluent that should be used for the reconstitution? _____

How long is the medication stable at room temperature? _____

How long is the medication stable in the refrigerator? _____

What is the trade name for the medication? _____

What is the generic name? _____

How should the medication be stored before reconstitution? _____

What total volume of medication is present when the reconstitution is complete for IM use? _____

What volume of medication is necessary to administer 250 mg? _____

What is the powder volume? _____

10.

TO PATIENT:
Shake well before using.
Keep tightly closed. Store in refrigerator and discard unused portion after ten days. Oversize bottle provides shake space.
TO THE PHARMACIST:
When prepared as directed, each 5 mL teaspoonful contains erythromycin ethylsuccinate equivalent to 200 mg of erythromycin in a cherry-flavored suspension.
Bottle contains erythromycin ethylsuccinate equivalent to 8 g of erythromycin.
Usual Dose: See package outsert.
Store at room temperature in dry form.
Child-Resistant closure not required; Reference: Federal Register Vol.39 No.29.
DIRECTIONS FOR PREPARATION: Slowly add 140 mL of water and shake vigorously to make 200 mL of suspension.
BARR LABORATORIES, INC.
Pomona, NY 10970
R11-90

BARR LABORATORIES, INC.

Erythromycin Ethylsuccinate
for Oral
Suspension, USP

200 mg of erythromycin activity per 5 mL reconstituted

Caution: Federal law prohibits dispensing without prescription.

200 mL (when mixed)

NDC 0555-0215-23
NSN 6505-00-080-0653

SAMPLE

Exp. Date:
Lot No.:

Pretest, cont.

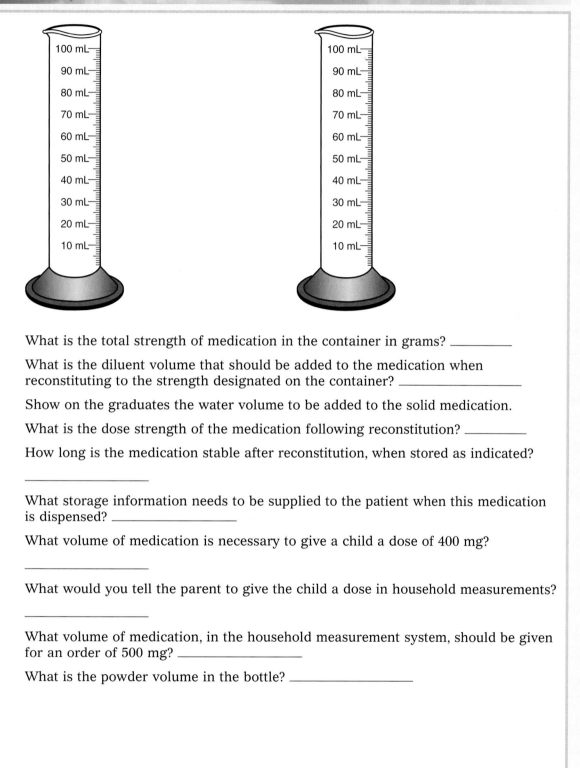

What is the total strength of medication in the container in grams? _____

What is the diluent volume that should be added to the medication when
reconstituting to the strength designated on the container? _____

Show on the graduates the water volume to be added to the solid medication.

What is the dose strength of the medication following reconstitution? _____

How long is the medication stable after reconstitution, when stored as indicated?

_____

What storage information needs to be supplied to the patient when this medication
is dispensed? _____

What volume of medication is necessary to give a child a dose of 400 mg?

_____

What would you tell the parent to give the child a dose in household measurements?

_____

What volume of medication, in the household measurement system, should be given
for an order of 500 mg? _____

What is the powder volume in the bottle? _____

INTRODUCTION

When medications that may require storage over a length of time in liquid form and are unstable, they are often shipped to the pharmacy in powder or crystalline (**lyophilized**) form requiring reconstitution before administration. Medications such as pediatric antibiotics, injectable antibiotics, or immunization agents are some of the most frequently found medicines in this form. These drugs must have liquid added before their use—liquids in the form of water when the medications are for oral use or in the form of sterile solutions such as sterile water for injection, saline for injection, or **diluents** supplied by the manufacturer when the medicine is used for parenteral administration. Dissolving the powdered medication in the liquid is called **reconstitution**.

The dry drug form may be found in single-dose or multidose containers for oral or injectable use. The label on the medication will tell the type of diluent to be used and the amount of the diluent for the desired dosage strength or, in some cases, concentration. The directions on the side of the label should be read carefully to prevent errors in the reconstitution process.

RECONSTITUTION OF POWDERS INTO LIQUID MEDICATIONS

Medications that are unstable in liquid form for extended periods of time are manufactured in either a powder or crystalline (lyophilized) form for reconstitution before use. To reconstitute a medication, care must be taken to follow the instructions on medication label *exactly*. Before using the medication, care must be taken that the dry ingredients are completely dissolved or suspended into liquid form by adding a diluent.

When used as an injectable medication, single-dose vials/ampules or multidose vials are available. Available multidose containers are used when a number of doses may be used from the same container within the amount of time that is with the safe time limit after reconstitution. The diluent used for reconstitution for injectable medications must be sterile and may come in a single-dose vial, as for reconstitution of immunizations that are single doses, or in multidose vials such as sterile water for injection used for multiple doses of antibiotics. To reconstitute injectable medications, sterile syringes are used in the appropriate size for the amount of diluent necessary for the manufacturer's label.

Most oral preparations are found in bottles that are larger than the medication volume present. This allows space for shaking medications before administration. Because the usual **vehicle** for reconstitution of oral medications is distilled water, **graduates** are used to measure the quantity of liquid to be added (Figure 9-1). In some pharmacies, a computerized dispenser for distilled water, such as a Fillmaster electronic pharmaceutical water dispenser, is available. When indicating the correct amount of water to be dispensed, this machine provides one half of the necessary diluent, stops and allows time for mixing the powder medication with the diluent, and then dispenses the remainder of the water on demand.

> **TECH NOTE**
> Flavorings are available to add to reconstituted medications to make them more palatable.

The label on the medication provides the needed information for the necessary volume of diluent to be mixed with the powder to provide the desired dosage per volume. Most oral liquid products are described in dosage strengths that indicate the amount of medication in 1 teaspoonful (5 mL) of medication, whereas the strength described on injectable products varies with the medication and the manufacturer's instructions based on the intended route of administration. If the medication is a single-strength, single-dose vial,

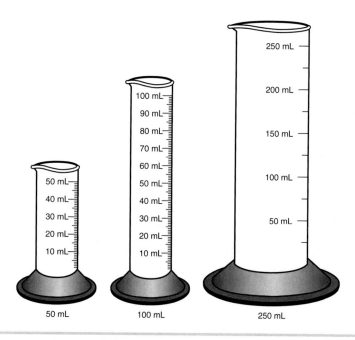

FIGURE 9-1 Examples of graduated cylinders.

the reconstitution is accomplished by adding the amount of diluent indicated on the label. On the other hand, if the medication vial may be prepared at multiple strengths or concentrations, such as found with antibiotics, the diluent must be adjusted to meet the strength necessary to meet the physician's order. When reconstituting multiple-strength doses, check the label on the vial for the options available for the route desired and then choose the one closest to that of the physician's ordered strength for the intended route of administration.

Vials of the same drug may require different volumes and types of diluent for different routes of administration when given parenterally. The directions on the label should be followed exactly to ensure that the correct type and amount of diluent have been used. Some medications may even require specific diluents be added for intramuscular use, such as small amounts of anesthetics to prevent discomfort with administration.

When powders are dissolved in the liquid, the weight or strength of the medication will always remain the same as the amount given on the label. For example, if a label for amoxicillin states that the container holds a total of 2.5 g as a powder, the total weight or strength of the medication will be 2.5 g after reconstitution has occurred. When medications are supplied in dry powder or crystalline form for stability, the space occupied by the powder is known as **powder volume** or **powder displacement**. The total liquid volume of the medication will be that of the amount of medication plus the amount of liquid. In the label shown in Figure 9-2, the final volume of the bottle is 100 mL when reconstituted with 78 mL of water (Figure 9-3). So with this reconstitution the powder volume or displacement is 22 mL (100 mL total volume − 78 mL diluent = 22 mL powder volume). Powder volume (Pv) is the difference between the final volume (Fv) and the diluent volume (Dv). This can be shown with the formula Pv = Fv − Dv.

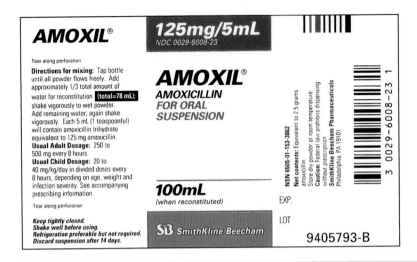

FIGURE 9-2 This label for Amoxil specifies that the total liquid volume of the medication will be 100 mL when reconstituted with 78 mL of water.

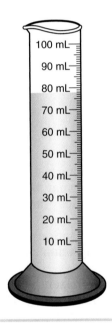

FIGURE 9-3 Graduated cylinder shows amount of water necessary (78 mL) for the reconstitution of the powder in Figure 9-2.

EXAMPLE 9-1

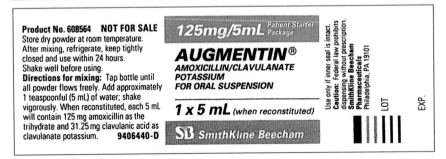

On the Augmentin label, the instructions state to add 1 teaspoon (approximately 5 mL) of water for a dose of 125 mg/5 mL. On this label, the difference or powder volume would be related to the approximate amount of water added. However, if the label is read as stated, Pv = 5 mL (Fv) – 5 mL (Dv) = 0 (Pv) or Pv = 0. This is not truly correct as the powder volume would be the difference found after adding the 5 mL of water. There is always a powder volume.

TECH NOTE

Be sure to calculate the total volume in container prior to calculating "Pv."

EXAMPLE 9-2

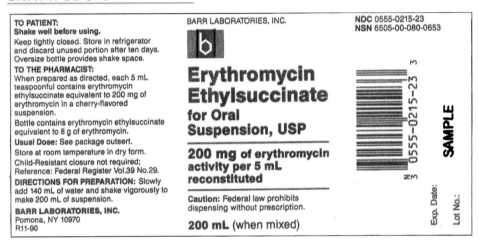

In this example, the bottle of erythromycin will contain 200 mL total (or final) volume with a dose strength of 250 mg/mL after reconstitution with 140 mL of distilled water (Dv).

$$Pv = 200\ mL\,(Fv) - 140\ mL\,(Dv)$$

$$Pv = 60\ mL$$

EXAMPLE 9-3

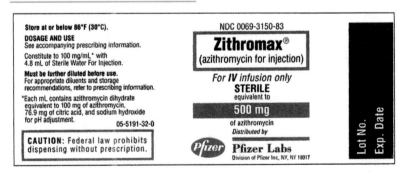

The label for Zithromax for injection shows a reconstituted strength of 100 mg/mL. The total dosage in the vial is 500 mg. Therefore the vial contains 5 mL after reconstitution. The directions for reconstitution state to add 4.8 mL of sterile water for injection.

$$Pv = 5\ mL\,(Fv) - 4.8\ mL\,(Dv)$$

$$Pv = 0.2\ mL$$

The total weight of the drug, as well as the total volume, are important when preparing the medication for dispensing when reconstitution is needed. The amount dispensed must be adequate to provide the dosage prescribed by the physician and must be in a volume appropriate for the ordered route of administration and the characteristics of the patient for whom the drug was ordered. The manufacturer determines the amount of diluent that should be added to each drug powder in the specific container for the desired dose. With oral medications, the container is usually sufficient for the usual volume of medication for the usual length of time the medication is prescribed, such as 10 to 14 days for antibiotics. However, in some instances, such as unavailability of drug in the needed dosage for the physician's order, it is not uncommon to partially fill a prescription with a smaller container and provide the remainder when the pharmacy obtains the balance of the needed supply. In other situations, a drug normally intended for pediatric use will be needed to provide adult dosing, and more than one bottle of the selected medication liquid may be needed to fill an entire adult prescription for the desired length of time.

TECH NOTE

Be aware that medications for intramuscular (IM) and intravenous (IV) use are not interchangeable. The label on the medication will give its exact use. Some medications will indicate that IM or IV use is acceptable but will usually show a difference in the amount of diluent to be added. Many medications for IV use may not be given directly from the vial, but require even further dilution in intravenous fluid prior to administration. Some medications are manufactured to be used for only one route of administration. As a pharmacy technician, you must read the product label closely to be sure the correct route as well as the correct medication and its concentration has been selected for the amount prescribed before reconstitution. Remember that after reconstitution, many of the medications have short expiration dates—some products even expire in hours, not days.

Practice Problems A

Calculate the powder volume using each of the labels that follow.

1.
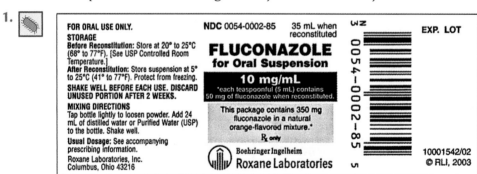

What is the powder volume for this medication? _____

2.
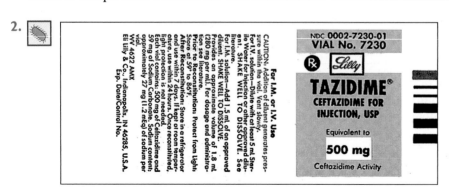

What is the powder volume for this medication given intramuscularly?

_____

3.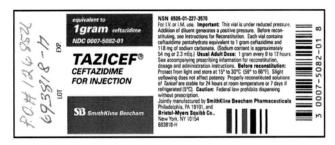

RECONSTITUTION

Single Dose Vials:

For I.M. injection, I.V. direct (bolus) injection, or I.V. infusion, reconstitute with Sterile Water for injection according to the following table. The vacuum may assist entry of the diluent. SHAKE WELL.

Table 5

Vial Size	Diluent to Be Added	Approx. Avail. Volume	Approx. Avg. Concentration
Intramuscular or Intravenous Direct (bolus) Injection			
1 gram	3.0 ml.	3.6 ml.	280 mg./ml.
Intravenous Infusion			
1 gram	10 ml.	10.6 ml.	95 mg./ml.
2 gram	10 ml.	11.2 ml.	180 mg./ml.

Withdraw the total volume of solution into the syringe (the pressure in the vial may aid withdrawal). The withdrawn solution may contain some bubbles of carbon dioxide.

NOTE: As with the administration of all parenteral products, accumulated gases should be expressed from the syringe immediately before injection of 'Tazicef'.

These solutions of 'Tazicef' are stable for 18 hours at room temperature or seven days if refrigerated (5∞C.). Slight yellowing does not affect potency.

For I.V. infusion, dilute reconstituted solution in 50 to 100 ml. of one of the parenteral fluids listed under COMPATIBILITY AND STABILITY.

What is the powder volume for intramuscular use? _____

What is the powder volume for intravenous infusion at 1 gm dosage?

_____

What is the powder volume for intravenous infusion at 2 gm dosage?

_____

4.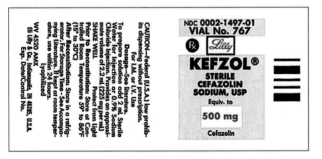

What is the powder volume of this medication? _____

Hint: Be sure to calculate total volume of medication first.

5.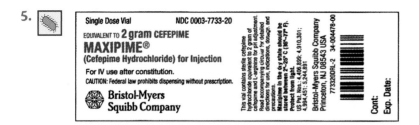

What is the powder volume for this medication? _____

Basic Principles of Reconstitution

Think of reconstitution as a means of mixing a powdered form of chocolate flavoring into a glass of milk. You have the powder and you add the milk (or the diluent) a little at a time to prevent the powder from clumping as the liquid is added. The same steps are used with the reconstitution of medication powders.

 TECH ALERT

Always remember to tap the vial or the bottle of medication to be reconstituted to loosen any medication that may be attached to the side of the container.

The most important step in reconstituting the powder is to read the label or package insert directions carefully because these provide the road map for correct reconstitution. The label tells you the total quantity of the drug in the container, the volume and type of diluent (usually in milliliters) to use for reconstitution, and the final strength (weight) or concentration of the medication following the reconstitution process. The information also includes the length of time the medication is stable and the storage needs following reconstitution. These directions must be read carefully and followed exactly each time a medication is reconstituted.

 TECH ALERT

Never assume the directions are the same as previously found on the same medication—READ the label directions every time medication is reconstituted.

TECH NOTE
- Never take for granted that you know the type and amount of diluent to be added to any medication.
- The amount of diluent will never equal the total volume of reconstituted medication because the powder occupies some space in the final volume of medication or powder volume.

The usual diluent for mixing a powder for an oral medication is either distilled water or, if different, as indicated by the manufacturer. The diluent with injectable medications may vary with each drug. Some injectable powders come with the diluent in two separate chambers, one for the powder and another for the diluent as with Solu-Medrol (methyl-prednisolone sodium succinate) or hydrocortisone sodium succinate (Figure 9-4). This system is called the Act-O-Vial system. In this case when the plunger is dislodged by pushing, the diluent drops from the upper chamber into the lower chamber which contains the powder. In other cases when a special diluent is necessary, this diluent may be packaged separately and supplied with the medication such as with some immunization agents. In these cases, finding the designated diluent is not necessary, because the manufacturer has included it.

In cases where the diluent is not supplied, reconstitution of the powder will use a diluent required by the manufacturer. With injectable medications the manufacturer may

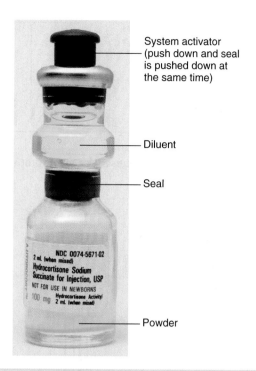

FIGURE 9-4 An Act-O-Vial.

choose to use either sterile water for injection or sterile normal saline. Some drugs may use bacteriostatic water for injection when used for IM injections. Some parenteral medications may even require the use of dextrose 5% in water for reconstitution. If the solution for reconstitution is not indicated, most medications can be mixed safely with sterile water. If the directions for reconstituting the medicine are not available, consult a drug reference.

Once the label has been read and the diluent of choice is known, the amount of diluent for the desired dosage must be verified. In single-dose vials, the amount of diluent will be one volume because a single dose will be given. In multidose vials, multiple instructions for different strengths following reconstitution may be possible and will be indicated on the label, each showing the amounts necessary for reconstituting to a particular strength (Figure 9-5). Read the possible concentrations or strengths following reconstitution, because typically the desired strength per volume should be the closest to the amount of the order and should also match the intended route of administration. Decide on the amount of diluent that will be added and prepare this for use. Remember that when adding diluent, the less fluid added to a specific container of medication, the more concentrated the medication—or "less is more" (Figure 9-6).

TECH NOTE

When reconstituting medications with multiple strengths possible, choose the strength closest to the physician's order or the strength that will provide a dose with the least chance for error.

After injecting diluent, the mixing process for an injectable medication should be accomplished by inverting the container slowly, unless otherwise specifically indicated by the manufacturer. Shaking the container may decrease the effectiveness of the medication and may also cause the liquid to foam. Foaming will prevent the correct amount of medication from being withdrawn for injection and may even prevent the medication from being drawn from the vial.

Be sure you know the length of time that the medication is stable and the directions for storage for both before and after the reconstitution. After the powder has been mixed,

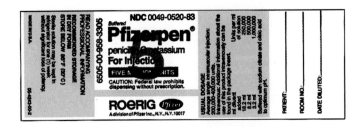

FIGURE 9-5 Label showing the volume of diluent necessary for reconstituting to a particular strength when multiple dosages are a possibility.

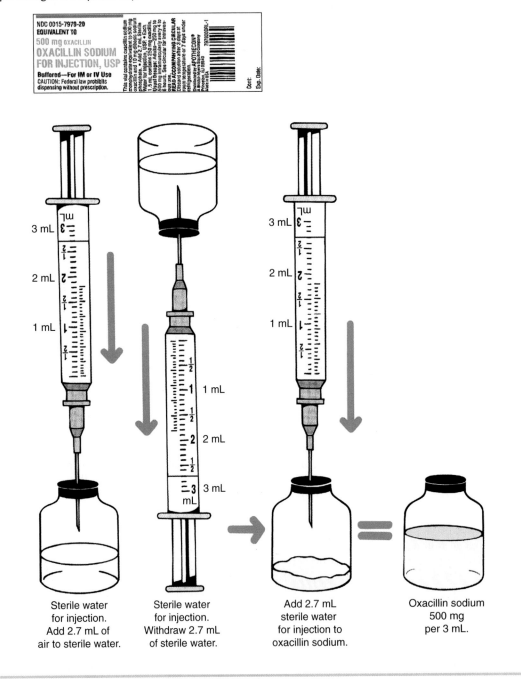

Sterile water for injection. Add 2.7 mL of air to sterile water.

Sterile water for injection. Withdraw 2.7 mL of sterile water.

Add 2.7 mL sterile water for injection to oxacillin sodium.

Oxacillin sodium 500 mg per 3 mL.

FIGURE 9-6 Diluting oxacillin sodium in sterile water for injection.

the person who did the reconstitution should add the following to the label if the container holds more than one dose and not all of the medication is used at time of reconstitution:

- His or her initials
- The date and time prepared
- The expiration date and time for injectable medications or length of time before expiration with oral medications
- The dose strength or final concentration after it has been mixed (e.g., 250 mg/5 mL) is important when preparing the medication dose for administration

Remember that the final volume of medication in the container will always be greater than the amount of diluent added because of powder volume. Thus the total volume prepared should always be checked to ensure there is an adequate amount for dispensing of the prescription or order; if not, be sure the correct medication strength has been chosen and reconstituted as required to meet the order. Usually the medication label also gives the total volume of medication after mixing according to indicated directions (e.g., see Figure 9-2, in which the label for Amoxil indicates the total amount of reconstituted medication is 100 mL).

TECH NOTE

Patient safety is of utmost importance and should be safeguarded throughout each step of handling medications, especially medications requiring reconstitution.

Practice Problems B

Answer the following questions and make necessary calculations as indicated.

1.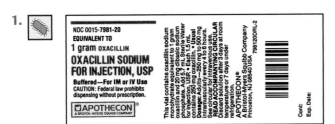

What is the total dosage of medication found in this container? _____

What volume of diluent is added to this medication for reconstitution? _____

What diluent is used for reconstitution? _____

What route(s) of administration is (are) appropriate for this vial of medication?

_____

What is the expiration time if this medication is stored at room temperature?

_____

What is the expiration time if this vial is stored under refrigeration? _____

What is the total volume of the vial of medication after reconstitution?

_____

What volume of medication is given for an order of 750 mg q6h IM? _____

How many vials of medication should be prepared for a 24-hour period? _____

What is the powder volume? _____

2.

NDC 0015-7339-99
NSN 6505-01-010-0832

Cefazolin for Injection, USP
1 gram

For IM or IV Use   **Rx only**

APOTHECON® PROTECT FROM LIGHT   10 SINGLE USE VIALS

PREPARATION OF SOLUTION: For IM Use - Add 2.5 mL Sterile Water for Injection. SHAKE WELL. Resulting solution provides an approximate volume of 3 mL (330 mg per mL).
For IV Use - See insert.
Discard unused solution 24 hours after reconstitution if stored at room temperature or within 10 days if stored under refrigeration, 2° to 8°C (36° to 46°F). Each vial contains cefazolin sodium equivalent to 1 gram cefazolin. The total sodium content is approximately 48mg (2.1 mEq sodium ion) per gram of cefazolin.
USUAL DOSAGE: 250 mg to 1 g every six to eight hours. See insert.
See package insert for detailed indications, IM or IV dosage and precautions.
Store dry powder at room temperature, 15° to 30°C (59° to 86°F).

What is the total dosage of medication in this vial? _____

What volume of diluent is added to this powder for IM administration? _____

What is the total volume in the vial following reconstitution? _____

What routes of administration can be used with this medication? _____

What is the medication strength per milliliter for IM route of administration?

_____

What diluent is used for reconstitution? _____

How many milliliters would the patient receive as a 500 mg dose? _____

If this medication is given at a dose of 500 mg at exactly the same time every day and the reconstituted medication is refrigerated, how many vials of medication would be necessary for 4 days? _____

What volume of medication is given if the dose is for 750 mg? _____

What is the powder volume? _____

3.

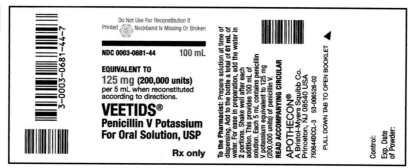

What is the total volume of medication after reconstitution? _____

What diluent is indicated to be added to powder for reconstitution?

_____

What volume of diluent is added to the powder? _____

Show the diluent volume on the graduate.

What special instructions are given for adding the diluent? _____

What is the metric strength of the solution in a dose after reconstitution? _____

What is the medication dose per 5 mL in units? _____

What volume of medication is necessary to provide 125 mg of medication? _____

What volume of medication in household measurements would be given for 62.5 mg? _____

How long would this medication last if 125 mg is given qid? _____

What is the powder volume? _____

4.

AUGMENTIN®
125mg/5mL

NSN 6505-01-340-0847
Directions for mixing:
Tap bottle until all powder flows freely.
Add approximately 2/3 of total water
for reconstitution (total = 67 mL);
shake vigorously to wet powder. Add
remaining water; again shake vigorously.
Dosage: See accompanying prescribing
information.

Keep tightly closed.
Shake well before using.
Must be refrigerated.
Discard after 10 days.

125mg/5mL
NDC 0029-6085-39

AUGMENTIN®
AMOXICILLIN/
CLAVULANATE POTASSIUM
FOR ORAL SUSPENSION
When reconstituted, each 5 mL contains:
AMOXICILLIN, 125 MG,
as the trihydrate
CLAVULANIC ACID, 31.25 MG,
as clavulanate potassium

75mL (when reconstituted)

SB SmithKline Beecham

LOT

EXP.

9405804-G

Use only if inner seal is intact.
Net contents: Equivalent to
1.875 g amoxicillin and
0.469 g clavulanic acid.
Store dry powder at room
temperature.
Caution: Federal law prohibits
dispensing without prescription.
SmithKline Beecham
Pharmaceuticals
Philadelphia, PA 19101

3 0029-6085-39 3

100 mL
90 mL
80 mL
70 mL
60 mL
50 mL
40 mL
30 mL
20 mL
10 mL

What two drugs are in this medication? _____

What diluent volume should be added? _____

On the graduate, show the volume of diluent to be added.

What special directions are necessary when adding the diluent? _____

On the label, what is the first direction necessary for reconstitution? _____

What is the total volume of medication available after reconstitution? _____

What is the volume of medication necessary for a dose of 250 mg? _____

What is the volume of a dose of medication given in household measurements?

_____

What instructions are given to the patient when dispensing? _____

What are the storage requirements prior to reconstitution? _____

What are the storage requirements after reconstitution? _____

How long is the reconstituted medication stable? _____

How many doses are available in this container if the child for whom it is prescribed receives 125 mg tid? _____

What is the powder volume? _____

5.

NDC 0049-1201-83

Cefobid®
(cefoperazone for injection)

equivalent to

1 g

of cefoperazone

Sterile
For IM or IV Use

Pfizer Roerig
Division of Pfizer Inc, NY, NY 10017

DOSAGE AND USE
See accompanying prescribing information.
RECOMMENDED STORAGE: Store at or below 25°C (77°F) and protect from light.
Before Reconstitution:
FOR IM USE: See "Preparation For Intramuscular Injection" in the RECONSTITUTION section of package insert.
FOR IV USE: First reconstitute with approximately 5 mL of a diluent given in the package insert. Withdraw the entire contents of the vial and further dilute with a recommended diluent.
For Intermittent Infusion: Dilute in 20 to 40 mL of diluent per gram and administer over a 15-30 minute time period.
For Continuous Infusion: Dilute to a final cefoperazone concentration range of 2 to 25 mg/mL.
After Reconstitution: Solutions may be stored for 24 hours at room temperature and under normal lighting conditions. See package insert for refrigerator and freezer storage. Discard solutions stored beyond recommended periods.

MADE IN USA

Rx only

PATIENT NAME
LOCATION
DATE PREPARED
TIME

05-4869-32-2

The instructions state 1.6 mL of diluent is used for IM use (1 gm = 2 mL).

What is the total medication dosage in the vial? _____

What diluent volume should be added to the vial for IM use? _____

How long is the medication stable after reconstitution? _____

What routes of administration may be used with this medication? _____

What volume of medication is given for an order for 0.5 g IM q12h? _____

Would one vial of medication be adequate for a single day? Explain your answer.

_____

How many vials of medication could be reconstituted at a time for a 5-day order?

_____

What is the powder volume of this medication? _____

6.   Order: Ampicillin 250 mg IM tid

NDC 0015-7404-20
NSN 6505-00-993-3518

EQUIVALENT TO
1 gram AMPICILLIN

**Ampicillin
for Injection, USP**
Formerly known as
Sterile Ampicillin Sodium, USP
For IM or IV Use
Rx only

For IM use, add 3.5 mL diluent (read accompanying insert). Resulting solution contains 250 mg ampicillin per mL.
Use solution within 1 hour.
This vial contains ampicillin sodium equivalent to 1 gram ampicillin.
Usual Dosage: Adults—250 to 500 mg IM q. 6h.
READ ACCOMPANYING INSERT for detailed indications, IM or IV dosage and precautions.

APOTHECON®
A Bristol-Myers Squibb Company
Princeton, NJ 08540 USA

7404230RL-3
34-001448-01

Cont:
Exp. Date:

What diluent volume is added to the container for IM use? _____

What is the dosage in the container? _____

What dosage of medication is found in 1.5 mL of reconstituted medication?

_____

How long would the medication be stable at room temperature? _____

How long would the medication be stable in the refrigerator? _____

What is the total number of vials of medication required for a day's supply for 250 mg tid? _____

What volume is given in a single dose? _____

How many vials of medication are necessary for a 2-day supply? _____

Can all of the medication for the day be reconstituted at the same time? _____
Explain your answer _____

What is the powder volume? _____

7.

NDC 0049-0530-83

Buffered

Pfizerpen ®

penicillin G potassium

For Injection

TWENTY MILLION UNITS **20**

FOR INTRAVENOUS INFUSION ONLY

CAUTION: Federal law prohibits dispensing without prescription.

ROERIG *Pfizer*

A division of Pfizer Inc. N.Y., N.Y. 10017

RECOMMENDED STORAGE IN DRY FORM STORE BELOW 86°F (30°C) Buffered with sodium citrate and citric acid to optimum pH. AFTER RECONSTITUTION, SOLUTION SHOULD BE REFRIGERATED. DISCARD UNUSED SOLUTION AFTER 7 DAYS. MADE IN U.S.A. 4

BULK PHARMACY PACKAGE READ ACCOMPANYING PROFESSIONAL INFORMATION USUAL DOSAGE 6 to 40 million units daily by intravenous infusion only Approx. units per ml of solution

ml diluent added	Approx. units per ml of solution
75 ml	250,000 u/ml
33 ml	500,000 u/ml
11.5 ml	1,000,000 u/ml

DATE/TIME PREPARED

BY

What is the total medication dosage found in the container? _____

If 75 mL of diluent is added to the container, what is the dosage per mL? _____

If 11.5 mL of diluent is added to the container, what is the dosage per mL?

_____

What is the route of administration for this medication? _____

What diluent is used to reconstitute this medication? _____

How long is the medication stable in the refrigerator after reconstitution? _____

If the medication is reconstituted to 250,000 units/mL, how many milliliters would be necessary for 375,000 units? _____

If reconstituted to 1,000,000 units/mL, how many milliliters would be necessary for 2,500,000 units? _____

What is the powder volume for 1,000,000 units/mL? _____

What is the powder volume for 250,000 units/mL? _____

What is the powder volume for 500,000 units/mL? _____

8.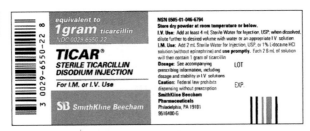

What is the total medication dosage in this vial? _____

What diluent volume is used for IM medications? _____

What diluent volume is used for IV medications? _____

How long is the medication stable if reconstituted for IM use? _____

What is the total volume of medication in the container after reconstitution for IM use? _____

What dose is necessary to supply 500 mg of medication IM? _____

How many vials are necessary to supply the medication if ordered 500 mg q8h IM for a day? _____

What is the powder volume when administered intramuscularly? _____

9.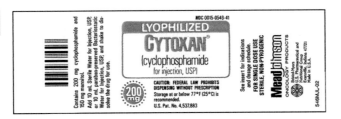

What is the total medication dosage in the vial? _____

What diluent is added to the vial? _____

What volume of diluent should be added to the vial? _____

How many doses are found in the vial? _____

10.

NDC 0002-5057-68
150 mL (When Mixed)   M-5057

Rx   *Lilly*

CECLOR®
CEFACLOR FOR
ORAL SUSPENSION, USP
125 mg
per 5 mL

CAUTION—Federal (USA) law
prohibits dispensing without
prescription.

0002-5057-68
PULL
N 3   4

150 mL CECLOR CEFACLOR FOR ORAL SUSPENSION, USP
125 mg per 5 mL
SHAKE WELL BEFORE USING
Control No.

Eli Lilly and Company
Indianapolis, IN 46285, USA
Expiration Date
WV 6465 AMX

Usual Dose—Pediatric patients, 20 mg per kg a day (40 mg per kg in otitis media) in three divided doses. Adults, 250 mg three times a day. See literature for complete dosage information.
Contains Cefaclor Monohydrate equivalent to 3.75 g anhydrous Cefaclor in a dry pleasantly flavored mixture.
Prior to Mixing, Store at Controlled Room Temperature 59° to 86°F (15° to 30°C).
Directions for Mixing—Add 90 mL of water in two portions to the dry mixture in the bottle. Shake well after each addition.
Each 5 mL (Approx. one teaspoonful) will then contain: Cefaclor Monohydrate equivalent to 125 mg anhydrous Cefaclor.

[graduated cylinder marked: 100 mL, 90 mL, 80 mL, 70 mL, 60 mL, 50 mL, 40 mL, 30 mL, 20 mL, 10 mL]

What is the total medication dosage in the bottle? _____

What diluent is used for reconstitution? _____

What diluent volume is added for reconstitution? _____

Show the amount of diluent on the graduate provided.

What special directions are necessary for reconstitution? _____

What is the medication strength after reconstitution? _____

Why is the container oversized? _____

What storage directions must be given to the patient? _____

How long can the medication be kept without loss of potency? _____

What is the total volume in the bottle after reconstitution? _____

What metric dose of medication would be in a teaspoonful? _____

How many total milliliters would be necessary for 375 mg/d? _____

How long would this container of medication last when given to the previous order?

_____

How long would the container of medication last if 250 mg bid were the order?

_____

What is the powder volume? _____

REVIEW

Reconstitution is necessary when a medication is unstable for storage in a liquid form. Most medications that need reconstitution come in powders, but some are in a crystalline form. When the medication will be used for injectable routes, the diluent may be sterile water for injection, bacteriostatic water for injection, 0.9% sodium chloride (normal saline) injectable, or a special solution provided with the medication by the manufacturer. If the medication is for oral use, distilled water is the common vehicle for reconstitution. After reconstitution, these medications require special storage because of the instability of the liquid medication. Some medications can be diluted to different strengths or concentrations as directed by the manufactures, whereas others have only one-strength dilution. Some drugs are found in single-dose vials for reconstitution, and others are found in multidose vials. Because of the variances in the reconstitution of these medications, their labels must be read closely by the pharmacy technician with each reconstitution so he or she can choose the correct diluent and the amount that will provide the nearest dosage to the physician's order for the route of administration. Always read labels of drugs for reconstitution; never assume that the label will be the same for the amount of diluent as previously prepared, because changes to product formulations may result in new directions for reconstitution.

Several steps are necessary in preparing reconstituted medications:

1. Read all of the directions on the medication label before starting the procedure.
2. Tap the bottle to loosen the powder in the bottle or vial.
3. Use the diluent that is designated by the manufacturer in the amount that is appropriate for the concentration or strength of medication necessary for the physician's order. If this information is not on the vial or bottle, use a drug reference for the appropriate diluent and amount.
4. After reconstitution of injectable label the medication with the initials of the person who reconstituted the medication, the date and time of reconstitution, the strength of the medication, and the expiration date and time for oral medications, be sure the time of expiration is excluded on the container label.
5. Remember that the final volume of the reconstituted powder will always be greater than the amount of diluent added because of the powder volume ($Pv = Fv - Dv$).

Posttest

Before taking the Posttest, retake the Pretest to check your understanding of the materials presented in this chapter. All dose measurements should be in a measurable volume, especially with injectable medications.

1.

NDC 0002-5136-18
75 mL (When Mixed)   M-5136

℞ Lilly

LORABID®
LORACARBEF
FOR ORAL
SUSPENSION, USP

200 mg
per 5 mL

CAUTION—Federal (USA)
law prohibits dispensing
without prescription.

0002-5136-18
PULL
N 3

75 mL   LORABID® LORACARBEF FOR ORAL SUSPENSION, USP
200 mg per 5 mL. Oversize bottle provides extra space for shaking. Store at room temperature (USP to 86°F). May be kept for 14 days without significant loss of potency. Keep Tightly Closed. Discard unused portion after 14 days.
SHAKE WELL BEFORE USING

WW 4581 AMX
Eli Lilly and Company
Indianapolis, IN 46285, USA

Control No.   Expiration Date

Usual Dose—Pediatric patients, 15 mg per kg per day (30 mg per kg per day). See literature for complete dosage information. Prior to Mixing, Store at Controlled Room Temperature 59° to 86°F (15° to 30°C).
Directions for Mixing—Add 45 mL of water in two portions to the dry mixture in the bottle. Shake well after each addition.
Contains Loracarbef equivalent to 3 g of activity in a dry pleasantly fla-vored mixture.
Each 5 mL (Approx. one teaspoonful) will then contain: Loracarbef equivalent to 200 mg of activity.

What is the total dosage of medication in the container? _____

What is used as the diluent for reconstitution? _____

What volume of diluent is added? _____ Show the volume of diluent on the graduate.

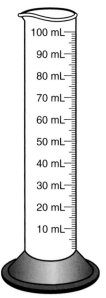

What is the medication concentration after reconstitution? _____

What volume of medication is necessary in the metric system to give 400 mg?

_____

What volume would 200 mg be in household measurements? _____

What are the storage requirements before reconstitution? _____

What are the storage requirements after reconstitution? _____

Posttest, cont.

How long is the medication potent after reconstitution? _____

What is the total volume in the container after reconstitution? _____

What is the route of administration of the medication? _____

How many total doses are in the container if 400 mg is given bid? _____

What is the powder volume? _____

2.

What is the total strength of medication in the vial? _____

If a physician orders a dose of 750 mg q6h, what volume of medication is given with each dose for IM use? _____

How many vials of medication would be given for a 24-hour supply of 750 mg q6h IM?

_____

Could all of the medication for the day be reconstituted at the same time? _____

Explain your answer using refrigeration as a guide. _____

_____

What volume of diluent is added to the powder for IM use? _____

What strength of medication would be found in 1 mL when reconstituted for IV use?

_____

What volume of diluent is added for IV use? _____

Continued

Posttest, cont.

3.

NDC 0015-7979-20
EQUIVALENT TO
500 mg OXACILLIN
OXACILLIN SODIUM
FOR INJECTION, USP
Buffered—For IM or IV Use
CAUTION: Federal law prohibits
dispensing without prescription.

What is the total strength of medication in the vial? _____

What is the strength of medication in each milliliter after reconstitution? _____

What volume of diluent is added for IM use? _____

How much medication would be found in 1.5 mL of medication? _____

If the physician orders oxacillin 750 mg IV q8h, how many vials of medication would be necessary in 1 day? _____

Could the entire day's supply be reconstituted at one time for this order? _____

Could a 3-day supply for a weekend be reconstituted on Friday? _____ Explain your answer. _____

How many milliliters of oxacillin are necessary to give 300 mg IM? _____

4. The physician orders Lorabid 200 mg po for a dose.

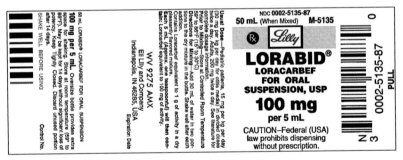

NDC 0002-5135-87
50 mL (When Mixed)   M-5135
Lilly
LORABID®
LORACARBEF
FOR ORAL
SUSPENSION, USP
100 mg
per 5 mL
CAUTION—Federal (USA)
law prohibits dispensing
without prescription.

0002-5135-87   PULL

How many milliliters of medication are administered for a dose? _____

What is the volume in household measurements? _____

What volume of diluent is added to the bottle of medication? _____ Show the volume of diluent that should be added on the appropriate graduate.

Posttest, cont.

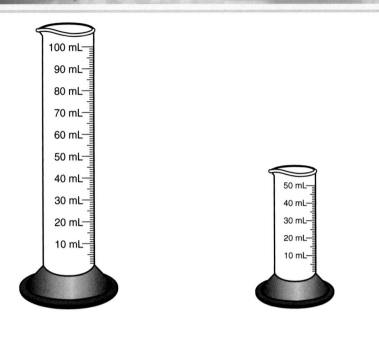

What diluent is used? _____

With the physician's order, how long would this medication last if it is given bid?

_____

How long is the medication stable after reconstitution? _____

What are the storage requirements after reconstitution? _____

What are the storage requirements before reconstitution? _____

How many bottle(s) of medication would be necessary for an order for 10 days if 200 mg is administered bid? _____

What is the powder volume? _____

Continued

Posttest, cont.

5.

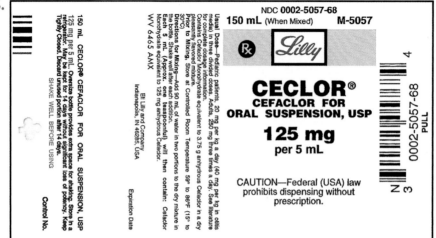

NDC 0002-5057-68
150 mL (When Mixed)   M-5057

℞   Lilly

CECLOR®
CEFACLOR FOR
ORAL SUSPENSION, USP
125 mg
per 5 mL

CAUTION—Federal (USA) law
prohibits dispensing without
prescription.

N 3 0002-5057-68 PULL 4

Usual Dose—Pediatric patients, 20 mg per kg a day (40 mg per kg in otitis media) in three divided doses. Adults, 250 mg three times a day. See literature for complete dosage information.
Contains Cefaclor Monohydrate equivalent to 3.75 g anhydrous Cefaclor in a dry pleasantly flavored mixture.
Prior to Mixing, Store at Controlled Room Temperature 59° to 86°F (15° to 30°C)
Directions for Mixing—Add 90 mL of water in two portions to the dry mixture in the bottle. Shake well after each addition.
Each 5 mL (Approx. one teaspoonful) will then contain: Cefaclor Monohydrate equivalent to 125 mg anhydrous Cefaclor.

Eli Lilly and Company
Indianapolis, IN 46285, USA

Expiration Date

150 mL CECLOR® CEFACLOR FOR ORAL SUSPENSION, USP
125 mg per 5 mL. Oversize bottle provides extra space for shaking. Store in a refrigerator. May be kept for 14 days without significant loss of potency. Keep Tightly Closed. Discard unused portion after 14 days.

SHAKE WELL BEFORE USING

WV 6465 AMX

Control No.

If a physician orders Ceclor 62.5 mg po for a child, what is the dose volume?

_____

What volume of diluent is added to this powder? _____ Show the volume of diluent on the appropriate graduate.

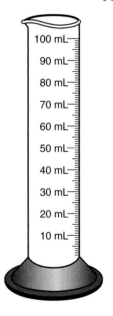

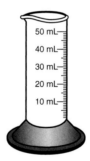

What volume of medication, in household units, would you tell the parent to give this child at home? _____

What are the specific directions for the reconstitution of this medication?

_____

Posttest, cont.

How long would the medication last if an adult receives Ceclor 250 mg tid?

_____

What are the storage requirements for this medication after reconstitution including the steps necessary to prepare the medication for administration? _____

What is the powder volume? _____

6.

Sterile
Streptomycin Sulfate, USP
Equivalent to 5.0 g of Streptomycin Base

5.0 g

FOR INTRAMUSCULAR USE ONLY

CAUTION: Federal law prohibits dispensing without prescription.

ROERIG *Pfizer*
A Division of Pfizer Inc., N.Y., N.Y. 10017

RECOMMENDED STORAGE
IN DRY FORM
STORE BELOW 86° F (30° C.)

Usual Daily Dosage
Adults: Varies with infection—
consult package insert.
Adult average single injection:
0.5 to 1.0 g
ml Diluent added
9.0 ml

mg/ml of Solution
400 mg/ml

The dry powder is dissolved by adding Water for Injection, USP or Sodium Chloride Injection, USP in an amount to yield the desired concentration.

PATIENT _____
ROOM NO. _____
DATE DILUTED _____

What is the total dosage in this vial? _____

What is the route of administration for this medication? _____

What volume of diluent is to be added to the medication? _____

If a physician orders streptomycin 500 mg daily to be given after dilution, what is the milliliter volume of medication in a dose? _____

How many days would this vial of medication last if the order is for a month?

_____

How long is the medication stable after reconstitution? _____

What is the powder volume? _____

Continued

Posttest, cont.

7. A physician orders Mandol 500 mg to be given qid in equal doses.

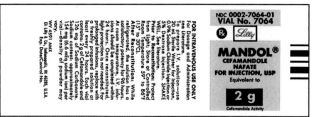

What volume of diluent is added to this vial of medication? _____

What diluent should be used for reconstitution? _____

What is the total strength of medication found in the vial after reconstitution?

_____

What is the route of administration for this medication? _____

What is the length of potency if medication is refrigerated after reconstitution?

_____

What is the length of potency if the medication is stored at room temperature?

_____

When used for this order, how many doses are found in the container? _____

8. A physician orders potassium phosphate 7.5 mM IV in 100 mL D-5-NS to be given today in previously ordered IV fluids.

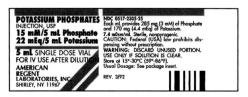

What is the total strength of potassium and phosphates in this vial of medication?

_____

What volume of medication is added to IV fluids to fulfill the physician's order?

_____

How should the unused portion of medication be stored? _____

How many total doses of medication are in the vial? _____

Posttest, cont.

9. A physician orders Tagamet 150 mg IV in D-5-W 100 mL q6h.

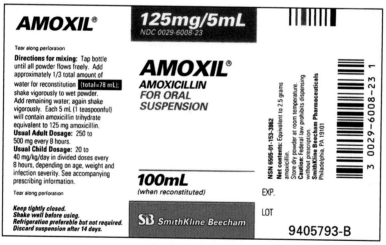

What is the total strength of medication, in grams, found in this vial? _____

How many milliliters of cimetidine HCl should be added to the fluids for the order?

_____

What routes of administration can be used to give the medication in the vial?

_____

What is the base fluid for the medication in the vial? _____

How should this medication be stored? _____

10.

What is the strength of this medication following reconstitution? _____

What diluent should be used for this medication? _____

What total volume of diluent should be added to the medication for reconstitution?

_____

Show the volume of diluent on the appropriate graduate.

Continued

Posttest, cont.

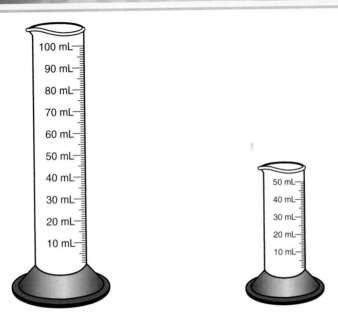

What volume of diluent should be used with the first addition for reconstitution?

_____

If the physician orders Amoxil 500 mg tid for an adult, how many milliliters of medication are administered with each dose?_____

If the medication dose is given tid, how many days would this bottle of medication

last? _____

How many containers of medication are necessary to fill an order for a 10-day supply? _____

What are the storage requirements for the medication after reconstitution?

_____

What is the powder volume? _____

REVIEW OF RULES

Reconstitution of Powdered Medications

- Before reconstituting any powdered medication for dispensing, carefully read all directions on the medication.

- Use the exact diluent designated by the manufacturer in the amount that is appropriate for the desired concentration or strength of medication. If this information is not available on the label, use a drug reference for the appropriate diluent and amount. Be sure that the diluent does not have an expiration date that falls before its use date.

- After reconstitution, label the medication with the initials of the person who did the reconstitution, the strength of the medication as reconstituted, and the expiration date and time for parenteral medications. For reconstituted oral medications, the length of time before expiration or the date of expiration should be noted.

- Remember that the volume of medication after reconstitution will always be greater than the diluent added because of powder volume.

- Powder volume may be calculated by subtracting diluent volume from the total or final volume ($Pv = Fv - Dv$).

SECTION IV
Special Medication Calculations

CHAPTER 10

Calculation of Medications for Special Populations Based on Body Weight and Patient Age

OBJECTIVES

- Calculate doses of medications for children and adults using body weight
- Calculate doses of medications for children using Clark's rule
- Calculate doses of medication for special populations based on body surface area
- Calculate doses of medication for infants using Fried's rule
- Calculate doses of medication for children using Young's rule

KEY WORDS

Adolescence From 13 through 17 years of age, some professionals consider to age 20

Body surface area (BSA) Means of calculating doses of medication on the basis of weight and height using a nomogram

Clark's rule Means of calculating a dose of medication for a child from an adult dose using as the basis the child's weight in pounds

Early childhood From 1 through 5 years of age

Fried's rule Means of calculating a dose of medication for an infant from an adult dose using the infant's age in months as the basis

Infant From age 1 month to 1 year

Late childhood From age 6 years through 12 years

Neonate From birth to 1 month

Nomogram A graph, diagram, or chart that shows a relationship between numerical variables, such as height and weight

Young's rule Means of calculating a dose of medication for a child based on the child's age

331

Pretest

Complete the following calculations for pediatric patients on the basis of age and body weight. The nomogram necessary for calculating some of these exercises can be found on p. 359. Show your calculations. Show your answers in tenths for strengths calculated for weights in the metric, apothecary or household system unless otherwise noted. Be sure your answer is a measurable dose for solids or volume measurements as appropriate unless otherwise noted.

1. The adult dose of amoxicillin is 500 mg tid.

   What is the dose for a child who is 2 years old? _____

2. The adult dose for Augmentin is 500 mg tid.

   How many mg per dose should be administered to a child who is 10 months old?

   _____

3. A child weighing 54 lb is to take phenobarbital. The physician orders 1 mg/kg tid.

   What is the dose to be given? _____

4. An 8-month-old infant is ordered Demerol following surgery. The normal adult dose is meperidine 50 mg.

   What dose should the infant receive? _____

Pretest, cont.

 5. A child weighs 55 lb and has an order for acetaminophen on the basis of body weight. The adult dose is 325 mg.

What is the dose for the child? _____

6. A child has an order for digoxin based on 8 mcg per kilogram of body weight. The child weighs 35 lb.

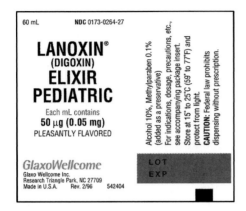

What is the exact volume dose (in hundredths) for the child using the label provided? _____

How many mcg of Lanoxin should be administered to the child? _____

What is the measurable volume of Lanoxin to be administered? _____

Continued

Pretest, cont.

7. An 8-year-old child is to receive phenobarbital, and the adult dose is phenobarbital gr s̄s̄.

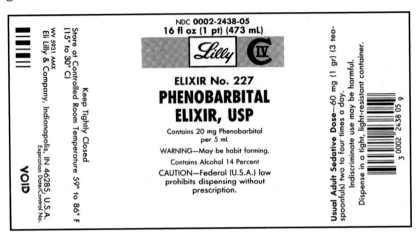

What would be the child's dose in the metric system? _____

If the phenobarbital available is the label shown, what volume of medication would the child receive? _____

Show the correct volume of medication to be provided on the measuring device.

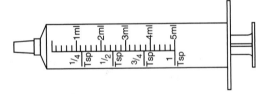

8. A physician orders Zantac syrup for a 10-month-old child. The adult dose is 150 mg bid.

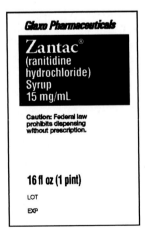

Pretest, cont.

What is the dose for the child? _____

What volume of medication should be given to the child using the label provided in hundredths? _____

What is the measurable dose? _____

Show the correct volume of medication to be provided on the measuring device.

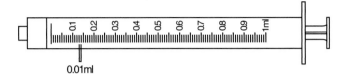

0.01ml

9. A child weighs 66 lb and is of normal height for weight. The physician orders Benadryl elixir to be given based on body surface area. The adult dose is 50 mg q8h prn.

N 0071-2220-17 ELIXIR **Benadryl**® (Diphenhydramine Hydrochloride Elixir, USP) Caution—Federal law prohibits dispensing without prescription. **4 FLUIDOUNCES** **PARKE-DAVIS** Div of Warner-Lambert Co Morris Plains, NJ 07950 USA	Elixir P-D 2220 for prescription dispensing only. **Contains**—12.5 mg diphenhydramine hydrochloride in each 5 mL. Alcohol, 14%. **Dose**—Adults, 2 to 4 teaspoonfuls; chil- dren over 20 lb, 1 to 2 teaspoonfuls; three or four times daily. See package insert. Keep this and all drugs out of the reach of children. **Store below 30°C (86°F). Protect from freezing and light.** Exp date and lot 2220G102

What is the measurable volume to be given using the provided label?

_____

What is the dose to be given in mg? _____

What is the dose in household measurements? _____

Continued

Pretest, cont.

10. A child 10 years old has bronchitis, and the physician orders Keflex suspension. The normal adult dose is 500 mg bid. Use age of the child and the normal adult dose as the basis for your answer.

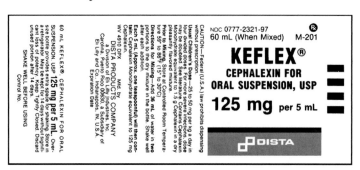

What dose should the child receive? _____

What volume of medication should be given if the label shown is used?

_____

What is the measurable dose? _____

11. A child age 5 years 4 months is ordered Colace syrup. The adult dose is Colace 100 mg hs.

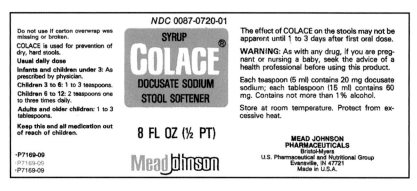

What is the dose for the child based on the child's age? _____

With the label shown, what is the volume of medication to be given?

_____

What is the measurable dose volume in household measurements?

_____

Is this an acceptable dose according to labeled manufacturer's dose?

_____

Pretest, cont.

12. A child weighs 88 lb, and the physician orders Compazine syrup 0.5 mg/kg tid.

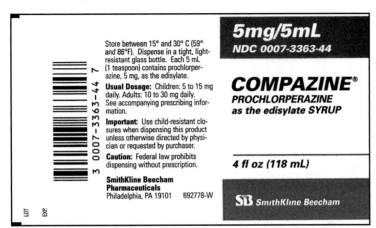

Store between 15° and 30° C (59° and 86°F). Dispense in a tight, light-resistant glass bottle. Each 5 mL (1 teaspoon) contains prochlorperazine, 5 mg, as the edisylate.

Usual Dosage: Children: 5 to 15 mg daily. Adults: 10 to 30 mg daily. See accompanying prescribing information.

Important: Use child-resistant closures when dispensing this product unless otherwise directed by physician or requested by purchaser.

Caution: Federal law prohibits dispensing without prescription.

SmithKline Beecham Pharmaceuticals
Philadelphia, PA 19101   692778-W

5mg/5mL
NDC 0007-3363-44

COMPAZINE®
PROCHLORPERAZINE
as the edisylate SYRUP

4 fl oz (118 mL)

SB SmithKline Beecham

What is the dose for the child based on body weight? _____

Using the measuring devices shown, what is the volume of medication to be administered per dose? _____

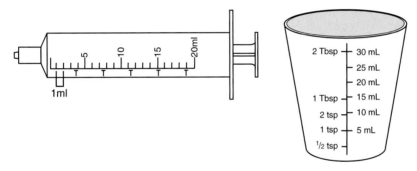

Pretest, cont.

13. A child weighs 84 lb. The physician orders Biaxin oral suspension 10 mg/kg bid in divided doses.

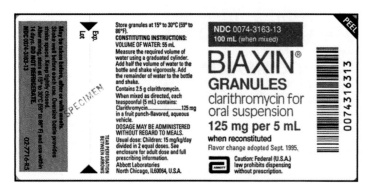

What is the dose of Biaxin for this child in hundredths? _____

Using the label given, what measurable volume of medication should be given to the child per dose? _____

Show the correct volume of medication to be provided on the measuring device.

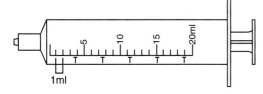

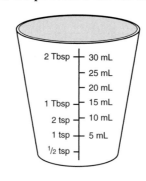

Pretest, cont.

14. A child weighs 56 lb and is 40″ tall. He has been diagnosed as having epilepsy. The physician orders Dilantin suspension for this child to be based on BSA. The normal adult dose is Dilantin 300 mg per day in three divided doses.

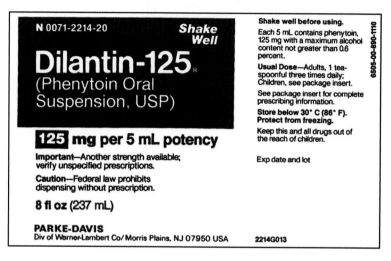

N 0071-2214-20   **Shake Well**

Dilantin-125 ®
(Phenytoin Oral Suspension, USP)

125 mg per 5 mL potency

Important—Another strength available; verify unspecified prescriptions.

Caution—Federal law prohibits dispensing without prescription.

8 fl oz (237 mL)

PARKE-DAVIS
Div of Warner-Lambert Co/ Morris Plains, NJ 07950 USA   2214G013

Shake well before using.
Each 5 mL contains phenytoin, 125 mg with a maximum alcohol content not greater than 0.6 percent.
Usual Dose—Adults, 1 tea-spoonful three times daily; Children, see package insert.
See package insert for complete prescribing information.
Store below 30° C (86° F). Protect from freezing.
Keep this and all drugs out of the reach of children.

Exp date and lot

6505-00-890-1110

What is the dose to be given for this child with each administration?

_____

What is the volume of medication to be given for this dose?

_____

Continued

Pretest, cont.

15. A 9-month-old child is to receive Dilantin according to the following label. The adult dose is Dilantin 100 mg.

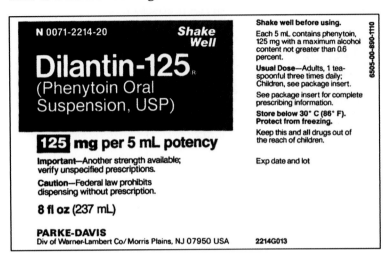

N 0071-2214-20   **Shake Well**

Dilantin-125 R
(Phenytoin Oral Suspension, USP)

125 mg per 5 mL potency

Important—Another strength available; verify unspecified prescriptions.

Caution—Federal law prohibits dispensing without prescription.

8 fl oz (237 mL)

PARKE-DAVIS
Div of Warner-Lambert Co/ Morris Plains, NJ 07950 USA   2214G013

Shake well before using.
Each 5 mL contains phenytoin, 125 mg with a maximum alcohol content not greater than 0.6 percent.
Usual Dose—Adults, 1 teaspoonful three times daily; Children, see package insert.
See package insert for complete prescribing information.
Store below 30° C (86° F). Protect from freezing.
Keep this and all drugs out of the reach of children.

Exp date and lot

6505-00-890-1110

What should be the dose for the infant? _____

What volume of medication should be administered? (Round to the nearest hundredth.) _____

What is the measurable dose to be administered? _____

Show the correct volume of medication to be provided on the measuring device.

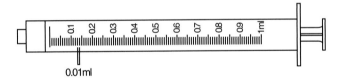

0.01ml

Pretest, cont.

 16. A child is 12 years old and is to receive Dilantin according to label A. The adult dose is Dilantin 200 mg qam.

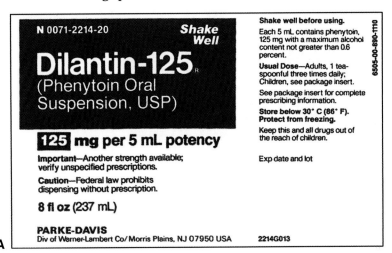

A

N 0071-2214-20   Shake Well

Dilantin-125ᴿ
(Phenytoin Oral Suspension, USP)

125 mg per 5 mL potency

Important—Another strength available; verify unspecified prescriptions.

Caution—Federal law prohibits dispensing without prescription.

8 fl oz (237 mL)

PARKE-DAVIS
Div of Warner-Lambert Co/ Morris Plains, NJ 07950 USA   2214G013

Shake well before using.

Each 5 mL contains phenytoin, 125 mg with a maximum alcohol content not greater than 0.6 percent.

Usual Dose—Adults, 1 teaspoonful three times daily; Children, see package insert.

See package insert for complete prescribing information.

Store below 30° C (86° F). Protect from freezing.

Keep this and all drugs out of the reach of children.

Exp date and lot

6505-00-890-1110

B

Pediatric Dose—
Initially, 5 mg/kg daily in two or three equally divided doses, with subsequent dosage individualized to a maximum of 300 mg daily.

See package insert for complete prescribing information.

Keep this and all drugs out of the reach of children.

0365G041

N 0071-0365-24

KAPSEALS®
Dilantin®
(Extended Phenytoin Sodium Capsules, USP)

30 mg

Caution—Federal law prohibits dispensing without prescription.

100 CAPSULES

PARKE-DAVIS
Div of Warner-Lambert Co
Morris Plains, NJ 07950 USA

Dispense in tight, light-resistant container as defined in the USP.

Store below 30°C (86°F). Protect from light and moisture.

NOTE TO PHARMACIST—Do not dispense capsules which are discolored.

Exp date and lot

What should be the dose for this child based on the adult dose? _____

What volume of medication should be administered to the child? _____

Using the dosage calculated, what dose should be approximated in the solid form of medication given in label B? _____ Explain your decision on the dose of solid medication to be administered. _____

Show the correct volume of medication to be provided on the measuring device.

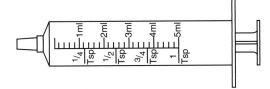

Continued

Pretest, cont.

17. A child weighing 75 lb has otitis media. The physician orders Keflex to be given tid.

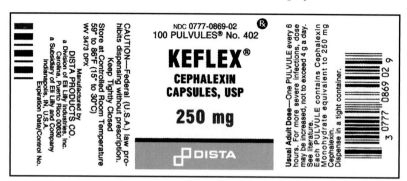

What is the dose to be administered if the adult dose is 500 mg/dose?

_____

Using the label, how many capsules should be given to the child with each dose?

_____

18. A child weighing 45 lb has been prescribed Lorabid 15 mg/kg/day in divided doses bid.

Round to the whole number for the total dosage per day.

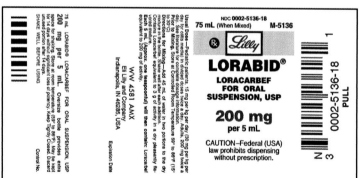

What is the strength of each dose for administration to the child using the Lorabid label shown? _____

What is the measurable volume of each dose of medication for administration?

_____

What is the total dosage of Lorabid to be given in a day? _____

Pretest, cont.

19. A child weighing 33 lb has an order for Epivir bid. The adult dose is Epivir 150 mg bid.

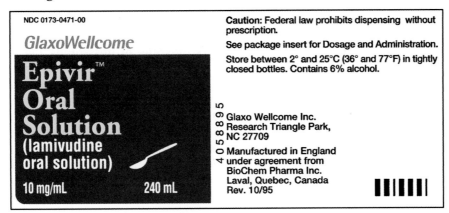

NDC 0173-0471-00

GlaxoWellcome

Epivir™ Oral Solution
(lamivudine oral solution)

10 mg/mL   240 mL

Caution: Federal law prohibits dispensing without prescription.

See package insert for Dosage and Administration.

Store between 2° and 25°C (36° and 77°F) in tightly closed bottles. Contains 6% alcohol.

59885045

Glaxo Wellcome Inc.
Research Triangle Park,
NC 27709

Manufactured in England under agreement from BioChem Pharma Inc.
Laval, Quebec, Canada
Rev. 10/95

What should be the strength per dose for the child aged 1½ years?

_____

Using the label shown, what volume of the medication should be given with each dose? _____

What measuring device could be used to best supply this amount of medication to a child of this age? _____

20. An 8-year-old child is being treated for a urinary tract infection. The usual adult dose for Furadantin is 100 mg.

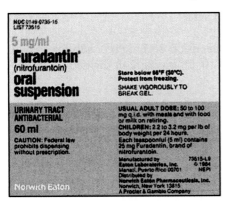

NDC 0149-0735-15
LIST 73515

5 mg/ml

Furadantin®
(nitrofurantoin)
oral suspension

URINARY TRACT ANTIBACTERIAL

60 ml

CAUTION: Federal law prohibits dispensing without prescription.

Norwich Eaton

Store below 86°F (30°C).
Protect from freezing.
SHAKE VIGOROUSLY TO BREAK GEL.

USUAL ADULT DOSE: 50 to 100 mg q.i.d. with meals and with food or milk on retiring.
CHILDREN: 2.2 to 3.2 mg per lb of body weight per 24 hours.
Each teaspoonful (5 ml) contains 25 mg Furadantin, brand of nitrofurantoin.

Manufactured by
Eaton Laboratories, Inc.   73515-L9
Manati, Puerto Rico 00701   © 1984 NEPI
Distributed by
Norwich Eaton Pharmaceuticals, Inc.
Norwich, New York 13815
A Procter & Gamble Company

What is the strength of the dose for the child? _____

What is the volume of medication that should be administered to the child?

_____

Show the correct volume of medication to be provided on the measuring device.

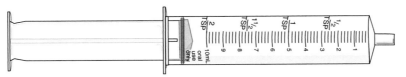

INTRODUCTION

Children are not small adults but rather distinct individuals who have different medication absorption, distribution, metabolism, and excretion rates compared with adults. The growth and development of the child, or the focus of the field of pediatrics, significantly affect the prescription for medication for the child. Pediatric patients include **neonates** or newborns—from birth to 1 month; **infants**—from 1 month to 1 year; **early childhood**—from age 1 to 5 years; **late childhood**—from age 6 to 12 years; and **adolescence**—from age 13 through 17 years or 20 years by some professionals. Geriatric persons also have differences in pharmacokinetics—drug absorption, metabolism, and excretion—thus requiring recalculation of drug dosages for many drugs. With toxic medications such as chemotherapeutics, even non-elderly adults with normal organ function may require use of **body surface area** (BSA) based on height and weight for drug calculations. Patients who have excessively low body weight or muscle mass (e.g., emaciated) or those who are obese may also require dose adjustments for some medications. Individuals with renal or liver dysfunction, whether adults or children, often also require dose adjustments of medications. All of these groups are considered special populations because of the need for special dosage calculations. These calculations may be based on height, weight, and overall physical condition for determining prescribed doses and dosages of a drug. Although as pharmacy technicians you will not be personally responsible for the calculation of the amount of medication to be given to these persons, you do need to understand how such determinations are made.

In these cases, the dose of the prescribed medication takes into account BSA which is based on patient height and weight relative to a typical adult. Remember that most usual dosages are provided in adult standards, so the dose for special populations must be altered to meet the patient's needs according to age and/or body weight/height.

> ### ! TECH ALERT
>
> Remember that if the manufacturer provides a pediatric dose/dosage for a medication, the dose/dosage indicated by the manufacturer should be used. Under these conditions, the dose/dosage does not need to be calculated using BSA or any of the specific rules for estimating dosage. If a physician's prescription does not agree with the manufacturer's indication, the physician should be consulted by the pharmacist.

CALCULATING MEDICATION DOSES BY BODY WEIGHT

Pediatric doses of medications may be calculated by using body weight or body mass. One method of calculation uses micrograms, milligrams, or grams of drug per kilogram of body weight. The formula therefore appears as mg (g or mcg)/kg. With this in mind, the child must be weighed with each visit to the hospital or physician's office to be sure the correct amount of medication can be ordered. Because most physician's office scales weigh in pounds, pounds must first be converted to kilograms before calculating the dose to be given.

To convert pounds to kilograms, 2.2 lb = 1 kg is the basis for the conversion. So to convert pounds to kilograms, the number of pounds is divided by 2.2 (or number of lb ÷ 2.2). For ratio and proportion, the formula is as follows for a child who weighs 22 lb:

$$2.2 \text{ lb} : 1 \text{ kg} :: 22 \text{ lb} : x$$

$$2.2 \text{ lb} : 1 \text{ kg} :: 22 \text{ lb} : x$$

$$2.2 \times x = 22 \times 1 \text{ kg} \quad \text{or} \quad 2.2x = 22 \text{ kg}$$

$$x = 22 \text{ kg} \div 2.2$$
$$x = 10 \text{ kg}$$

If an infant is weighed in pounds and ounces, the ounces must be converted to pounds. For example, an infant weighs 18 lb 4 oz. The first step in calculation is to convert ounces to pounds using 16 oz to 1 lb.

$$16 \text{ oz} : 1 \text{ lb} :: 4 \text{ oz} : x$$

Again, ounces may be canceled and the means and extremes multiplied or

$$16x = 4 \times 1 \text{ lb}$$

$$x = 4 \div 16 \quad \text{or} \quad 4\frac{4}{16} \text{ or } \frac{1}{4} \text{ lb} \quad (1.00 \div 4)$$

$$x = 0.25 \text{ lb or } 4 \text{ oz} = 0.25 \text{ lb}$$

Now convert total weight to kilograms for the child weighing 18.25 lb.

$$2.2 \text{ lb} : 1 \text{ kg} :: 18.25 \text{ lb} : x \text{ kg}$$

$$2.2x = 18.25 \text{ kg}$$

$$x = 18.25 \div 2.2$$

$$x = 8.3 \text{ kg}$$

Therefore kilograms used for calculating amount of medication for a child weighing 18 lb 4 oz would be 8.3 kg or 8 kg, depending on the policy of the place of employment and the desires of the prescriber.

Practice Problems A

Calculate the following problems and round to the nearest hundredth kilogram. Show all of your calculations.

1. A child weighs 65 lb; what is the weight in kilograms? _____

2. An infant weighs 8 lb 12 oz; what is the weight in kilograms? _____

3. A child weighs 75 lb; what is the weight in kilograms? _____

4. A child weighs 112 lb; what is the weight in kilograms? _____

5. A child weighs 48 lb; what is the weight in kilograms? _____

6. A child weighs 33 lb; what is the weight in kilograms? _____

7. An infant weighs 13 lb 6 oz; what is the weight in kilograms? _____

8. A child weighs 26 lb; what is the weight in kilograms? _____

9. A child weighs 56 lb; what is the weight in kilograms? _____

10. A child weighs 84 lb; what is the weight in kilograms? _____

After you have calculated the pounds to kilograms, the next step is to place number of kilograms into the expression "mg/kg," using the physician's order for the strength of the medication to be given. You may find that the physician may place the number of times per day or the amount per day that the medication is to be administered into the equation.

TECH NOTE

The "/" in the formula "mg/kg/dose" or "mg/kg/times a day" is the same as having a multiplication signs (×). Therefore the formula would read "mg × kg × dose" [(mg)(kg)(dose)] or "mg × kg × times a day" [(mg)(kg)(times a day)].

TECH NOTE

In the formula, substitute the "knowns" of milligrams provided by the physician's order and kilograms that are calculated from the patient's weight, and then multiply as indicated by "/".

The steps for calculating mg/kg are as follows:

1. Obtain the weight of the patient, and calculate that weight into kilograms.
2. Read the physician's order for the strength or weight of the medication that is to be provided to the patient.
3. Complete the calculation of medication of "mg/kg" by multiplying.
4. After obtaining the dose of medication to be administered, use the ratio and proportion, dimensional analysis, or formula method to calculate the dose in either solid tablets or capsules or volume of liquid medication as shown in Chapters 7 and 8. If the medication needs reconstitution, use the knowledge from Chapter 9 to reconstitute the medication.

Examples of the calculation of medication for children using medication strength (mg)/ body weight (kg) follow.

EXAMPLE 10-1

A child who has been diagnosed with epilepsy weighs 53 lb. The physician orders Dilantin 30 mg Kapseals to be given at 2.5 mg/kg/dose. What dose of the medication should be given to this child? _____

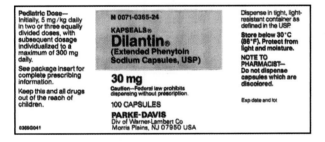

First you need to change pounds to kilograms:

$$2.2 \text{ lb} : 1 \text{ kg} :: 53 \text{ lb} : x$$

$$2.2 : 1 \text{ kg} :: 53 : x \quad \text{or} \quad \frac{2.2}{1} \bowtie \frac{53}{x}$$

$$2.2x = 53 \times 1 \text{ kg} \quad \text{or} \quad x = 53 \text{ kg} \div 2.2$$

$$x = 24.1 \text{ kg}$$

Now place the number of kilograms into the formula mg/kg, using the physician's order of 2.5 mg as the desired dose strength. The formula is then 2.5 mg/24.1 kg/1dose or (2.5 × 24.1 × 1), or 60.25 mg/dose. This weight of medication should be rounded to 60 mg as the amount of medication to be administered with each dose.

Now that you know the amount of medication to be administered is 60 mg, use the dimensional analysis, ratio and proportion, or formula method to calculate the desired dose of medication in a measurable dose. In this instance the calculation is by formula method, and the answer will be rounded to hundredths as would be found in most clinical situations.

$$\frac{60.25 \text{ mg (DD)}}{30 \text{ mg (DA)}} \times 1 \text{ Kapseal (Qty)} = DG$$

$$\frac{60.25 \text{ mg} \times 1 \text{ Kapseal}}{30 \text{ mg}} = DG \quad \frac{60.25 \text{ kap}}{30} = DG$$

DG = 2.01 Kapseals (The answer found was 2.008 Kapseals
when rounded to hundredths.)

Therefore the child should be administered 2 Kapseals with each dose of medication because this is the measurable dose as capsules (Kapseals) cannot be divided.

EXAMPLE 10-2

A physician orders amoxicillin 20 mg/kg/day to be given q8h to a child who weighs 42 lb. The concentration of amoxicillin is 125 mg/mL. What would be the dosage for the day? _____

What would be the strength of each dose? _____

What amount or volume of medication should be given as a dose? _____

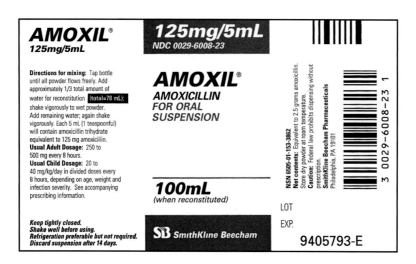

First convert the pounds to kilograms and round to the nearest kilogram.

2.2 lb : 1 kg :: 42 lb : x

2.2x = 42 kg   or x = 42 kg ÷ 2.2

x = 19.09

Now place the weight in kilograms into the formula for calculating the dosage of medication to be given in a day.

The dosage for the day would be 20 mg × 19.09 kg × 1 day = 381.8 mg/day.

The next step is to take the total amount of medication for the day and divide it by the number of doses to be given in a day. In this problem, a dose every 8 hours calculates to 3 doses daily (24 hours/day ÷ q8h = 3 doses/day).

The dose to be administered in strength would be 381.8 mg ÷ 3 doses = 127.27 mg/dose when rounded to the nearest hundredth.

The last step is to calculate the amount of medication related to the label on the available medication strength. The available medication is 125 mg/5 mL, so the 127.27 mg is the dose to be used.

$$\frac{127.27 \text{ mg (DD)}}{125 \text{ mg (DA)}} \times 5 \text{ mL (Qty)} = \text{Dose to be given (DG)}$$

$$\frac{127.27 \text{ mg}}{125 \text{ mg}} \times 5 \text{ mL} = \text{DG} \quad \text{or} \quad \frac{127.27}{125} \times 5 \text{ mL} = \text{DG}$$

DG = 5.09 mL per dose or 5.1 mL. In many cases, the measurable quantity will be 5 mL when using dose syringes or household measurements as the dose syringe is divided into 0.2 mL increments.

If you need to review the mathematical calculations for doses of liquid medications, refer to Chapter 8. If the medication is in a solid form, review Chapter 7 as needed.

If dimensional analysis is the preferred method for this calculation, one equation may be used to obtain the answer. Remember that with dimensional analysis, the final answer is the dose to be given.

EXAMPLE 10-3

A physician orders amoxicillin 20 mg/kg/day to be given q8h to a child who weighs 42 lb. The dosage strength of amoxicillin is as shown above at 125 mg/mL. (The q8h would be a 3-times-a-day dosage—therefore the use of 3 doses in the formula.)

What amount or what volume of medication would be given as a dose in household measurements?

$$\frac{42 \text{ lb}}{\text{DD}} \times \frac{1 \text{ kg}}{2.2 \text{ lb}} \times \frac{20 \text{ mg}}{\text{kg/day}} \times \frac{\text{day}}{3 \text{ dose}} \times \frac{5 \text{ mL}}{125 \text{ mg}} \times \frac{1 \text{ tsp}}{5 \text{ mL}} = \text{DG}$$

$$\frac{42 \text{ lb}}{\text{DD}} \times \frac{1 \text{ kg}}{2.2 \text{ lb}} \times \frac{20 \text{ mg}}{\text{kg/day}} \times \frac{\text{day}}{3 \text{ dose}} \times \frac{5 \text{ mL}}{125 \text{ mg}} \times \frac{1 \text{ tsp}}{5 \text{ mL}} = \text{DG}$$

$$\frac{42 \times 1 \times 20 \times 1 \times 5 \times 1 \text{ tsp}}{2.2 \times 1 \times 3 \times 125 \times 5 \text{ dose}} = \text{DG}$$

$$\frac{4200 \text{ tsp}}{4125 \text{ dose}} \quad \text{OR} \quad \frac{1.02 \text{ tsp}}{\text{dose}}$$

The dose answer rounded to hundredths, or 1.02, tsp should again be rounded to 1 tsp/dose because 1.02 tsp cannot be measured in any available oral medication dispensing device.

USE OF CLARK'S RULE FOR PEDIATRIC DOSAGE

The other method used for calculating pediatric dosage based on child's body weight or mass is **Clark's rule**. Although you may never use the following means of calculating a pediatric dose of medication, you should be familiar with its indications. With Clark's rule, as with others for children's dosages, the assumption is that the average adult weighs approximately 150 lb and that the adult dose indicated by the manufacturer is calculated on that adult weight. Because studies of body weight of the average adult have shown that the average adult now weighs more than 150 lb, Clark's rule is being phased out as the means for calculating pediatric doses.

Clark's rule:

$$\text{Child's dose} = \frac{\text{Child's weight in pounds}}{150} \times \text{Adult dose}$$

OR if weight in kilograms is to be used, the calculation formula would be

$$\text{Child's dose} = \frac{\text{Child's weight in kg}}{75} \times \text{Adult dose}$$

EXAMPLE 10-4

Now calculate a problem using Clark's rule in pounds.

A physician orders Cefzil for a child with an upper respiratory infection who weighs 38 lb. The adult dose for Cefzil is 500 mg q24h.

Using Clark's rule, the following equation would be appropriate:

$$\text{Child's dose} = \frac{38 \text{ lb (Child's weight)}}{150 \text{ (assumed pounds)}} \times 500 \text{ mg (Adult dose)}$$

$$\text{Child's dose} = \frac{38 \cancel{\text{ lb}} \times 50\cancel{0} \text{ mg}}{15\cancel{0}} \quad \text{or} \quad \frac{1900 \text{ mg}}{15} = 126.67 \text{ mg}$$

Now take the ratio and proportion, dimensional analysis, or formula method to calculate the dose necessary for the child. In this problem the ratio and proportion method is used.

125 mg (DA) : 5 mL (DF) :: 126.67 mg (DO) : Dose to be given (DG)

125 mg : 5 mL :: 126.67 mg : DG

125 DG = 126.67 × 5 mL   or   125 DG = 633.35 mL

$$DG = \frac{633.35 \text{ mL}}{125} = 5.07 \text{ mL}$$

Dose to be given = 5.07 or 5.1 mL as the dose when rounded to tenths.
In most cases the measurable dose will be 5 mL because a dosage syringe in tenths of mL is not as available. A 5 mL dosage syringe is in 0.2 mL increments.

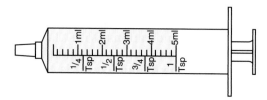

NOTE: Remember that this may be expressed in fractional units as follows and that cross-multiplication is necessary if this form of calculation is used:

$$\frac{125 \text{ mg (DA)}}{5 \text{ mL (DF)}} \overset{\nearrow}{\underset{\searrow}{\times}} \frac{126.67 \text{ mg (DO)}}{\text{Dose to be given (DG)}}$$

The child's dose to be given is 5.1 mL.

Now use Clark's rule using kilograms.

EXAMPLE 10-5

 A physician orders Amoxicillin tid for a child who weighs 20 kg. The adult dose is 500 mg tid. The available medication is 125 mg/5 mL.

$$\text{Child's dose} = \frac{20 \text{ kg (Child's weight)}}{75} \times 500 \text{ mg (Adult dose)}$$

Child's dose = 133.33 mg when rounded to the hundredth

Now using ratio and proportion figure the dose to be given.

125 mg (DA) : 5 mL (DF) :: 133.33 mg (DO) : Dose to be given (DG)

125 DG = 133.33 × 5 mL (666.65 mL)

DG = 5.33 mL when rounded to hundredth

Practice Problems B

In this chapter and subsequent chapters the practice problems are written with the desired medication and the necessary information for the pertinent calculation. When converting pounds to kilograms, you should round the answer to the nearest kilogram for ease in calculating the dosage and doses. Because Clark's rule is not a practice performed by pharmacy technicians, only a limited number of problems are included in the practice problems for you to gain understanding of the process for medication calculations using this rule. The calculation should be for a single dose unless otherwise stated in the question. This calculation should be rounded to tenth. Round all calculations to a measurable dose for the measuring device to be used in the final step of dose to be given. Show all of your calculations. Use a calculator as permitted by the instructor.

1. A physician orders Veetids 10 mg/kg q8h for a child who weighs 55 lb. The medication dosage is 250 mg/5 mL.

    What is the dosage strength for the child for the entire day? _____

    What is the strength of the medication for the child for a dose? _____

    What volume of medication should be given with each dose? _____

    Indicate the amount of medication to be administered on the following measuring devices.

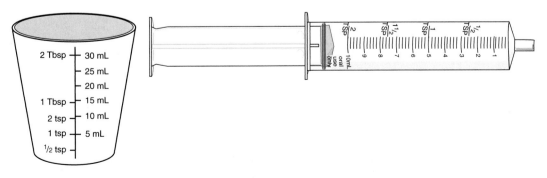

2. A physician orders Zithromax suspension 10 mg/kg per day as an initial dose for a child who weighs 44 lb with acute bronchitis. The medication dosage available is 200 mg/5 mL.

What is the dose strength for the child? _____

What is the volume of medication to be given to the child with this dose?

_____

What is the dosage for the child for this day? _____

Indicate the amount of medication to be administered on the following measuring devices.

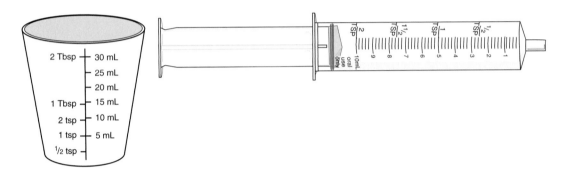

3. A physician orders Zyrtec syrup 0.1 mg/kg daily for a child with allergies who weighs 55 lb. The medication is available in 5 mg/5 mL.

What dosage strength is ordered for the child? _____

What volume of medication in the metric system should be given to the child with each dose? _____

What volume of medication in the household measurement system should be given to the child with each dose? _____

Indicate the amount of medication to be administered on the following measuring devices.

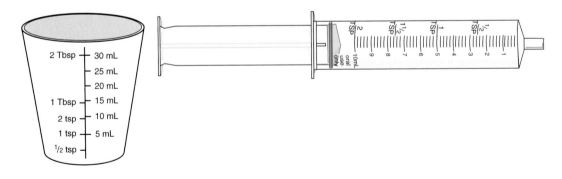

4. A physician orders Benylin syrup for a child weighing 30 lb. The normal adult dose of Benylin is 20 mg q6h. The medication on hand is Benylin syrup 15 mg/5 mL.

What is the dose strength for this child? _____

What is the volume of each dose of medication to be given in the metric system?

_____

What is the volume of each dose of medication in the household measurements?

_____

Indicate the amount of medication in household measurements on the dose syringe to provide the nearest correct dose for the child.

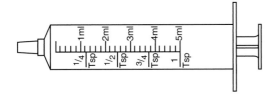

5. A physician orders Zarontin syrup 20 mg/kg/day given in divided doses bid for a child who has been diagnosed with seizures. The child weighs 54 lb. The medication available is Zarontin syrup 250 mg/5 mL.

What is the total strength of medication to be given in a day? _____

What is the strength of medication to be administered as a single dose?

_____

What is the volume of medication to be given to the child as a dose?

_____

Show the dose to be given to the child using the measuring device shown.

6. A physician orders sulfamethoxazole/trimethoprim suspension 8 mg/kg/day in divided doses q12h for a child with a urinary tract infection and otitis media. The child weighs 75 lb. The available medication is sulfamethoxazole 200 mg/ trimethoprim 40 mg/5 mL.

Hint: Calculate dosage on the strength of trimethoprim.

What is the total dosage of medication to be given to the child in a day?

_____

What strength of the medication should be given in a dose? _____

What volume of suspension should the child take with each dose?

_____

What is the dose in household measurements? _____

7. A physician orders digoxin elixir 8 mcg/kg/day for a child. The child weighs 55 lb. The available medication is 50 mcg/mL.

What is the dose strength of the medication for the child? _____

What volume of medication for a dose should be given to this child?

_____

Indicate the amount of medication to be administered on the correct measuring device.

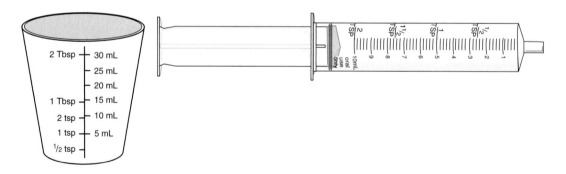

8. A child is prescribed Biaxin suspension for acute sinusitis. The child weighs 60 lb. The adult dose of Biaxin is 1 g daily, in divided doses bid. The medication available is 125 mg/5 mL.

What dose strength of medication should be given to the child? _____

What volume of medication should be given to the child? _____

9. [PA IN] A child has an order for meperidine syrup 1 mg/kg per dose for postoperative pain. The child weighs 88 lb. The medication available is meperidine 50 mg/5 mL.

What strength for each dose to be given to the child? _____

What volume of medication should be administered with each dose to this child?

_____

Indicate the amount of medication to be administered on the correct measuring device.

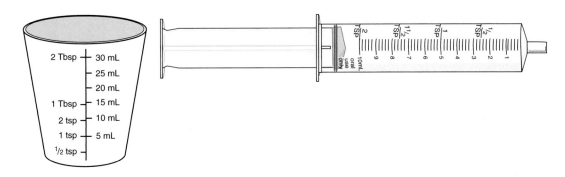

10. [PA IN] A physician wants a child who has a high fever and weighs 24 lb to have acetaminophen elixir gr s̄s̄ per kg q8h prn high fever and aching. The medication available is acetaminophen 325 mg/5 mL.

Hint: Be sure to do the conversions as needed to complete the problem.

What strength of medication should be given with each dose? _____

What volume of medication should be given with each dose? _____

11. [lungs icon] A physician orders diphenhydramine elixir q4h for a child who weighs 62 lb. The usual adult dose is 25 mg q4h. The available medication is diphenhydramine elixir 12.5 mg/5 mL.

What is the dose strength for the child? _____

What is the volume of medication to be given to the child? _____

Indicate the amount of medication to be administered on the correct measuring device.

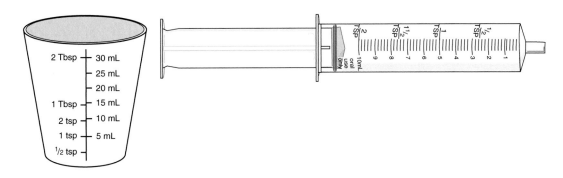

12. ▨ A physician orders erythromycin 10 mg/kg/q6h. The patient, a child who has cellulitis of the leg, weighs 88 lb. Available is erythromycin suspension 400 mg/5 mL and erythromycin 200 mg chewable tablets.

What strength of erythromycin should be given to the child q6h?

_____

What volume of the suspension should be given as a dose? _____

How many chewable tablets should be administered with each dose?

_____

13. ▨ A physician orders Tofranil 0.3 mg/kg hs for child with enuresis. The child weighs 70 lb. The available medication is 10-mg tabs.

What dose strength of medication should be administered to the child each bedtime?

_____

How many tablets should be administered to the child for each dose?

_____

14. ▨ A physician orders Ceclor 50 mg/kg/day to be administered in divided doses qid. The child weighs 38 lb. The available medications have concentrations of 250 mg/5 mL and 125 mg/5 mL.

Which available medication concentration should be chosen for this child?

_____

Explain your answer. _____

What calculated weight of medication should be administered to the child as a single dose? _____

What volume of medication should be administered to the child as a dose using the chosen strength of the medication? _____

For a dose, what volume of medication would have been administered to the child if the other medication strength had been chosen? _____

What is the measureable dose for the medication strength calculated in the aforementioned question? _____

15. A physician orders ampicillin 100 mg/kg/day in four divided doses for an infant who weighs 12 lb. The available medication is 125 mg/5 mL.

What strength of medication should be given to this child as a dose?

_____

What volume of medication should be given to this child as a dose?

_____

What would be the dose in household measurements? _____

What would be the dose, in household measurements, if the medication were available in 250 mg/5 mL? _____

16. A physician orders aminophylline 2.5 mg/kg/dose q8h for a child who weighs 40 lb. The available medication is aminophylline oral liquid 90 mg/5 mL.

What strength of medication should be administered to the child as a dose?

_____

What volume of medication should be administered as a dose with the available medication? _____

How many teaspoons of medication should be administered to the child with each dose? _____

Indicate the amount of medication to be administered on the following measuring devices.

17. [PA IN] A physician orders acetaminophen elixir 6 mg/kg for a child who weighs 45 lb. The available medication is an elixir containing 160 mg/5 mL.

What is the strength of medication that should be administered to the child?

_____

What volume of medication should be administered to the child? _____

What type of measuring device should be available for the parent to administer this medication at home? _____

18. [♥] A child weighing 25 lb has an order for furosemide 2 mg/kg IM as a stat dose. The available medication is Lasix 10 mg/mL.

What strength of the dose should be administered to the child? _____

What volume of medication should be injected to fill the physician's order?

_____

A syringe of what volume should be used to measure this dose? _____

19. [PA IN] A physician orders acetaminophen gr $\frac{1}{6}$/kg/q4-6h prn for a child who weighs 72 lb. The available medication is Tylenol 325 mg per tablet.

What is the calculated dose strength of medication to be administered to the child?

_____

How many tablets should be administered to the child as a dose?

_____

20. [PA IN] A physician order for meperidine 5 mg/kg/day IM to be given q6h prn for a child who weighs 44 lb. The available medication is 50 mg/mL.

What is the strength for each dose q6h? _____

What is the volume of medication to be given q6h? _____

CALCULATING DOSAGE USING BODY SURFACE AREA

The third method of drug calculations using body weight is BSA. BSA is based on weight compared to height of the person. This form of calculation is often used for pediatric patients, but it may also be used when preparing toxic medications such as chemotherapeutics for adults or for adult medication amounts for the elderly, who are not of height or weight to be classified as "average adult." This calculation provides the most accurate determination of the therapeutic dose to be administered on the basis of body weight/height. BSA refers to the total body area that is exposed to the environment and is expressed in square meters (m^2). To calculate BSA, or m^2 (meters squared), the weight and height of the person must be measured and then used for the calculations. These measurements may be accomplished either in the metric or English systems for use with the **nomogram**, a means of using a chart to plot height and weight and to provide the estimated square meters of BSA. The children's nomogram is seen in Figure 10-1. A nomogram specific for adults is also available for use with adults who fall outside what is considered normal weight for height or those who are being administered toxic medications (Figure 10-2). The nomogram to be used is based on the person's age or on the nomogram's limitation by height and weight.

To use a nomogram, find the height and the weight on the correct indication line of the chart. Notice that the metric system is on the left side of the height measurement column and on the right side of the weight measurement column on the child's nomogram. On the adult chart, the metric system is on the left side of both the height and weight columns. After finding the height and weight for either the child or the adult, draw a straight line between the two points to find the line where the straight line intersects the surface area (SA) line. The estimated BSA is the point where the line intersects the SA m^2 line. For the child who is of normal height and weight for age, the BSA may be calculated only by the child's weight. Notice that the nomogram has this added column within the center box that shows BSA indicated by weight in pounds for the child of normal height and weight. This box is not found on the adult nomogram.

Figure 10-3 shows the use of the nomogram; notice that the person is 41″ tall and weighs 36 lb. The intersection of the straight line on the SA line is 0.68, so the estimated BSA for this patient is 0.68 m^2.

Practice Problems C

Using the proper nomogram, calculate the following BSA as practice. Round to the nearest hundredth.

1. A child weighs 15 lb and is 24″ tall.

2. A child is 48″ tall and weighs 50 lb.

3. A child is 60 cm tall and weighs 5 kg.

4. A child is normal height for 40 lb.

5. A child weighs 20 kg and is 100 cm tall

After the BSA has been found, the following formula is used to calculate the dose of medication. The typical BSA for an adult is 1.7 m^2. Therefore this number is used in the formula to calculate doses for children. The formula is as follows:

$$\text{Desired dose (DD)} = \frac{\text{BSA (m}^2\text{)}}{1.7 \text{ m}^2} \times \text{Adult dose}$$

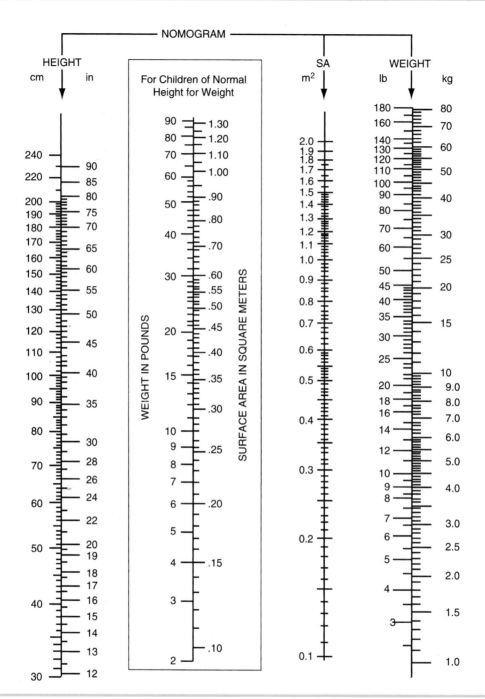

NOMOGRAM

FIGURE 10-1 Nomogram for measuring body surface area for a child.

Using the nomogram for a child, the formula is used for calculating dose to be administered based on the normal adult dose.

For calculating doses for adults, the BSA in m² (meters squared) is multiplied by the dose ordered (weight per dose [DO] × BSA = DD).

EXAMPLE 10-6

CA   If a physician orders Cytoxan 50 mg/m²/dose IV for an adult who is 55″ tall and weighs 160 lb, what dose should be given?

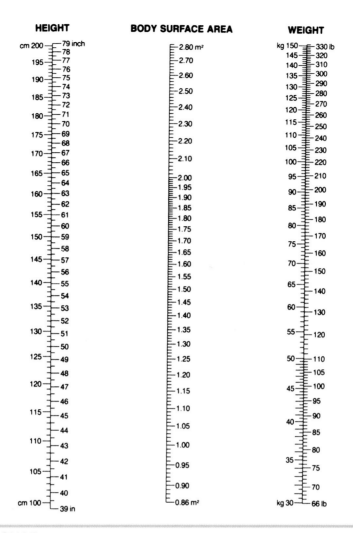

FIGURE 10-2 Nomogram for calculating body surface area for an adult.

The first step is to find the BSA in m² by plotting 55″ and 160 lb on the nomogram. The BSA is 1.75 m². Now all that needs to be done is to fill in the equation.

50 mg (DO) × 1.75 = DD, or 87.5 mg to be administered

If the medication is in a vial of 200 mg/10 mL, what would be the volume of medication?

$$\frac{87.5 \text{ mg (DD)}}{200 \text{ mg (DA)}} \times 10 \text{ mL (Qty)} = \text{Dose to be given}$$

87.5 mg × 10 mL ÷ 200 mg = 4.38 mL, or 4.4 mL to be administered

Now work a problem for a child's dosage of medication.

EXAMPLE 10-7

A physician orders amoxicillin tid for a child who weighs 50 lb and is 45″ tall. The normal adult dose is amoxicillin 500 mg tid.

What dose should be given to the child if the available medication is 250 mg/5 mL?

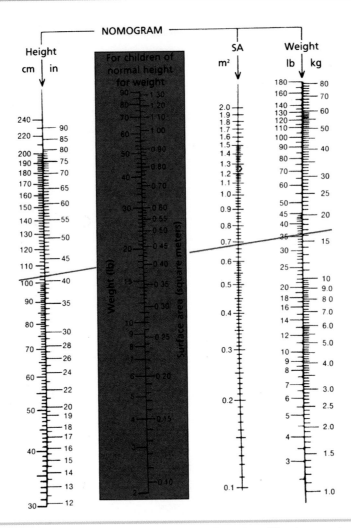

FIGURE 10-3 Reading an estimated body surface area at the point of line intersection on the SA (surface area) line.

First find the BSA of the child by using the nomogram. The height and weight calculate to a BSA of 0.86 m^2.

Now fill in the formula given earlier to obtain the desired strength of medication.

$$\frac{0.86 \text{ BSA (m}^2)}{1.7 \text{ m}^2} \times 500 \text{ mg} = \text{Child's dose}$$

$$0.86 \times 500 \div 1.7 = 252.94 \text{ for desired dose of medication}$$

Now the dose needs to be calculated.

$$\frac{252.94 \text{ mg (DD)}}{250 \text{ mg (DA)}} \times 5 \text{ mL (Qty)} = \text{Dose to be given}$$

$$\frac{252.94 \text{ mg}}{250 \text{ mg}} \times 5 \text{ mL} = \text{DG} \quad \text{or} \quad 5.06 \text{ mL}$$

The dose to be given will be 5 mL when the measurable dose is calculated.

TECH NOTE

> Other dose calculations may be accomplished using drug weight based on body weight such as mg/kg. Clark's rule bases calculations on the child's weight as it relates to the average adult weight (150 lb) and the adult medication dose. Fried's rule, used for infants up to 1 year of age, and Young's rule, for children aged 1 to 12 years, base dose calculations on the child's age in relation to normal adult doses. These formulas will be described later in the chapter.

Practice Problems D

Calculate the following problems using BSA. Remember to obtain the BSA and then insert this into the proper formula. Use the same formula for BSA for adults who do not meet the standard height/weight sizes. Show your calculations. Round to nearest hundredth for dosage. Round to nearest tenths for volume to be administered (measurable dose). Use a calculator as permitted by instructor.

1. A child is 25″ long and weighs 15 lb. The physician orders Lanoxin elixir daily. The adult dose of Lanoxin is 0.25 mg/day. The available medication is Lanoxin pediatric elixir 0.05 mg/mL.

   Indicate the BSA calculation. _____

   What is the daily dose strength of Lanoxin for the child? _____

   What volume of medication would be administered to the child? _____

2. A child weighs 50 lb and is 36″ tall. The physician orders Keflex qid for the child. The adult dose of Keflex is 500 mg qid. The available medication is Keflex suspension 250 mg/5 mL.

   Indicate the BSA calculation. _____

   What is the single dose strength for the child? _____

   What is the volume of medication per dose? _____

3. A child weighs 55 lb and is 42″ tall. The physician orders Tegretol for the child, who has epilepsy. The adult dose of the medication is 200 mg qid. The medication is available in Tegretol suspension 100 mg/5 mL.

   Indicate the BSA calculation. _____

   What is the single-dose strength for the child? _____

   What is the volume of medication per dose? _____

4. CA An adult is 64″ tall and weighs 120 lb. The physician has ordered Vancocin 600 mg/m² IV q12h. The available medication is 1 g/10 mL after reconstitution.

Hint: Be sure the metric designations are in the same weight equivalents before calculating the problem.

Indicate the BSA calculation. _____

What is the single-dose strength to be given, in mg? _____

What volume of medication should be prepared for administration of the infusion?

_____

5. 🦠 A child weighs 55 lb and is 35″ tall. The physician orders ampicillin for the child qid. The usual adult dose is 500 mg qid. The available dose is ampicillin 250 mg/5 mL.

Indicate the BSA calculation. _____

What is the dose of medication to be administered? _____

How many milliliters should be given to the child? _____

How much medication would the parent give in household measurements?

_____

6. EN DO A physician orders prednisone for a child for an allergic reaction. The child weighs 90 lb and is 62″ tall. The usual adult dose is 5 mg tid. The medication available is prednisone syrup 1 mg/1 mL.

Indicate the BSA calculation. _____

What strength of medication should be administered to the child for a dose?

_____

What volume of medication should be administered? _____

7. 🧠 A 40-lb child is of normal height for weight. The physician orders Dilantin suspension for the child for seizures. The available medication is Dilantin suspension 125 mg/5 mL. The normal adult dose is 100 mg tid.

Indicate the BSA calculation. _____

What is the dose to be administered to the child? _____

What is the volume of medication to be given to the child? _____

8.   A physician orders erythromycin oral suspension for a child with acute
      bronchitis who weighs 75 lb and is 48″ tall. The usual adult dose is
      erythromycin 250 mg qid. The medication is available in Ilosone oral suspension
      250 mg/5 mL.

      Indicate the BSA calculation. _____

      What strength of medication should be given to the child in a single dose?

      _____

      What is the volume of medication to be given in a dose? _____

      What volume of medication should be given per day if the child receives a dose qid?

      _____

9.   A child is 50″ tall and weighs 75 lb. A physician orders Zantac liquid tid for
      gastric irritation. The usual adult dose is 150 mg bid. The available medication
      is 15 mg/mL.

      Indicate the BSA calculation. _____

      What is the strength of the medication to be given to the child in a dose?

      _____

      What volume of medication should be given to the child in a dose?

      _____

      What total volume of medication should the child receive in a day?

      _____

10.   A child weighs 30 lb and is normal length for weight. The normal adult dose of
      doxycycline is 200 mg on the first day and then 100 mg per day. The available
      medication is doxycycline 50 mg/5 mL.

      Indicate the BSA calculation. _____

      What is the strength of the child's dose for the first day? _____

      What volume of medication should be given to the child on the first day?

      _____

      What is the strength of the dose on subsequent days? _____

      What is the volume of medication to be given as a dose on subsequent days?

      _____

11. A child with epilepsy weighs 48 lb and is of normal height for weight. The physician orders phenobarbital to control the seizures. The normal adult dose is 100 mg tid. The available medication is phenobarbital 20 mg/5 mL.

Indicate the BSA calculation. _____

What strength of medication should be given to the child for each dose?

_____

What volume of medication should be given to the child for each dose?

_____

12. A child weighs 46 lb, has a normal height for his age, and is suffering from rheumatic heart disease. The physician orders digoxin to be given daily to the child. The usual adult dose is 0.25 mg per day. The available medication is Lanoxin elixir 0.05 mg/mL.

Indicate the BSA calculation. _____

What strength of medication should be given to the child each morning?

_____

What is the volume of medication to be given with each dose? _____

13. A child weighs 44 lb and is 45″ tall. The child has a severe earache and has an order for Demerol po q6h prn severe pain. The usual adult dose is 50 mg q6h. The medication is available as 50 mg/5 mL.

Indicate the BSA calculation. _____

What dose should be administered to the child q6h? _____

What volume of medication should be given to the child? _____

14. An adult in the nursing home has lost weight and does not fit the weight/height indicators for normal adults. The patient, who has an acute cellulitis, weighs 93 lb and is 64″ tall. The normal adult dose of amoxicillin is 500 mg per dose. The medication is available in 250 mg/5 mL and 400 mg/5 mL.

Indicate the BSA calculation. _____

What strength of medication should be given to the nursing home patient in a single dose? _____

What volume of medication should be given if using the 250 mg/5 mL strength?

_____

What volume of medication should be given if using the 400 mg/5 mL strength?

_____

Which medication strength would be the best choice for administering the desired ordered dose to the patient? _____

15. **CA** An adult who weighs 150 lb and is 5′4″ tall has been diagnosed with a malignant neoplasm. The physician orders Oncovin 1.4 mg/m^2 IV for this patient. Oncovin is available as 1 mg/1 mL.

What is the BSA of this patient? _____

What dose should be given to the patient intravenously? _____

What volume of medication should be given to this patient? _____

16. An adult who weighs 125 lb and is 5′6″ tall has severe herpes zoster. The physician has ordered acyclovir 500 mg/m^2 for administration q8h. Zovirax is available in 400-mg tablets.

Indicate the BSA calculation. _____

What dose of medication should be given to the patient q8h? _____

How many tablets should be given to this person with each dose?

_____

17. A child has severe streptococcal pneumonia, and the physician orders Augmentin to be given q8h. The child weighs 45 lb and is of normal height for weight. The usual adult dose is 500 mg q8h. The medication is available in Augmentin pediatric chewable tablets 250 mg and Augmentin suspension 250 mg/5 mL.

Indicate the BSA calculation. _____

What amount of medication should be administered to the child with each dose?

_____

How many chewable tablets should be given to the child? _____

What volume of suspension should be given to the child for each dose?

_____

Which form of medication would be the most accurate for the child?

_____

18. A child who weighs 30 lb has a severe case of urticaria. The physician orders diphenhydramine 5 mg/kg/day in four divided doses. The elixir is available in 12.5 mg/5 mL.

What total strength of medication should be given to this child per day?

_____

What is the strength of medication for administration per dose? _____

What volume of medication should be administered with each dose?

_____

19. An emaciated adult has severe nausea. The person weighs 96 lb and is 5'5" tall. The physician orders Vistaril 35 mg/m^2 IM for this patient. The medication is available as Vistaril 25 mg/mL.

Indicate the BSA calculation. _____

What is the dose of medication that should be given to this patient?

_____

What volume of medication should be administered to this patient?

_____

20. A child who weighs 50 lb has been exposed to a severe case of influenza A. The physician wants to reduce any chance of infection affecting an older adult who lives in the same household. The child is of normal height for weight. The order is for amantadine 55 mg/m^2 bid as the prophylactic dose. The medication is available as amantadine syrup 50 mg/5 mL.

Indicate the BSA calculation. _____

What amount of medication should be given as a single dose? _____

What volume of medication should the child be given for each dose?

_____

CALCULATION OF MEDICATIONS FOR PEDIATRIC PATIENTS BASED ON AGE

Pediatric dosage may also be calculated by age using Fried's and Young's rules based on normal adult dose. **Fried's rule** is used for an infant up to 12 months based on the age in months times the adult dose divided by 150 (basis of normal adult weight). **Young's rule** is used to calculate medications for children 1 year of age to 12 years of age. The calculation is age in years times the adult dose divided by the age in years plus 12. Although these are not often used in pharmacy today, as a pharmacy technician you should be aware that these are possible means for providing a dose for a child based on age.

TECH NOTE

Again, remember that if the manufacturer has a suggested amount for a pediatric dose, that dose should be used when preparing medications for dispensing. More and more physicians are using only medications that have suggested manufacturer's dose limits rather than using age or body weight as the basis for calculating prescriptions for special populations.

The following formulas should be used for calculating doses using age. Included is a sample problem worked with each formula for your information. Because age is no longer considered a single valid criterion for determining pediatric dosing, only three problems are provided for practice.

Fried's Rule

Fried's rule is to be used with infants up to 1 year.

$$\text{Infant's dose} = \frac{\text{Age in months} \times \text{Adult dose}}{150}$$

EXAMPLE 10-8

 A physician orders amoxicillin for an infant 6 months old. The usual adult dose is 500 mg. Calculate the dose for the child.

$$\text{Infant's dose} = \frac{\text{Age in months} \times \text{Adult dose}}{150}$$

$$\text{Infant's dose} = \frac{6 \times 500}{150} \quad \text{or} \quad \frac{3000}{150}$$

$$\text{Infant's dose} = 20 \text{ mg}$$

If the medication available is amoxicillin 50 mg/mL, what dose would be given to the infant?

$$\text{Dose to be given (DG)} = \frac{\text{Dose desired (DD)}}{\text{Dosage on hand (DH)}} \times \text{Quantity}$$

$$DG = \frac{20 \text{ mg}}{50 \text{ mg}} \times 1 \text{ mL or } 2 \div 5 \times 1 \text{ mL}$$

$$DG = 0.4 \text{ mL}$$

The infant would receive amoxicillin 0.4 mL if the dose is based on age.

Young's Rule

Young's rule is to be used with children aged 1 to 12 years.

$$\text{Child's dose} = \frac{\text{Age in years} \times \text{Adult dose}}{\text{Age in years} + 12}$$

EXAMPLE 10-9

 A physician orders amoxicillin for a 5-year-old child. The adult dose is 500 mg per dose. What dose would be given to the child?

$$\text{Child's dose} = \frac{\text{Age in years} \times \text{Adult dose}}{\text{Age in years} + 12}$$

$$\text{Child's dose} = \frac{5 \times 500}{5 + 12} \quad \text{or} \quad \frac{2500}{17}$$

$$\text{Child's dose} = 147.1 \text{ mg}$$

The medication is available as amoxicillin suspension 400 mg/5 mL.

$$DG = \frac{147.1 \text{ mg (DD)}}{400 \text{ mg (DH)}} \times 5 \text{ mL (Qty)} \quad \text{or} \quad \frac{150 \times 5 \text{ mL}}{400} \quad \text{or} \quad 725.5 \div 400$$

$$DG = 1.81 \text{ mL or } 1.8 \text{ mL}$$

Practice Problems E

Calculate the following doses of medication. Show your calculations being sure that you round to nearest hundredth for dosing calculations. Round to the nearest tenth when providing volume calculations, unless otherwise noted. Use a calculator as permitted by instructor.

1. A physician orders Milk of Magnesia for a 3-year-old child. The adult dose for Milk of Magnesia is 30 mL.

   What volume of Milk of Magnesia should be given to the child? _____

2. A physician wants a 6-month-old child to have phenobarbital. The usual adult dose is phenobarbital 30 mg. Medication is available in an elixir of 20 mg/5 mL.

   What dose of the medication should be given to the child? _____

   What volume of medication should be administered with each dose?

   _____

3. A physician orders phenobarbital for a 4-year-old child for seizures. The adult dose for phenobarbital is 30 mg. The medication is available as phenobarbital elixir 20 mg/5 mL.

   What dose of medication should be given with each dose? _____

   What volume of medication should be given to the child with each dose?

   _____

   What is the measurable dose to be administered? _____

4. **PAIN** A 6-month-old infant has an order for Demerol q4h. The usual adult dose is Demerol 50 mg per dose. The medication is available as meperidine 50 mg/5 mL.

What dose should be given to the child? _____

What volume of medication should be administered with each dose?

_____

5. A 6-year-old child has a severe case of hives. The physician wants the child to have prednisone for relief. The adult dose is 20 mg. The available medication is prednisone oral solution 5 mg/5 mL.

What dose should be given to the child? _____

What volume of medication should be administered to the child with each dose?

_____

What type of measuring device should be supplied with the medication to provide accurate dosing? _____

6. An 8-month-old infant has a severe staphylococcal infection. The physician wants this child to have cephalexin. The adult dose is 500 mg q12h. The available medication is cephalexin 125 mg/5 mL.

What dose of medication should be given to the infant? _____

What would be the calculated volume of medication that would be administered to the infant q12h? _____

What is the measurable dose of medication to be administered? _____

What measuring device should be provided to ensure the proper dose is administered? _____

REVIEW

Medications for children and those medications that have a high toxicity level may require special calculations for doses to be given safely and accurately. In the past with children's doses, age has been used as a means of estimating a dose calculation. In most cases today, BSA calculated using the nomogram is the basis for children's dosage calculations. An adult nomogram for calculating BSA is also used, especially for medications with highly toxic side effects. With other medications, the physician may write adult or children's dosages to be given on the basis of the amount of medication related to the body weight found in such measurements as milligrams/kilogram. In all cases, the manufacturer's suggested dosage should be the guideline for the amount of medication that is administered to children and adults, in particular those patients who have special dosage needs.

! TECH ALERT

Remember that "normal" for an adult is not always "normal" but must be adjusted for certain characteristics of patients, such as body weight, disease to be treated, organ function, and other parameters.

Posttest

Before taking the Posttest, retake the Pretest to check your understanding of the materials presented in this chapter.

Calculate the following problems using the correct formula for each situation provided. If measuring devices for administration are included, indicate the volume of medication on the appropriate measuring device(s). Show all of your calculations. Prior to the final answer, dosing calculations should be rounded to the nearest hundredth. Round to the nearest tenth for your final answer as appropriate, being sure that you have a measurable dose (as allowed by measuring device). If the volume of medication is less than a mL, the answer should be provided in hundredths of mL. Remember that you will be calculating for a dose unless otherwise specified. Use a calculator as permitted by your instructor.

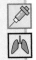

1. A child weighs 66 lb, and the physician orders Benadryl elixir 0.4 mg per kilogram of body weight.

N 0071-2220-17 ELIXIR **Benadryl**® (Diphenhydramine Hydrochloride Elixir, USP) **Caution**—Federal law prohibits dispensing without prescription. 4 FLUIDOUNCES **PARKE-DAVIS** Div of Warner-Lambert Co Morris Plains, NJ 07950 USA	Elixir P-D 2220 for prescription dispensing only. **Contains**—12.5 mg diphenhydramine hydrochloride in each 5 mL. Alcohol, 14%. **Dose**—Adults, 2 to 4 teaspoonfuls; children over 20 lb, 1 to 2 teaspoonfuls; three or four times daily. See package insert. Keep this and all drugs out of the reach of children. **Store below 30°C (86°F). Protect from freezing and light.** Exp date and lot 2220G102

What is the strength of medication to be given? _____

What dose should be given using the Benadryl label? _____

What would be the dose in household measurements? _____

Posttest, cont.

2. A child weighs 88 lb, and the physician orders Compazine syrup 0.5 mg/kg tid.

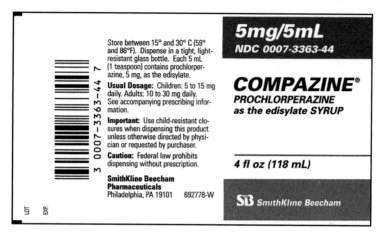

5mg/5mL
NDC 0007-3363-44

COMPAZINE®
PROCHLORPERAZINE
as the edisylate SYRUP

4 fl oz (118 mL)

SB SmithKline Beecham

Store between 15° and 30° C (59° and 86°F). Dispense in a tight, light-resistant glass bottle. Each 5 mL (1 teaspoon) contains prochlorperazine, 5 mg, as the edisylate.
Usual Dosage: Children: 5 to 15 mg daily. Adults: 10 to 30 mg daily. See accompanying prescribing information.
Important: Use child-resistant closures when dispensing this product unless otherwise directed by physician or requested by purchaser.
Caution: Federal law prohibits dispensing without prescription.

SmithKline Beecham Pharmaceuticals
Philadelphia, PA 19101   692778-W

What is the volume dose for the child? _____

Using the label shown, what volume of medication should be administered?

_____

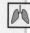

3. A child weighs 55 lb and is normal height for weight. The physician orders amoxicillin for this child. The normal adult dose is amoxicillin 500 mg tid. The medication is available as amoxicillin 125 mg/5 mL and 250 mg/5 mL.

What is the BSA? _____

What dosage strength should be given to this child? _____

What is the most acceptable strength of medication available to be administered to the child? _____

What volume of the chosen medication should be administered? _____

4. A child is 27″ tall and weighs 30 lb. The physician wants this child to have Claritin for hay fever. The normal adult dose is 10 mg. The available medication is 1 mg/1 mL.

What is the BSA? _____

What dosage strength should be given to the child? _____

What volume of medication should be administered to the child? _____

Continued

Posttest, cont.

5. The recommended dose for a child for meperidine is 6 mg/kg/day for pain. The physician orders this to be given every 4 hours for a child who weighs 66 lb. The medication is available as 50 mg/5 mL.

What is the total amount of medication that the child can receive in a day?

_____

If the child could receive six doses a day, what is the maximum strength of medication that should be given with each dose? _____

What volume of medication would be required to provide that dose of medication?

_____

6. An emaciated adult who weighs 100 lb has an order for aminophylline to be given 3 mg/kg/dose every 8 hours as a maintenance dose. The medication is available as aminophylline oral liquid 105 mg/5 mL.

What strength of medication should be given to this patient every 8 hours?

_____

What volume of medication should be administered for each dose?

_____

7. A 6-year-old child has an order for Tofranil. The usual adult dose is Tofranil 50 mg. The medication is available in 10-mg scored tablets.

What strength of medication should be administered to the child?

_____

How many tablets should be given to the child? _____

8. A 10-year-old child has an order for ibuprofen for elevated temperature. The usual adult dose is 400 mg q6h. Ibuprofen is available as 100 mg/5 mL.

What strength of medication should be given to this child? _____

What volume of medication should be administered for each dose?

_____

If the medication is available in 50-mg chewable tablets, could these be used to administer the exact dose of medication ordered? _____

If so, how many tablets would be given? _____

Posttest, cont.

 9. A 6-month-old infant is to be given acetaminophen q4h for a high fever related to cellulitis. The usual adult dose is 325 mg q4-6h. The medication is available as acetaminophen 160 mg/5 mL.

What strength of medication should be given to the infant? _____

What volume of medication should be given to the infant? _____

Choose the correct measuring device for use with the medication and mark the amount on the chosen measuring device.

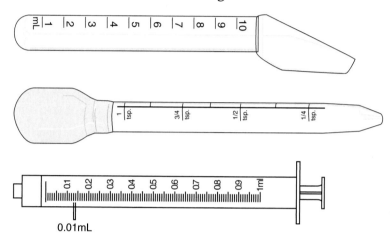

 10. A 9-year-old child has a severe allergic reaction to a bee sting. The physician orders Decadron for the child. The normal adult dose is Decadron 4 mg. The medication is available as dexamethasone elixir 0.5 mg/5 mL.

What strength of medication should be administered to the child?

_____

What volume of medication should be administered to the child? _____

How could this be given in household measurements for the closest possible dose?

_____

Continued

Posttest, cont.

11. A child weighs 48 lb and is normal height for weight. A physician orders dexamethasone for the child once daily. The normal adult dose is Decadron 4 mg per day. The medication is available as Decadron oral solution 4 mg/1 mL.

What is the BSA? _____

What strength of medication should be administered to the child?

_____

What is the calculated volume of medication in hundredths needed to supply the dose? _____

What measureable volume of medication should be administered to the child?

_____

What volume of medication would be administered if the physician ordered the same dose IM and the available injection is Decadron 10 mg/mL?

_____

Show the dosage for the oral medication and the injectable on the correct measuring devices.

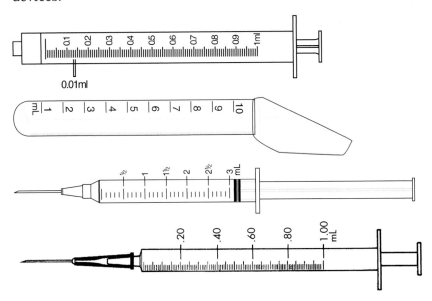

12. A child who weighs 48 lb has an order for dexamethasone 0.08 mg/kg to be given every 12 hours. The medication is available as dexamethasone oral liquid 0.5 mg/5 mL and dexamethasone injectable 4 mg/mL.

What strength of medication should be given to the child with each dose?

_____

What volume of medication should be given to the child orally? _____

What volume of medication should be administered parenterally?

_____

Posttest, cont.

Select the correct measuring devices, and mark the appropriate dose for the oral administration and the exact dose for the parenteral administration.

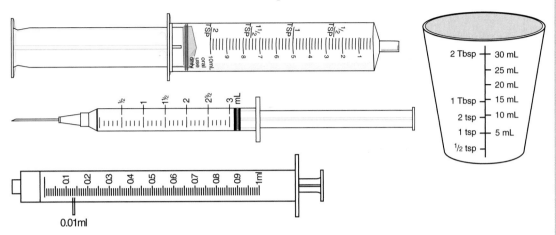

 13. A 7-year-old child weighing 78 lb is being treated for status epilepticus with diazepam. The recommended dose for this age child is 0.3 mg/kg. The medication available is diazepam oral solution 5 mg/5 mL, injectable 5 mg/mL, and 10-mg tablets. At present the child is not having a seizure but has had multiple seizures throughout out the day.

What strength of the medication should be administered to the child?

_____

What volume of medication should be administered if the oral solution is used?

_____

What is the calculated volume of medication that should be administered to the child parenterally? _____

What is the measurable volume of medication to be administered parenterally?

_____

Can this medication be given orally with the solid medication supplied?

_____

If so, what is the dose for administration? _____

If the child were having a seizure, would you prepare the medication for oral administration? _____

If a diazepam 5-mg rectal gel and a diazepam 15-mg rectal gel were available, which medication would you prepare for administration? _____

Number of rectal gel doses to be administered for the dosage would be

_____ .

Continued

Posttest, cont.

 14. A male patient who is 5'11" tall weighing 185 lb is being treated with cisplatin IV for testicular cancer. The dosage for cisplatin is 20 mg/m² per day × 5 days of each cycle, in cyclic doses. The medication is available in a powder found in 10- and 50-mg vials. The medication is reconstituted to a concentration of 1 mg/mL.

What strength of medication should be administered to the patient each day a dose is due? _____

Which vial of medication should be chosen to be used for reconstitution to provide the ordered dose? _____

What is the volume of reconstituted medication to be administered?

_____

Show the amount of medication to be administered.

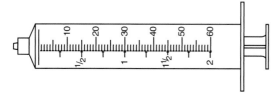

 15. A patient is being treated for Hodgkin's disease with doxorubicin 65 mg/m². The person is 5'5" tall and weighs 140 lb. The medication is available in 20-, 50-, 100-, and 150-mg vials with a strength of 20 mg/mL.

What is the BSA? _____

What strength of medication should this patient receive with each treatment?

_____

What volume of medication would be used to provide the patient's dose?

_____

Which vial of medication would be the best choice for use? _____

Show the amount of medication to be administered.

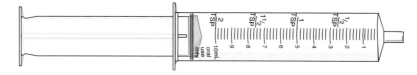

 16. A child weighing 56 lb has an order for azithromycin oral suspension to prevent complications of influenza. The amount of medication to be given is 10 mg/kg/day for the first day and 5 mg/kg/day for the next 3 days. Use the label shown for the calculations of doses to be given.

Posttest, cont.

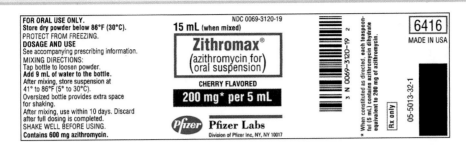

FOR ORAL USE ONLY.
Store dry powder below 86°F (30°C).
PROTECT FROM FREEZING.
DOSAGE AND USE
See accompanying prescribing information.
MIXING DIRECTIONS:
Tap bottle to loosen powder.
Add 9 mL of water to the bottle.
After mixing, store suspension at
41° to 86°F (5° to 30°C).
Oversized bottle provides extra space
for shaking.
After mixing, use within 10 days. Discard
after full dosing is completed.
SHAKE WELL BEFORE USING.
Contains 600 mg azithromycin.

NDC 0069-3120-19
15 mL (when mixed)

Zithromax®
(azithromycin for
oral suspension)
CHERRY FLAVORED
200 mg* per 5 mL

Pfizer **Pfizer Labs**
Division of Pfizer Inc, NY, NY 10017

6416
MADE IN USA

* When constituted as directed, each teaspoonful (5 mL) contains azithromycin dihydrate equivalent to 200 mg of azithromycin.

Rx only

05-5013-32-1

What strength of medication should be given to the child on the first day?

_____

What volume of medication should be given on the first day in a measurable amount? _____

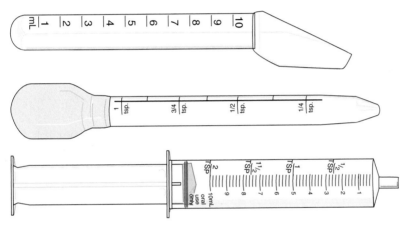

What strength of medication should be given to the child for doses on subsequent days? _____

What volume of medication should be given to the child on subsequent days?

_____

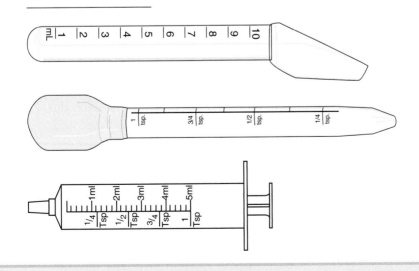

Continued

Posttest, cont.

 17. A 4-month-old child is being treated with ampicillin for a strep infection. The normal adult dose is ampicillin 500 mg per dose. The medication is available as an oral suspension 125 mg/5 mL.

What strength of medication should be administered to this child?

_____

What volume of medication should be ordered for the child? _____

What is the measurable dose of medication to be administered? _____

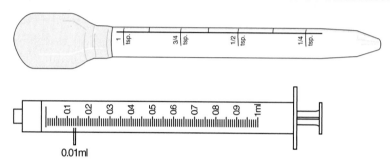

 18. A 4-year-old child with a severe case of bacterial pneumonia has an order for kanamycin to be administered tid IV. The ordered dose is kanamycin 15 mg/kg/day in three divided doses. The child weighs 60 lb. The medication is available as shown on the following label.

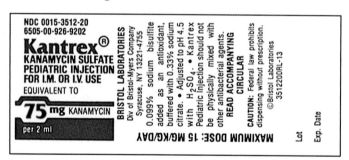

What total strength of medication should be administered to this child over the entire day? _____

What strength of medication should be administered to this child for each dose?

_____

What volume of medication should be prepared for administration to the child with each dose? _____

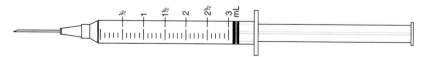

Posttest, cont.

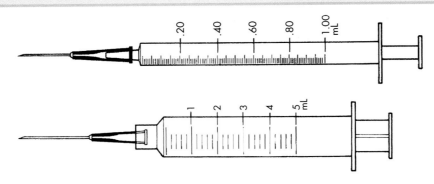

19. A 7-year-old child has a prescription for penicillin V potassium to be given q8h. The normal adult dose is penicillin V potassium 500 mg q8h. Use the following label for calculations.

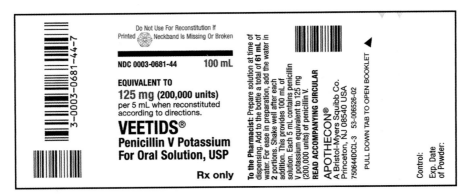

What strength of medication should be administered with each dose?

_____

What is the volume of medication to be administered with each dose?

_____

What is the measurable volume of medication to be administered?

_____

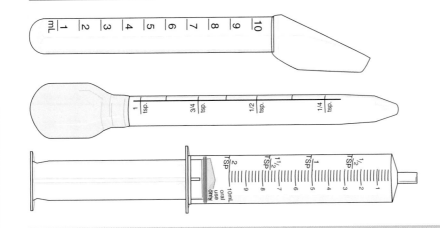

Continued

Posttest, cont.

PA IN

20. A child who weighs 52 lb is of normal height for weight. A physician orders codeine to be given q6h for a severe aching related to influenza. The dose is 15 mg/m²/dose but not to exceed 60 mg per day. The medication is available as 15 mg/5 mL and as 15-mg tablets.

What is the BSA of the child? _____

What strength of medication should be administered to the child with each dose?

_____

What volume of medication should be administered with each dose if the oral liquid

is used? _____

If the tablets can be administered as approved by the physician as an approximate

dose, how many tablets can be given with each dose? _____

Is the dosage within acceptable range if the child receives the medication every 6

hours? _____

What would be the total weight of medication per day if using tablets?

_____

What would be the total weight of medication per day if using liquid?

_____

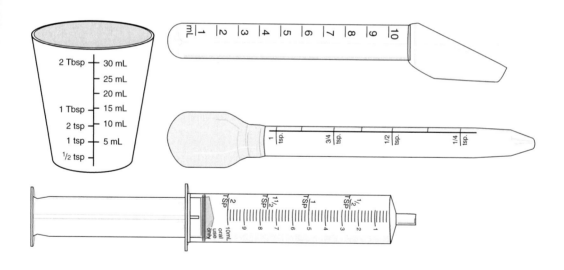

REVIEW OF RULES

Calculation of Medication Doses Based on Age or Weight

- Medications for special populations may require special calculations based on either weight, age, or BSA.

- Medications may be ordered in the drug strength to be given for the weight in kilograms (strength/kg/time period [such as day or hours]). To calculate these problems, weight in pounds must be converted to kilograms before performing the calculation. To calculate kilograms, divide the number of pounds by 2.2 (2.2 lb = 1 kg). This calculation may be easily accomplished using the ratio and proportion method. (If dimensional analysis is the preferred method of calculation, this conversion is not necessary because it may be done as a step in the problem.) After the kilograms have been calculated, complete the formula of mg/kg by substituting the order and the calculation of kilograms.

- Doses calculated on age are not generally used because age alone as the criterion for calculations is not considered to be singularly valid for this determination.

- Clark's rule may be used to calculate a pediatric dose of medication by inserting the known information into the following formula:

$$\text{Child's dose} = \frac{\text{Child's weight in pounds}}{150 \text{ lb}} \times \text{Adult dose}$$

- BSA is based on the nomogram to find the meters squared (m^2) of the body's external area. The nomogram is available for either children or adults, and the correct nomogram must be used when calculating medications.

- To use the nomogram, find the height in either inches or centimeters in the height column. Then find the weight in either pounds or kilograms in the weight column. Finally, draw a line connecting the height point and the weight point of the child. The number on the m^2 line where the line intersects the surface area (SA) column is the BSA.

- After finding the BSA, use the following formula and fill in the known amounts to calculate the dose for special populations.

$$\text{Desired dose (DD)} = \frac{\text{BSA } (m^2)}{1.7 \text{ m}^2} \times \text{Adult dose}$$

- Age may also be used to calculate medication dosages for children.

- For infants (ages birth to 12 months), Fried's rule may be used:

$$\text{Infant's dose} = \frac{\text{Age in months} \times \text{Adult dose}}{150}$$

- For children between 1 and 12 years old, Young's rule may be used:

$$\text{Child's dose} = \frac{\text{Age in years} \times \text{Adult dose}}{\text{Age in years} + 12}$$

After the dose for the child has been calculated, the formula or ratio/proportion must be used to complete the calculation for the desired dose.

Calculation of Medications Measured in Units, Milliequivalents, and Percentages of Concentration

OBJECTIVES

- Calculate doses of antibiotic medications measured in units
- Calculate insulin doses measured in units
- Calculate anticoagulant doses measured in units
- Calculate medications measured in milliequivalents
- Interpret dosage when the medication is expressed as a percentage
- Interpret dosage of solutions expressed in ratio strength
- Calculate weight of active ingredients expressed in percentage or ratio and proportion

KEY WORDS

Anticoagulant Substance that stops or delays the clotting of blood

International units System of measure for international technical and scientific work based on metric system

Milliequivalent One thousandth of a chemical equivalent; represents the number of grams of solute (usually electrolytes in pharmacology) dissolved in a milliliter of solution or the chemical combining power of the substance

Patent, Patency State in which an object is open or evident

Unit Basic measurement used to indicate the strength of some medications; the unit describes a standardly agreed upon amount of an individual drug that can produce a given biological effect and is specific to that drug alone. The units of one substance are not equivalent to the same number of units of another substance.

384

Pretest

Calculate the following problems. If syringes are included, indicate the volume of medication to be administered on the correct syringe, based on the route of administration, to give the most accurate dose. Show your calculations in all instances. Round to the nearest hundredth, as appropriate.

1. A physician orders Acthar Gel 50 units IM stat. The medication on hand has a label reading Acthar Gel 80 units/mL.

   What measureable volume of medication should be given to the patient?

   _____

   What type of syringe should be used to administer this medication?

   _____

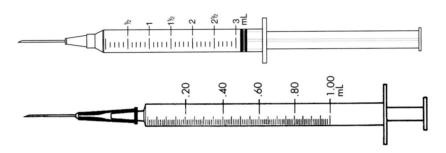

   Interpret the physician's order. _____

Continued

Pretest, cont.

2. A physician orders heparin sodium 1500 units subcutaneously stat. Use the label provided for calculations.

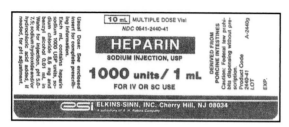

Interpret the medication order. _____

What is the measurable volume of medication that should be given to the patient?

_____

What type and size of syringe should be used to prepare this medication?

_____

What is the total volume of medication in the vial? _____

What is the total strength of heparin in the vial? _____

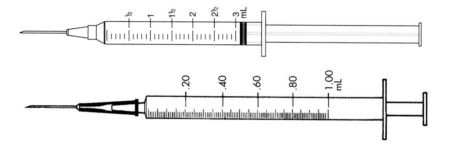

Pretest, cont.

3. A physician orders 750,000 units of penicillin G IM stat for a male teenager who has pneumonia. Use the following label to calculate this information. The medication is reconstituted to 500,000 units/mL.

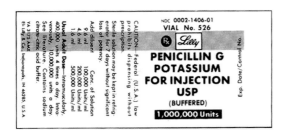

What volume of medication should be given to the teen? _____

What is the recommended route of administration? _____

What is the volume of diluent that was added to the vial? _____

How long would the medication be potent after reconstitution? _____

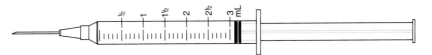

4. A physician orders penicillin G potassium 500,000 units IM for an adult. Add 1.8 mL of sterile water and use the label provided to answer questions.

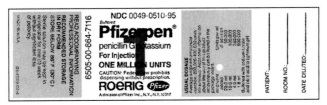

What is the strength of medication per milliliter? _____

What volume of medication should be administered to the patient?

_____

What total volume of medication is in the vial after reconstitution?

_____

What type of syringe should be used to administer the medication?

_____

Continued

Pretest, cont.

5. A physician orders potassium chloride 2 mEq to be added to IV fluids for a patient in electrolyte imbalance. Using the following label, calculate the necessary dose.

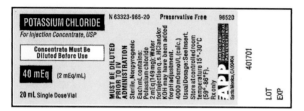

What volume of medication should be added to the IV fluids for this patient?

_____

What is the milliequivalent per milliliter in this vial? _____

What is the total volume of medication of the vial? _____

What is the total strength of medication in the vial? _____

How many doses of medication are in this vial if the patient receives the same amount of medication for each dose? _____

6. A physician orders 500,000 units of penicillin G IM stat and q6h. The available medication is penicillin G 250,000 units/mL in a 10-mL vial.

Interpret the order. _____

What volume of medication should be administered to the patient with each dose?

_____

What is the total strength of the medication in the vial? _____

How many doses of medication can be administered from a single vial if the dosage remains the same? _____

7. A physician orders 2500 units of heparin sodium subcutaneously. The medication available is 10,000 units/mL in a 1 mL vial.

What volume of medication would the patient receive? _____

What volume of medication would be available in the vial after this dose has been prepared? _____

Pretest, cont.

Which syringe should be used to provide the most accurate dose of medication?

_____

Indicate the dose that would be drawn for this order.

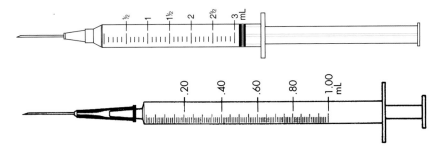

8. A physician orders Humulin R 50 units in IV fluids to make an insulin infusion.

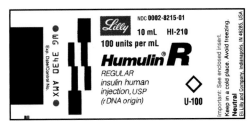

Using an unopened vial of medications, what volume of medication should be added to the fluids? _____

What volume of medication would be available in the vial after the dose of insulin has been prepared? _____

Choose the syringe that would provide the most accurate dose of medication and indicate the desired volume.

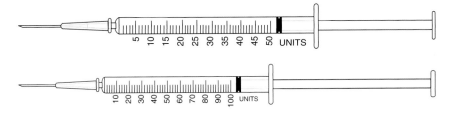

Continued

Pretest, cont.

9. A physician orders Humulin R 35 units subcutaneously stat. The available medication is shown on the previous label.

What volume of medication should be prepared to meet the order? _____

Which syringe would you choose to provide the most accurate dose to administer this medication? _____

Indicate the dose that would be drawn for this order.

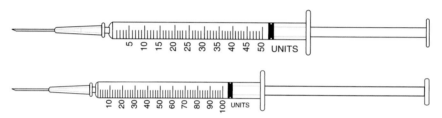

10. A physician orders procaine penicillin G 1,000,000 units IM. The medication available is a 10-mL vial of procaine penicillin G 250,000 units/mL.

What volume of medication should be given for this order? _____

Which syringe should you choose for the order? _____

What is the total concentration of the medication in the vial? _____

Indicate the volume of medication on the correct syringe.

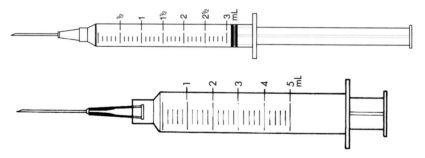

Pretest, cont.

11. A physician orders Lantus insulin glargine 55 units subcutaneously to be given daily at bedtime. The medication available is shown on the following label.

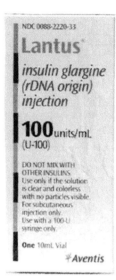

Can this medication be mixed with other insulin preparations? _____
Indicate on the syringe the amount of medication that should be shown to the patient for appropriate administration at home.

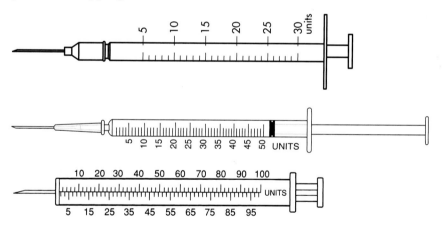

Continued

Pretest, cont.

12. A physician orders 17,000 units of heparin sodium subcutaneously as a stat dose. The available medications are shown on the following labels.

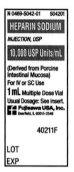

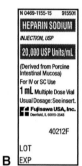

Which label strength of medication would be optimal to prepare the medication order? _____

What volume of medication should the patient receive when using the selected vial of medication? _____

Which syringe would be appropriate for administration of the medication? _____

Indicate the amount of medication on the appropriate syringe.

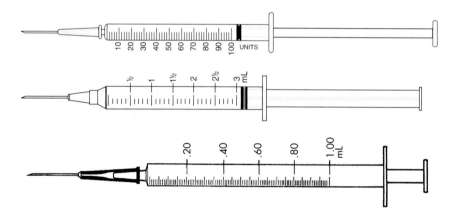

Pretest, cont.

13. A physician orders heparin sodium 750 units subcutaneously as a stat dose. Available are the following labels for preparing the medication for the order.

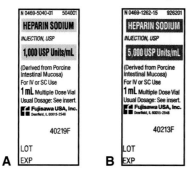

Which vial of medication should be made available for administration?

_____

Which syringe should be used for administration? _____

Indicate the amount of medication on the correct syringe.

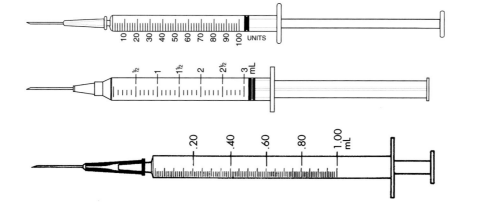

Continued

Pretest, cont.

14. A physician orders a heparin sodium flush 45 units to be administered q12h to keep an intravenous site **patent**. The available medications are shown on the following labels.

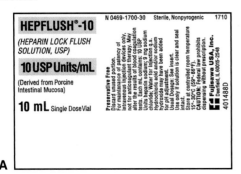
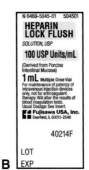

A   **B**

Choose the appropriate medication for completing the order. _____

What volume of medication should be administered to the patient using the appropriate medication label? _____

Indicate the correct amount of medication to be administered to prepare this order on the correct syringe.

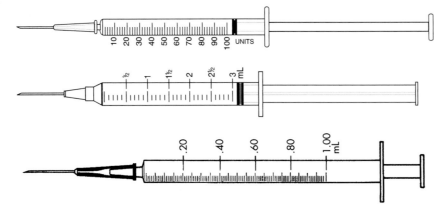

Pretest, cont.

15. A physician orders penicillin G potassium 10,000,000 units to be given IV stat. Use the following label to complete this order.

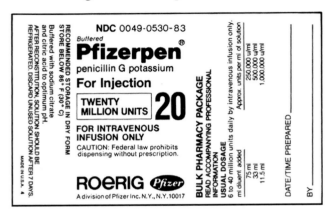

If 11.5 mL of diluent is added to this vial, what is the strength of the medication per milliliter? _____

For what length of time would the medication be acceptable for use after reconstitution? _____

What volume of medication should be added to IV fluids to complete this order as diluted above? _____

Indicate the needed documentation for the label following reconstitution using today's date and time and initials as appropriate. _____

Choose the appropriate syringe that is necessary to add the penicillin to the fluids.

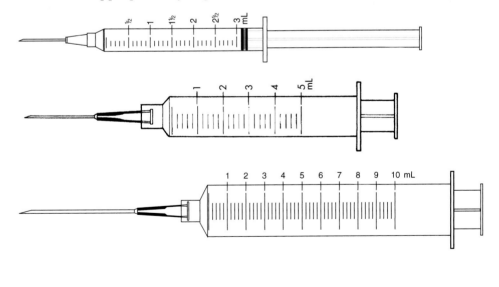

Continued

Pretest, cont.

16. A physician orders V-Cillin K suspension 300,000 units q6h. The available medication is V-Cillin K suspension 200,000 units/5 mL.

What volume of medication should be administered? _____
On the following measuring device(s), show the volume of medication that should be administered.

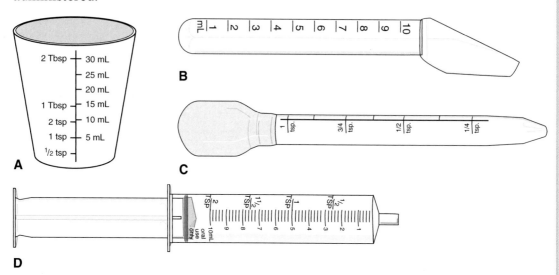

17. A physician orders Mycostatin oral suspension 250,000 units to be swished and swallowed. The medication is available as shown in the following label.

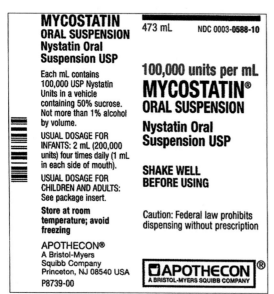

What volume of medication should be administered? _____

Which oral measuring device(s) could be used to administer this medication?

_____

Pretest, cont.

Indicate the amount to be administered on the correct measuring device(s).

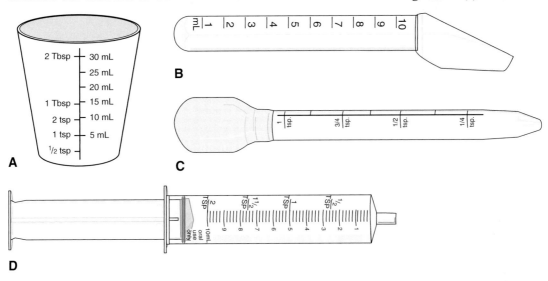

18. A physician orders Kaon-Cl 40 mEq po qam. The available medication is Kaon-Cl 40 mEq/15 mL.

What volume of medication should be administered? _____

Which measuring device(s) should be used to administer this medication?

_____

How could this be administered using a household measuring device? _____

Indicate the amount to be administered on the correct utensil.

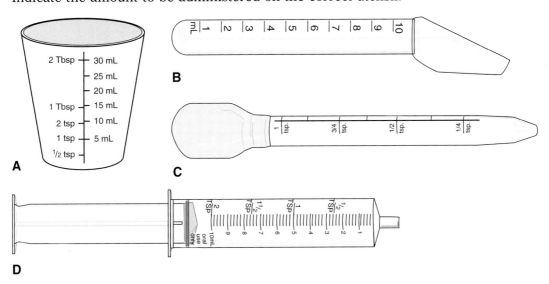

Continued

Pretest, cont.

 19. A physician orders Klor-Con (KCl) 10 mEq daily. The available medication is Klor-Con 20 mEq scored tablet.

How many tablet(s) should be administered to fulfill this order?

_____

20. A physician provides a new prescription for Humulin R 12 units and Humulin N 35 units subcutaneously qam. Use the following labels to calculate the medication for this order.

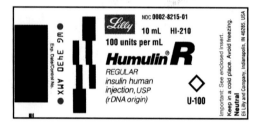 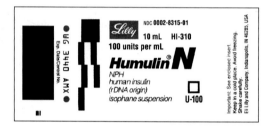

How many units of medication would be available in each vial for future use when this dose of medication has been prepared? _____

Using the syringes that follow, show the amount of regular insulin on one syringe, the amount of Lente insulin on another syringe, and the total amount of insulin on the final syringe.

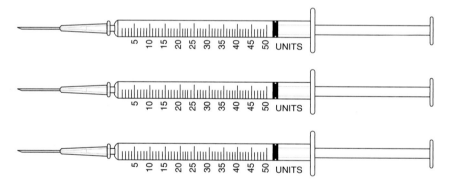

Posttest, cont.

2. A physician orders potassium bicarbonate powder 15 mEq to be dissolved in water for administration. The available potassium bicarbonate powder is 10 mEq per packet to be dissolved in 5 mL.

How many milliliters should be used to dissolve two packets before preparing the necessary dose? _____

How many milliliters of prepared medication, after dissolution, should be administered for the dose ordered? _____

3. A physician orders heparin sodium 7500 units subcutaneously stat.

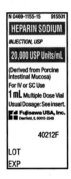

What volume of medication should be administered? _____

Continued

Posttest, cont.

4. A physician orders Humalog 12 units ac.

Which vial of medication should be used to fill this medication order?

_____

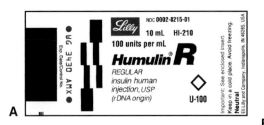

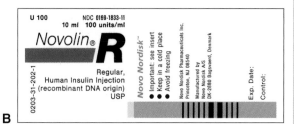

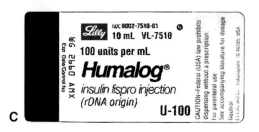

Which syringe should be used to administer this medication?

_____

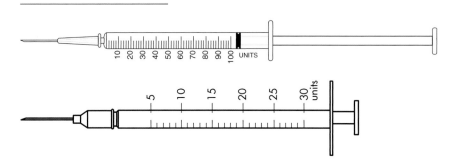

Posttest, cont.

5. A physician orders Duracillin A.S. 600,000 units IM bid for a patient with a severe infection. The available medication is shown on the following label.

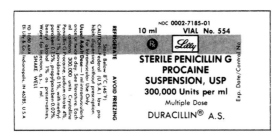

What volume of penicillin should be administered to this patient?

_____

6. A physician orders Fragmin 5000 International units subcutaneously.

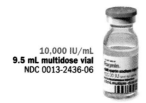

10,000 IU/mL
9.5 mL multidose vial
NDC 0013-2436-06

What volume of medication should be given to this patient? _____

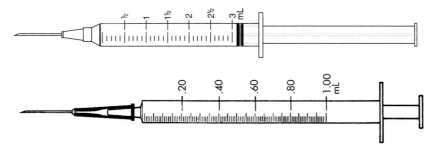

Continued

Posttest, cont.

7. A physician orders penicillin V oral suspension 275,000 units po qid. The medication available is penicillin V oral suspension 400,000 units/5 mL.

What volume of medication should be administered to the patient?

_____

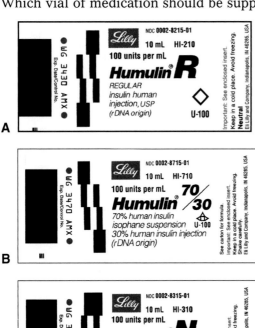

8. A physician orders Humulin 70/30 19 units qam for an elderly patient.

Which vial of medication should be supplied to the patient? _____

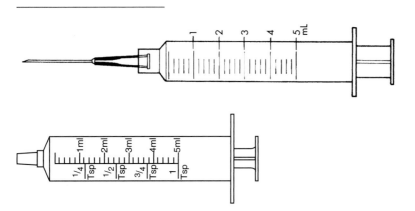

Posttest, cont.

Which syringe(s) should be supplied to fill the order? _____

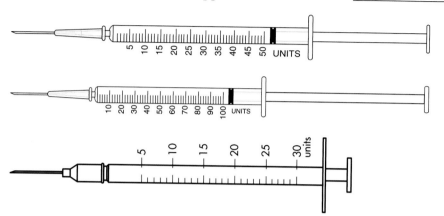

Explain why this choice was made for an elderly patient. _____

What is meant by Humulin 70/30? _____

9. A physician orders potassium chloride 12 mEq IV. The label reads 8 mEq/5 mL.
   What volume of medication should be administered to the patient?

   _____

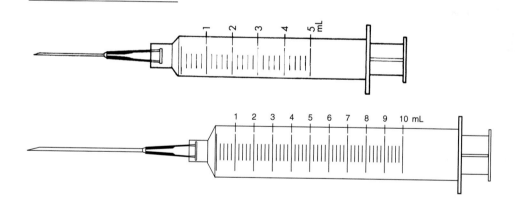

Continued

Posttest, cont.

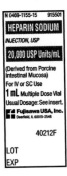

10. A physician orders heparin sodium 12,000 units subcutaneously stat.

N 0469-1155-15   915501
HEPARIN SODIUM
INJECTION, USP
20,000 USP Units/mL
(Derived from Porcine
Intestinal Mucosa)
For IV or SC Use
1 mL Multiple Dose Vial
Usual Dosage: See insert.
■■ **Fujisawa USA, Inc.**
■■ Deerfield, IL 60015-2548

40212F

LOT
EXP

What volume of medication should be administered to the patient?

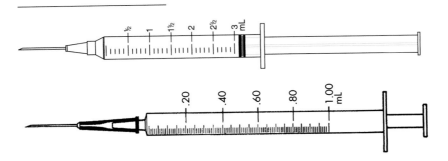

Posttest, cont.

EN DO

11. A physician orders Humulin N 21 units and Humulin R 36 units qam.

Which vials of medication should be used to fill this order? _____

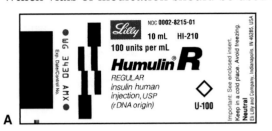

A

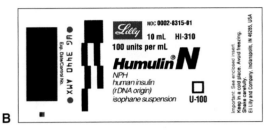

B

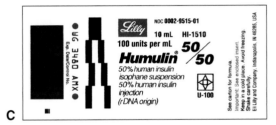

C

Which syringe(s) should be used to administer this medication?

_____

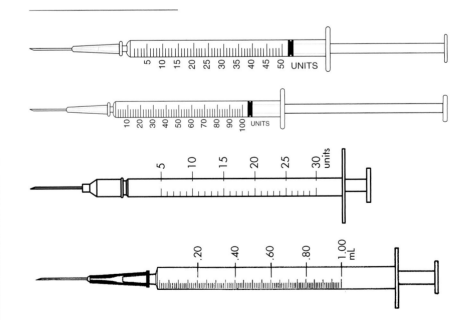

Continued

Posttest, cont.

EN DO **12.** A physician orders Humulin 70/30 26 units and Humulin R 14 units qam 30 min ac breakfast.

Which bottles of medication should be used to fill the prescription?

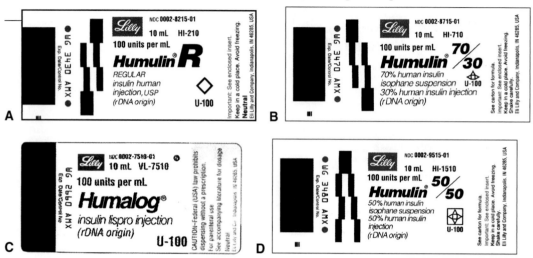

How many total units of regular insulin would be administered every morning?

_____

How many units of NPH would be administered every morning? _____

Show the amount of medication for each type of insulin on the correct syringe.

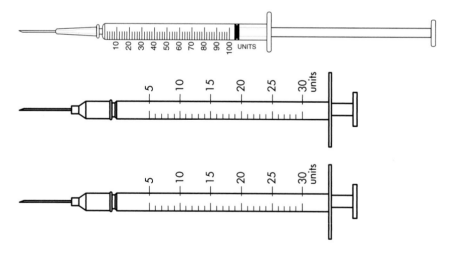

Posttest, cont.

 13. A physician orders KCl 25 mEq to be added to 1000 mL D-5-W.

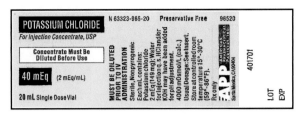

How many milliliters of KCl would need to be added to the fluids for this order?

_____

Continued

Posttest, cont.

14. A physician orders penicillin G potassium 250,000 units IM bid for a patient with strep throat.

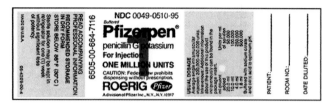

How many milliliters of diluent should be added to the vial to prepare the solution to 500,000 units per milliliter IM? _____

Show the amount of diluent addition on the correct syringe.

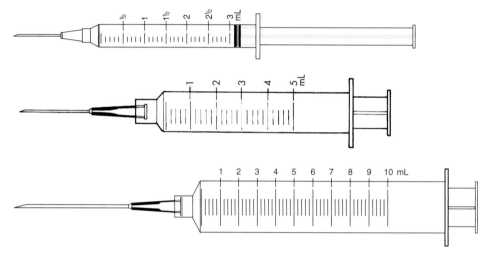

What would be the dose volume to be administered to the patient bid after dilution?

_____

Show the amount of medication to be administered on the correct syringe.

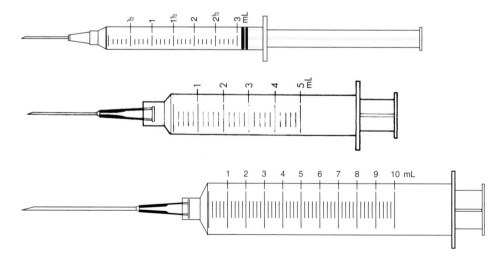

Posttest, cont.

15. A patient is to receive Fragmin 2500 international units subcutaneously daily. The label reads Fragmin 10,000 international units/mL.

What amount of medication should the patient receive daily?

_____

Show the amount of medication on the correct syringe.

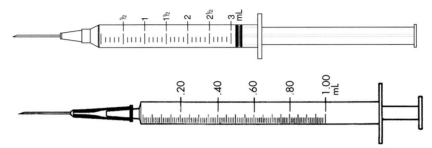

16. A physician orders Humulin N 30 units for a patient qam. The vial of medication contains 10 mL. No insulin syringe is available to measure this amount of medication today, but a tuberculin syringe is available and can be used because no insulin syringe is available for immediate use. The physician has approved use of a tuberculin syringe.

Show on the tuberculin syringe the amount of medication that should be drawn into the tuberculin syringe.

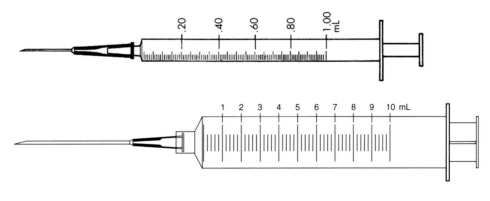

Continued

Posttest, cont.

 17. A physician orders KCl 30 mEq daily for a patient who is taking Lasix daily. The medication available is KCl 10 mEq tablets.

How many tablets should be given to this patient as a single dose?

_____

 18. A physician orders Duracillin 500,000 units IM. A 10-mL vial of Duracillin 300,000 units/mL is the medication on hand.

Using the above reconstitution, what volume of medication should be given to the

patient? _____

Show the amount to be administered on the correct syringe.

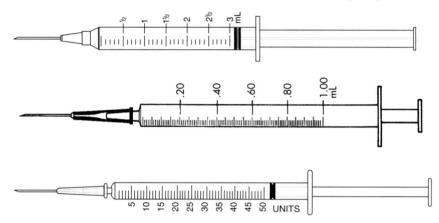

 19. A physician orders regular insulin 70 units to be added to a liter of D-5-W.

Choose the correct syringe and indicate the volume to be added to the fluids.

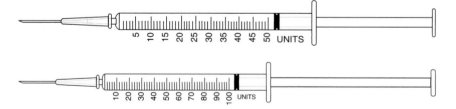

Posttest, cont.

20. A physician orders penicillin G procaine 750,000 units IM stat and then 600,000 units bid. The following label is the medication available for this order.

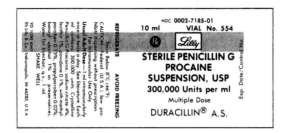

What volume of medication should be administered to the patient stat?

_____

What volume of medication should be administered bid? _____

Indicate on the correct syringe the volume to be given stat.

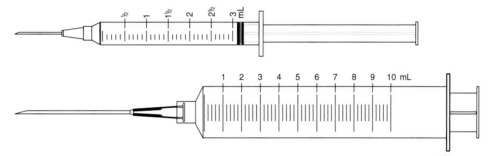

Indicate on the correct syringe the volume to be given bid.

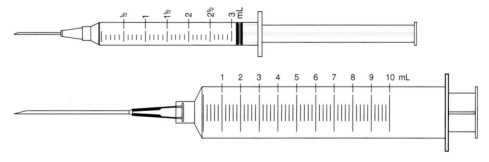

REVIEW OF RULES

Calculations of Medications Measured in Units and Milliequivalents

- Medications found in units are expressed as the number of units per liquid volume.

- Medications in milliequivalents may be shown as the number of milliequivalents per liquid or solid measure.

- Labels on medications given in units/volume must be read carefully and interpreted for the strength of the medication.

- Use either formula (Dose desired/Dose available × quantity = Dose to be given), dimensional analysis method, or ratio and proportion to calculate medications in units.

Interpreting Medications in Percentage and Ratio Concentrations

- Percentage and ratio solutions are expressed to indicate the weight of solute found in the solvent.

- The solute is an active ingredient found in either a solid or liquid solvent.

- The percentage would be amount of solute found in 100 mL or 100 g of solvent.

- The ratio would be the amount of medication found in a total prepared volume of solution, usually milliliters.

- Percentage is expressed using % as an indication of the amount of active ingredient in a medication. The ratio is divided by a colon (:) to separate the solute and solvent.

- To calculate the amount of drug in the prepared solution, write the solution strength as a ratio to show the amount of medication found in the total solution. (Refer to Chapter 2 if necessary to review percentage and ratio.)

- To calculate the ratio in a medication preparation, whether solid, semi-solid, or liquid, the total amount of prepared medication minus the amount of solute equals the amount of solvent that should be added for the total volume desired.

- The following formula expresses the actual mathematical formula that would be used to provide a percentage relationship:

$$\text{Percentage} = \frac{\text{Weight or volume of solute (grams or milliliters of solute)}}{\text{Volume/100 millimeters of prepared solution}}$$

- The formula below shows the mathematical calculation for medications expressed as ratios:

$$\text{Ratio} = \text{Weight or volume of solute} : \text{Amount of prepared medication}$$

CHAPTER 12

Calculation of Medications Used Intravenously

OBJECTIVES

- Interpret orders for volume of medications to be administered as intravenous (IV) fluids
- Calculate dosages of IV solutes in IV fluids including those expressed as percentages
- Calculate IV flow rates in drops per minute (gtts/min)
- Calculate time needed to infuse an ordered volume of IV fluids

KEY WORDS

Continuous infusion Introduction of a substance such as IV fluids or interstitial fluids over period of time without interruption of therapy

Conversion factor, time Factor needed to change from one unit of time to another such as hours to minutes

Conversion factor, volume Factor needed to change from one unit of volume to another between measuring systems or within a measuring system, such as liters to milliliters

Dose time Amount of time needed to administer medication

Dose volume Volume of medication administered at a given time

Drop factor Size of drop from the drip chamber found on IV tubing (drops/mL)

Flow rate Speed at which IV medications are infused depending on physician's order; usually drops/minute

Intravenous Within vein

Macrodrip infusion sets Infusion sets used for measuring rate of IV fluids; macrodrip sets provide large drops (10 to 20 drops/mL) of fluid called macrodrops

Maintenance therapy Using IV fluids to provide necessary nutrients to meet daily needs for water, electrolytes, and glucose

Microdrip infusion sets Infusion sets used for measuring rate of IV fluids; microdrip sets supply small drops (e.g., 60 drops/mL) called microdrops; other microdrip sets provide 50, 100, or 150 drops/mL

Piggyback Special coupling for primary IV lines to allow supplementary solutions to be added for administration into current IV administration set

Prophylaxis Using biological, chemical, or mechanical agent to prevent disease to prevent entrance of infectious organisms into the body

Replacement therapy The process of providing fluids and electrolytes to the body, when a deficit of fluids or electrolytes is present, in order to meet physiologic needs

Restorative therapy Day-by-day restoration of vital fluids and electrolytes using IV therapy

Solute Substance dissolved in a solution or semisolid

Solvent Substance in which a solute is dissolved, either liquid or semisolid

TECH NOTE

The medications found in this chapter are capitalized because that is how IV medications are designated when used for IV medication therapy.

Pretest

Answer the following problems to determine your level of ability in calculating medication orders for IV administration of fluids. In final answers round to the nearest drop or nearest milliliter (if less than one, round to the nearest tenth). Measurements for total volume in containers (such as liters) should be rounded to the nearest hundredth. Weight measurements should be carried to the nearest hundredth as appropriate unless otherwise stated. Time measurements should be to the closest minute or hour as indicated. Show your work. When adding volumes of medication to fluids, the volume of medication(s) added should be included when calculating the total volume of fluids.

1. A physician orders a continuous infusion of 1000 mL D-5-W with 20 mEq KCl/L q8h.

   How many milliequivalents of POTASSIUM CHLORIDE are found in each 100 mL of the fluids? _____

   How many milliequivalents of KCl should the patient receive each hour?

   _____h

   How many milliliters of fluids should be administered every hour? _____

2. A physician orders 500 mL D-5-1/2 NS q8h as a continuous infusion to be administered to a patient. The physician wants the pharmacy technician to calculate the total amount of DEXTROSE and SODIUM CHLORIDE the patient will receive.

   How many grams of DEXTROSE would the patient receive every 8 hours?

   _____

   How many grams of SODIUM CHLORIDE would the patient receive every 8 hours?

   _____

3. A physician orders 1 L of D-5-NS to be infused over 8 hours.

   How many mL/hr should the patient receive for the order to last the desired time?

   _____

   If using a macrodrip infusion set at 20 gtts/mL, how many milliliters per minute should the patient receive? _____

   How many gtt(s)/min should be administered? _____

Pretest, cont.

4. A physician orders 3000 mL LACTATED RINGER'S solution to infuse over 16 hours. The drop factor is 10 gtts/mL.

   How many gtt(s)/min should the patient receive for this order? _____

   How many mL/hour should be administered? _____

   How many mL/min should be administered? _____

5. A physician orders ANCEF 1g in 100 mL D-5-W IVPB to be infused over 1 hour.

   How many mL/min does the patient receive? _____

   If the drop factor is 20 gtts/mL, how many gtt(s)/min should the patient receive?

   _____

6. A container of fluids contains 550 mL, and the drop rate for the infusion set is 20 gtts/mL.

   How long do the fluids take to be infused if the infusion flow rate is 15 mL/min?

   _____

   How many gtt(s)/min should be administered? _____

7. A physician orders 1500 mL 0.45% NaCl IV over 24 hours. The drop factor on the infusion set is 20 gtts/mL.

   What is the weight in grams of SODIUM CHLORIDE in the total solution?

   _____

   What is the weight in grams of SODIUM CHLORIDE in 500 mL of solution?

   _____

   How many milliliters of solution should be administered to the patient q8h?

   _____

   How many mL/min should be administered so the fluids will last the time indicated by the physician? _____

   How many gtt(s)/min should the patient receive? _____

Continued

Pretest, cont.

8. A physician orders 1000 mL of D-10-W to be administered over 6 hours. The infusion set supplies 10 gtts/mL.

What are the total drops in the solution using the given infusion set? _____

What number of gtt(s)/min would be necessary to complete the order?

_____

What is the metric weight of DEXTROSE in the solution? _____

How many mL/min should be administered? _____

9. A physician orders LACTATED RINGER'S solution to be administered with a 20 gtts/min infusion set. The physician wants the pharmacy to decide the amount of fluid that should be necessary over a 24-hour period if the medication is administered at 2 mL/min.

How many liters of fluids would be necessary to fulfill this order?

_____

How many milliliters of fluids would the patient receive in a day?

_____

How many 1000 mL containers of fluids are needed to fulfill this order? _____

10. A physician orders D-5-NS q24h. The drop factor is 20 gtts/mL, and the flow rate is 50 mL/hr.

How many liters of fluids would be necessary to provide the fluids for this order?

_____

How many mL/hr should be given to the patient? _____

What is the total metric weight of SODIUM CHLORIDE that this person would receive in a 24-hour period? _____

How many milliliters per minute should the patient receive? _____

Pretest, cont.

 11. An order is given for a patient to receive D-5-NS as a continuous infusion until further orders. The drop factor is 20 gtts/mL, and the flow rate is 40 mL/hr.

How many 1000-mL containers of fluids would be necessary each 24 hours to fill this order? _____

How many gtt(s)/min should be administered to the patient? _____

What is the total metric weight of SODIUM CHLORIDE this person would receive daily in the fluids? _____

How many mL/min should the patient receive? _____

What is the total amount of IV fluids to be administered each 24 hours? _____

12. How many grams of DEXTROSE are in the fluids for the label shown?

_____

If the drop factor is 15 gtts/mL, and the flow rate is 20 mL/min, how long would these fluids need for infusion? _____

How many gtt(s)/min should be administered? _____

LOT   EXP

 ⊙   ⊙   2B2073
                                NDC 0338-0125-03   —**1**

Lactated Ringer's
and 5% Dextrose   —**2**
Injection USP

500 mL   —**3**

EACH 100 mL CONTAINS   5 g DEXTROSE HYDROUS USP
600 mg SODIUM CHLORIDE USP   310 mg SODIUM LACTATE
30 mg POTASSIUM CHLORIDE USP   20 mg CALCIUM CHLORIDE USP
pH 5.0 (4.0 TO 6.5) mEq/L SODIUM 130 POTASSIUM 4 CALCIUM 2.7
CHLORIDE 109 LACTATE 28 HYPERTONIC OSMOLARITY 525 mOsmol/L   —**4**
(CALC) STERILE NONPYROGENIC SINGLE DOSE CONTAINER NOT FOR USE
IN THE TREATMENT OF LACTIC ACIDOSIS   ADDITIVES MAY BE INCOMPATIBLE
CONSULT WITH PHARMACIST IF AVAILABLE   WHEN INTRODUCING ADDITIVES USE
ASEPTIC TECHNIQUE   MIX THOROUGHLY   DO NOT STORE   DOSAGE
INTRAVENOUSLY AS DIRECTED BY A PHYSICIAN   SEE DIRECTIONS   CAUTIONS
SQUEEZE AND INSPECT INNER BAG WHICH MAINTAINS PRODUCT STERILITY
DISCARD IF LEAKS ARE FOUND   MUST NOT BE USED IN SERIES CONNECTIONS
DO NOT ADMINISTER SIMULTANEOUSLY WITH BLOOD   DO NOT USE UNLESS
SOLUTION IS CLEAR   FEDERAL (USA) LAW PROHIBITS DISPENSING WITHOUT
PRESCRIPTION   STORE UNIT IN MOISTURE BARRIER OVERWRAP AT ROOM
TEMPERATURE (25°C/77°F) UNTIL READY TO USE   AVOID EXCESSIVE HEAT
SEE INSERT

Baxter   Viaflex® CONTAINER
BAXTER HEALTHCARE CORPORATION   PL 146® PLASTIC
DEERFIELD IL 60015 USA   FOR PRODUCT INFORMATION
MADE IN USA   CALL 1-800-933-0303

Continued

Pretest, cont.

13. How many grams of SODIUM CHLORIDE are in the fluids shown in the following label? _____

The fluids are to infuse for 24 hours at a rate of 30 gtts/min. How many bags of fluids would be necessary for the order as written if the drop factor is 15 gtts/mL?

_____

What is the total volume of IV fluids to be received in 24 hours? _____

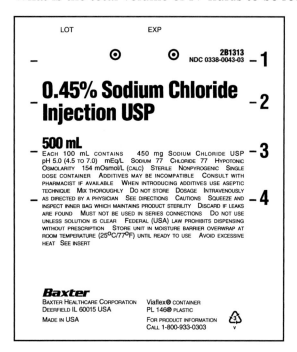

14. One L of D-5-NS is to infuse at 8 mL/min, and the drop factor is 20 gtts/mL.

How many gtt(s)/min should the patient receive? _____

How long would it take to infuse 1 L? _____

Which container of fluids should be used for the patient? _____

Pretest, cont.

A

LOT   EXP

2B1064
NDC 0338-0089-04   **1**

5% Dextrose and 0.9% Sodium Chloride Injection USP   **2** **3**

1000 mL   **4**

EACH 100 mL CONTAINS   5 g DEXTROSE HYDROUS USP
900 mg SODIUM CHLORIDE USP   pH 4.0 (3.2 TO 6.5)
mEq/L   SODIUM 154   CHLORIDE 154   HYPERTONIC
OSMOLARITY 560 mOsmol/L (CALC)   STERILE NONPYROGENIC
SINGLE DOSE CONTAINER   ADDITIVES MAY BE INCOMPATIBLE
CONSULT WITH PHARMACIST IF AVAILABLE   WHEN INTRODUCING
ADDITIVES USE ASEPTIC TECHNIQUE   MIX THOROUGHLY   DO NOT
STORE   DOSAGE   INTRAVENOUSLY AS DIRECTED BY A PHYSICIAN
SEE DIRECTIONS   CAUTIONS   SQUEEZE AND INSPECT INNER BAG
WHICH MAINTAINS PRODUCT STERILITY   DISCARD IF LEAKS ARE
FOUND   MUST NOT BE USED IN SERIES CONNECTIONS   DO NOT
USE UNLESS SOLUTION IS CLEAR   FEDERAL (USA) LAW PROHIBITS
DISPENSING WITHOUT PRESCRIPTION   STORE UNIT IN MOISTURE
BARRIER OVERWRAP AT ROOM TEMPERATURE (25ºC/77ºF) UNTIL
READY TO USE   AVOID EXCESSIVE HEAT   SEE INSERT   **5** **6** **7**

Baxter   **8**
BAXTER HEALTHCARE CORPORATION   Viaflex® CONTAINER
DEERFIELD IL 60015 USA   PL 146® PLASTIC
MADE IN USA   FOR PRODUCT INFORMATION
CALL 1-800-933-0303   **9**

B

LOT   EXP

2B0064
NDC 0338-0017-04   **1**

5% Dextrose Injection USP   **2** **3**

1000 mL   **4**

EACH 100 mL CONTAINS   5 g DEXTROSE HYDROUS USP
pH 4.0 (3.2 TO 6.5)   OSMOLARITY 252 mOsmol/L (CALC)
STERILE   NONPYROGENIC   SINGLE DOSE CONTAINER   ADDITIVES
MAY BE INCOMPATIBLE   CONSULT WITH PHARMACIST IF AVAILABLE
WHEN INTRODUCING ADDITIVES USE ASEPTIC TECHNIQUE   MIX
THOROUGHLY   DO NOT STORE   DOSAGE   INTRAVENOUSLY AS
DIRECTED BY A PHYSICIAN   SEE DIRECTIONS   CAUTIONS   SQUEEZE
AND INSPECT INNER BAG WHICH MAINTAINS PRODUCT STERILITY
DISCARD IF LEAKS ARE FOUND   MUST NOT BE USED IN SERIES
CONNECTIONS   DO NOT ADMINISTER SIMULTANEOUSLY WITH BLOOD
DO NOT USE UNLESS SOLUTION IS CLEAR   FEDERAL (USA) LAW
PROHIBITS DISPENSING WITHOUT PRESCRIPTION   STORE UNIT IN
MOISTURE BARRIER OVERWRAP AT ROOM TEMPERATURE
(25ºC/77ºF) UNTIL READY TO USE   AVOID EXCESSIVE HEAT   SEE
INSERT   **5** **6** **7**

Baxter   **8**
BAXTER HEALTHCARE CORPORATION   Viaflex® CONTAINER
DEERFIELD IL 60015 USA   PL 146® PLASTIC
MADE IN USA   FOR PRODUCT INFORMATION
CALL 1-800-933-0303   **9**

C

LOT   EXP

2B1073
NDC 0338-0085-03   **1**

5% Dextrose and 0.45% Sodium Chloride Injection USP   **2**

500 mL   **3**

EACH 100 mL CONTAINS   5 g DEXTROSE HYDROUS USP   450 mg SODIUM
CHLORIDE USP   pH 4.0 (3.2 TO 6.5)   mEq/L   SODIUM 77   CHLORIDE 77
HYPERTONIC   OSMOLARITY   406 mOsmol/L (CALC)   STERILE
NONPYROGENIC   SINGLE DOSE CONTAINER   ADDITIVES MAY BE INCOMPATIBLE
CONSULT WITH PHARMACIST IF AVAILABLE   WHEN INTRODUCING ADDITIVES USE
ASEPTIC TECHNIQUE   MIX THOROUGHLY   DO NOT STORE   DOSAGE   **4**
INTRAVENOUSLY AS DIRECTED BY A PHYSICIAN   SEE DIRECTIONS   CAUTIONS
SQUEEZE AND INSPECT INNER BAG WHICH MAINTAINS PRODUCT STERILITY
DISCARD IF LEAKS ARE FOUND   MUST NOT BE USED IN SERIES CONNECTIONS
DO NOT USE UNLESS SOLUTION IS CLEAR   FEDERAL (USA) LAW PROHIBITS
DISPENSING WITHOUT PRESCRIPTION   STORE UNIT IN MOISTURE BARRIER
OVERWRAP AT ROOM TEMPERATURE (25ºC/77ºF) UNTIL READY TO USE
AVOID EXCESSIVE HEAT   SEE INSERT

Baxter
BAXTER HEALTHCARE CORPORATION   Viaflex® CONTAINER
DEERFIELD IL 60015 USA   PL 146® PLASTIC
MADE IN USA   FOR PRODUCT INFORMATION
CALL 1-800-933-0303

Continued

Pretest, cont.

15. A physician orders KEFZOL 1 g IVPB; the KEFZOL is to be mixed in 100 mL D-5-W to infuse over 1 hour. The drop factor is 50 gtts/mL.

What is the rate in gtt(s)/min necessary to fulfill the order? _____

How many milliliters should be infused within 30 minutes? _____

How many milligrams of KEFZOL would be administered in 15 minutes? _____

16. Three L of D-10-W are to infuse over a 24-hour period.

How many mL/hr should the patient receive? _____

How many milliliters (in tenths) per minute should the patient receive?

_____

If the drop factor is 10 gtts/mL, how many gtt(s)/min would the patient receive?

_____

17. A liter of D-5-NS is infusing at the rate of 45 gtts/min. The drop factor is 15 gtts/mL.

How many mL/hr would the patient receive? _____

How long in hours would it take for the fluids to infuse? _____

18. A physician orders PEPCID (FAMOTIDINE) 20 mg IVPB q12h. The medication is available in 10 mg/mL vials. The medication is to be added to 100 mL LACTATED RINGER'S solution and is to infuse over 30 minutes.

How many milliliters of FAMOTIDINE are added to each IVPB? _____

How many milliliters (in tenths) per minute would the patient receive?

_____

If the drop factor is 20 gtts/mL, how many gtt(s)/min are infused?

_____

Pretest, cont.

19. A physician orders AMPHOTERICIN B 40 mg IV in 500 mL of D-5-W daily to be infused over 12 hours. After reconstitution, the medication contains 50 mg/10 mL. The drop factor is 25 gtts/mL.

How many milliliters of AMPHOTERICIN B would be added to each 500 mL of fluids? _____

How many milliliters are administered every hour? _____

How many milliliters are administered every minute to fulfill the order?

_____

How many gtt(s)/min are administered? _____

1 vial   NDC 0003-0437-30
NSN 6505-01-084-9453

50 mg

FUNGIZONE®
INTRAVENOUS

Amphotericin B
for Injection USP

FOR INTRAVENOUS INFUSION
IN HOSPITALS ONLY

Caution: Federal law prohibits
dispensing without prescription

Read all sides

☐ APOTHECON®
A BRISTOL-MYERS SQUIBB COMPANY

20. A physician orders AMPICILLIN 2 g IVPB. After mixing in 500 mL of D-5-1/2 NS, it will be administered over 2 hours using a drop factor of 10 gtts/mL. The available medication is AMPICILLIN 1 g vials to be reconstituted with 2.5 mL NS in each vial.

How many milliliters per hour should be given to the patient? _____

How many gtt(s)/min should be administered? _____

What fluids should be chosen for adding the AMPICILLIN? _____

How many milliliters per minute should be administered for the ordered time and amount of fluids? _____

Continued

Copyright © 2013, 2007 by Saunders, an imprint of Elsevier Inc.

Pretest, cont.

A

LOT   EXP

2B1073
NDC 0338-0085-03 — 1

5% Dextrose and 0.45% Sodium Chloride Injection USP — 2

500 mL — 3

Each 100 mL contains 5 g Dextrose Hydrous USP 450 mg Sodium Chloride USP pH 4.0 (3.2 to 6.5) mEq/L Sodium 77 Chloride 77 Hypertonic Osmolarity 406 mOsmol/L (calc) Sterile Nonpyrogenic Single dose container Additives may be incompatible Consult with pharmacist if available When introducing additives use aseptic technique Mix thoroughly Do not store Dosage Intravenously as directed by a physician See directions Cautions Squeeze and inspect inner bag which maintains product sterility Discard if leaks are found Must not be used in series connections Do not use unless solution is clear Federal (USA) law prohibits dispensing without prescription Store unit in moisture barrier overwrap at room temperature (25°C/77°F) until ready to use Avoid excessive heat See insert — 4

Baxter
Baxter Healthcare Corporation
Deerfield IL 60015 USA
Made in USA

Viaflex® container
PL 146® plastic
For product information
Call 1-800-933-0303

B

LOT   EXP

2B1313
NDC 0338-0043-03 — 1

0.45% Sodium Chloride Injection USP — 2

500 mL — 3

Each 100 mL contains 450 mg Sodium Chloride USP pH 5.0 (4.5 to 7.0) mEq/L Sodium 77 Chloride 77 Hypotonic Osmolarity 154 mOsmol/L (calc) Sterile Nonpyrogenic Single dose container Additives may be incompatible Consult with pharmacist if available When introducing additives use aseptic technique Mix thoroughly Do not store Dosage Intravenously as directed by a physician See directions Cautions Squeeze and inspect inner bag which maintains product sterility Discard if leaks are found Must not be used in series connections Do not use unless solution is clear Federal (USA) law prohibits dispensing without prescription Store unit in moisture barrier overwrap at room temperature (25°C/77°F) until ready to use Avoid excessive heat See insert — 4

Baxter
Baxter Healthcare Corporation
Deerfield IL 60015 USA
Made in USA

Viaflex® container
PL 146® plastic
For product information
Call 1-800-933-0303

C

LOT   EXP

2B1163
NDC 0338-0095-03 — 1

10% Dextrose and 0.9% Sodium Chloride Injection USP — 2

500 mL — 3

Each 100 mL contains 10 g Dextrose Hydrous USP 900 mg Sodium Chloride USP pH 4.0 (3.2 to 6.5) mEq/L Sodium 154 Chloride 154 Osmolarity 813 mOsmol/L (calc) Hypertonic May cause vein damage Sterile Nonpyrogenic Single dose container Additives may be incompatible Consult with pharmacist if available When introducing additives use aseptic technique Mix thoroughly Do not store Dosage Intravenously as directed by a physician See directions Cautions Squeeze and inspect inner bag which maintains product sterility Discard if leaks are found Must not be used in series connections Do not use unless solution is clear Federal (USA) law prohibits dispensing without prescription Store unit in moisture barrier overwrap at room temperature (25°C/77°F) until ready to use Avoid excessive heat See insert — 4

Baxter
Baxter Healthcare Corporation
Deerfield IL 60015 USA
Made in USA

Viaflex® container
PL 146® plastic
For product information
Call 1-800-933-0303

INTRODUCTION

The definition of **intravenous** is to administer a medication and/or fluid directly into a vein. All medications administered intravenously must be in liquid form and must be sterile. IV fluids may be given in large volumes for **continuous infusion** in such basic fluids in 1000 mL amounts as sterile water or normal saline with dextrose added to meet caloric needs. Medications, such as electrolytes or antibiotics, may also be added to these containers to supply drugs or nutritional needs over a period of time. The physician's order will include the type and total fluid volume to be administered over a total period of time. In other cases, medications may be added to small volumes of fluids for administration on an intermittent basis either through an injection port in the tubing or a secondary line called IV **piggyback** (IVPB).

Intravenous medication prescriptions (intermittent, IVPB) specify the drug (solute), the dose to be given, and frequency of dosing but do not commonly state infusion rate or infusion time. The pharmacy determines the **solvent**, solvent volume, and time to be infused while the physician's order provides the **solute** to be added. This information from both the physician's order and the determinations made by the pharmacy is the information to be included on the label added to the parenteral fluid container for the specific person.

Fluids may be given as replacements for electrolytes or lost fluids such as with patients who have dehydration. **Maintenance therapy** provides the nutrients necessary to meet the daily needs for water, electrolytes, and glucose. With a deficit of fluids and electrolytes over a period of time, usually 48 hours, **replacement therapy** may be necessary to meet the fluid and electrolyte needs of the person. Finally, **restorative therapy** is a day-by-day restoration of vital fluids and electrolytes. With this therapy, the types of fluids being lost are those that are replaced. Often, several different types of fluids will be ordered for the patient on the same day.

Fluids may also be ordered as a means for transporting medications needing rapid absorption in the body. With the addition of drugs, the infusion is used as **prophylaxis** or therapeutically for disease processes.

Intravenous solutions are available in 50-mL to 1000-mL containers (commonly in flexible plastic bags) with each containing solutes and solvents prescribed for the patient's specific needs. The reason for therapy dictates the type of fluid and rate of infusion ordered. Fluids given to keep a vein open are given slowly, whereas replacement fluids are usually given at a rate that will provide the necessary fluids while preventing an overload on the vascular system. The rate of flow depends on the patient's physical condition. Most IV fluids are found in percentages of solutes (solids) in the total volume of solvent (solution) such as D-5-W, which is 5% dextrose in water. As learned in Chapter 11, this means that 5 g of dextrose are dissolved in every 100 mL of sterile water, or 50 g of dextrose are found in 1000 mL of water. While most IV fluids are infused by pump today, it is still important to be conscious of selecting the correct fluids for the IV infusion and ensuring an infusion is administered at the prescribed rate.

This chapter will focus on how to determine **flow rates** in drops per minute and determining the infusion time. You may need to determine the total time necessary for an amount of fluid to be administered as ordered, or you may need to calculate the flow rate when a total time of administration has been specified in the physician's order.

Persons allowed to prepare and administer IV fluids are regulated by state law and the regulations of the facility where the fluids are to be administered. In some states, technicians may prepare the IV fluids for infusion, whereas in others this preparation must be done by the pharmacist. As a pharmacy technician, you must always be cognizant of the laws of your state of practice and regulations of the place of employment.

Pharmacy technicians who work in retail pharmacy may find that they do not use this chapter often, because IV infusion preparation is rarely performed in a community pharmacy. On the other hand, IV fluids are often used in the hospital setting. Understanding the calculations related to IV infusions is important for the hospital pharmacy technician but is also necessary for the retail pharmacy technician, who might one day practice in the hospital setting.

INTERPRETING AMOUNTS OF SOLUTES IN INTRAVENOUS FLUIDS

To provide patients with continuous medications or for fluid replacement over a period of time, IV fluids are often administered to them rather than requiring them to undergo repeated injections by other parenteral routes. The medications found in fluids may be standard medications found in prepared IV fluids, such as dextrose or sodium chloride, or they may be added in the pharmacy to fill the physician's orders, such as antibiotics or electrolyte replacements. In some instances medications may be prepared by manufacturers as commonly seen with premixed IV piggyback solutions containing antibiotics found in routinely used volumes such as 50-mL containers. The health care professional must have the ability to read the physician's order and select the correct fluids and additives for the patient's needs. Remember that once the fluids have been injected into the vein, the medications cannot be retrieved because the medication circulates throughout the body instantaneously. Therefore it is imperative for patient safety that the correct fluids with the correct additives (medications) are used at a safe flow rate depending on the patient's physical condition and the medication being administered. Calculations for IV medications are performed using either ratio and proportion, formula (Dose desired/Dose on hand × Quantity = Dose to be given), or dimensional analysis, depending on method of choice.

In most cases the physician will use common abbreviations for ordering IV fluids. These are shown in Table 12-1. Notice fluids are labeled with a percentage of solute in the container of fluids or the amount of solute found in the solvent. D-5-W indicates that 5% dextrose is available in the solvent (sterile water). Remember that percentage is based on 100. So if the percentage is shown in 100 mL of solution, the 5% indicates that 5 g of dextrose is found in 100 mL of fluid. However, if the 5% is shown in 500 mL of a solvent such as water, then the total weight of the solute must be calculated. The easiest method for calculating the weight of solute is ratio and proportion (Known solute:Known volume::Desired-to-know solute:Desired-to-know volume). To review percentage and ratio and proportion, see Chapter 2.

TABLE 12.1 Abbreviations for Common Intravenous Solutions

ABBREVIATION	SOLUTION
NS	Normal saline; 0.9% sodium chloride
½ NS	Half-normal saline; 0.45% sodium chloride; or ½ strength normal saline
D-5-W or 5% D/W	Dextrose 5% in water
D-5-LR	Dextrose 5% in lactated Ringer's
RL or LR	Ringer's lactate solution or lactated Ringer's
D-5-NS	Dextrose 5% in 0.9% sodium chloride; dextrose 5% in normal saline
D-5-½ NS	Dextrose 5% in ½ normal saline or 0.45% sodium chloride
D-2.5-½ NSt	2.5% dextrose in 0.45% sodium chloride
D-2½-W	2½% dextrose in water

TECH NOTE

Remember that when interpreting fluid solutes, 1 mL of water has a weight of 1 gram.

EXAMPLE 12-1

A physician orders 500 mL 5% D/W to be given to a patient. What is the metric weight (in grams) of the dextrose in this bag of fluids? Remember, 5% means that 5 g (solute) of dextrose is found in 100 mL of water (solvent).

Known   Unknown

$5 \text{ g} : 100 \text{ mL} :: x : 500 \text{ mL}$

$5 \text{ g} : 100 \text{ mL} :: x : 500 \text{ mL}$

$5 \text{ g} : 100 :: x : 500$

$100x = 5 \text{ g} \times 500$ or 2500

$x = 2500 \div 100$

$x = 25 \text{ g of DEXTROSE in } 500 \text{ mL of the above fluids}$

In some cases it is necessary to calculate the amount of medication a patient has received when the entire amount of ordered fluids is not infused.

EXAMPLE 12-2

A 1000-mL container of D-5-W contains 80 mEq KCl. The patient has received 650 mL of the fluids when it is discontinued. How many mEq KCl has the patient received?

Known   Unknown

$80 \text{ mEq} : 1000 \text{ mL} :: x : 650 \text{ mL}$

$80 \text{ mEq} : 1000 \text{ mL} :: x : 650 \text{ mL}$

$1000x = 650 \times 80 \text{ mEq}$ or $52{,}000 \text{ mEq}$

$x = 52{,}000 \text{ mEq} \div 1000$ or $52{,}000 \div 1000$

$x = 52 \text{ mEq of KCl were received by the patient}$

Practice Problems A

Calculate the solute volume found in the IV fluids. Use the method of choice for the calculations. Round answers to the nearest tenth. In some cases, the answer must be shown in hundredths; these will be noted with an asterisk. Supply answers in metric weight such as grams, unless otherwise noted. Show all of your work.

1. What is the weight of SODIUM CHLORIDE in these fluids? _____

What is the weight of DEXTROSE in these fluids? _____

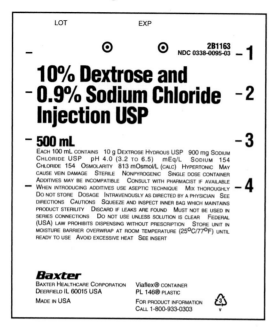

2. What is the weight of DEXTROSE in these fluids? _____

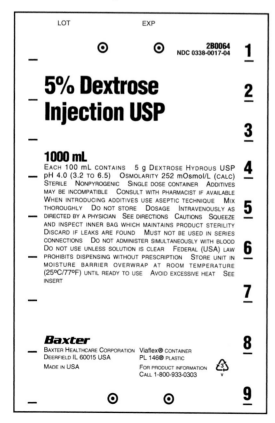

3. 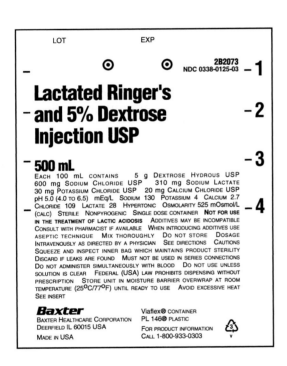 A 50-mL IVPB contains PENICILLIN 1.5 million units. The patient has received 35 mL of the medication.

How many units of PENICILLIN has the patient received? _____

4. What is the weight in grams of SODIUM CHLORIDE in the fluids shown in the following illustration? _____

What is the weight in grams of DEXTROSE in the fluids shown in the following illustration? _____

```
LOT              EXP

        ⊙        ⊙      2B2073      — 1
                      NDC 0338-0125-03

  Lactated Ringer's
— and 5% Dextrose              — 2
  Injection USP

— 500 mL                       — 3
  EACH 100 mL CONTAINS      5 g DEXTROSE HYDROUS USP
  600 mg SODIUM CHLORIDE USP    310 mg SODIUM LACTATE
  30 mg POTASSIUM CHLORIDE USP  20 mg CALCIUM CHLORIDE USP
  pH 5.0 (4.0 TO 6.5) mEq/L SODIUM 130 POTASSIUM 4 CALCIUM 2.7
  CHLORIDE 109 LACTATE 28 HYPERTONIC OSMOLARITY 525 mOsmol/L   — 4
  (CALC) STERILE NONPYROGENIC SINGLE DOSE CONTAINER NOT FOR USE
  IN THE TREATMENT OF LACTIC ACIDOSIS   ADDITIVES MAY BE INCOMPATIBLE
  CONSULT WITH PHARMACIST IF AVAILABLE   WHEN INTRODUCING ADDITIVES USE
  ASEPTIC TECHNIQUE   MIX THOROUGHLY   DO NOT STORE   DOSAGE
  INTRAVENOUSLY AS DIRECTED BY A PHYSICIAN   SEE DIRECTIONS   CAUTIONS
  SQUEEZE AND INSPECT INNER BAG WHICH MAINTAINS PRODUCT STERILITY
  DISCARD IF LEAKS ARE FOUND   MUST NOT BE USED IN SERIES CONNECTIONS
  DO NOT ADMINISTER SIMULTANEOUSLY WITH BLOOD   DO NOT USE UNLESS
  SOLUTION IS CLEAR   FEDERAL (USA) LAW PROHIBITS DISPENSING WITHOUT
  PRESCRIPTION   STORE UNIT IN MOISTURE BARRIER OVERWRAP AT ROOM
  TEMPERATURE (25°C/77°F) UNTIL READY TO USE   AVOID EXCESSIVE HEAT
  SEE INSERT

  Baxter                    Viaflex® CONTAINER
  BAXTER HEALTHCARE CORPORATION  PL 146® PLASTIC
  DEERFIELD IL 60015 USA    FOR PRODUCT INFORMATION   ⟁
  MADE IN USA               CALL 1-800-933-0303         ᵥ
```

5. *What is the weight of SODIUM CHLORIDE in grams found in the fluids shown below? _____

LOT   EXP

                    ⊙   ⊙   2B1313
                                        NDC 0338-0043-03   — **1**

0.45% Sodium Chloride   — **2**
Injection USP

500 mL   — **3**
Each 100 mL contains   450 mg Sodium Chloride USP
pH 5.0 (4.5 to 7.0) mEq/L Sodium 77 Chloride 77 Hypotonic
Osmolarity 154 mOsmol/L (calc) Sterile Nonpyrogenic Single
dose container Additives may be incompatible Consult with
pharmacist if available When introducing additives use aseptic
technique Mix thoroughly Do not store Dosage Intravenously   — **4**
as directed by a physician See directions Cautions Squeeze and
inspect inner bag which maintains product sterility Discard if leaks
are found Must not be used in series connections Do not use
unless solution is clear Federal (USA) law prohibits dispensing
without prescription Store unit in moisture barrier overwrap at
room temperature (25°C/77°F) until ready to use Avoid excessive
heat See insert

Baxter
Baxter Healthcare Corporation   Viaflex® container
Deerfield IL 60015 USA   PL 146® plastic
Made in USA   For product information
                                 Call 1-800-933-0303

6. A physician orders PENICILLIN G POTASSIUM 2.4 million units to be added to 1 L NS. You have on hand a vial of this medication that has been reconstituted to 1,000,000 units/mL.

How many milliliters of medication should be added to the fluids?

_____

If only 750 mL of fluids are administered, how many units of PENICILLIN G POTASSIUM has the patient received? _____

7. One liter of D-5-NS contains the POTASSIUM CHLORIDE as shown on the following label using the entire vial. The vein infiltrates after 900 mL have been infused.

How many milliequivalents of KCl were added to the fluids? _____

How many milliliters of KCl were added to the fluids? _____

How many grams of DEXTROSE did the patient receive before infiltration?

_____

How many grams of SODIUM CHLORIDE did the patient receive before infiltration?

_____

How many milliequivalents of KCl did the patient receive before the infusion was discontinued? _____

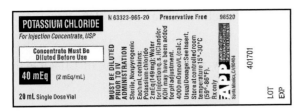

8. A physician orders FUROSEMIDE 100 mg in 200-mL NS. The patient receives 150 mL of the medication. Available medication is FUROSEMIDE 10 mg/mL.

*What total amount of SODIUM CHLORIDE did the patient receive?

_____

What amount of FUROSEMIDE did the patient receive? _____

9. **PAIN** A physician orders FENTANYL CITRATE 50 mcg to be added to D-5-W 500 mL. The medication is available as 10 mcg/mL.

How many milliliters of FENTANYL should be added to the fluids?

_____

If the patient receives 400 mL of the fluids, how many grams of dextrose has the patient received? _____

*How many milligrams of FENTANYL has the patient received? (Do not round this answer.) _____

10. A physician orders 1 L of DEXTROSE 3% to be administered over 6 hours.

If the complete bag of fluids is administered, how many grams of DEXTROSE would the patient receive? _____

If the fluids run for 5 hours only and the patient is discharged, how many grams of DEXTROSE would the patient receive? _____

11. ♥ A physician desires that a patient receive LIDOCAINE 150 mg in D-5-W 200 mL IVPB. The available medication is 1% LIDOCAINE for injection.

*How many milligrams of LIDOCAINE are in each milliliter of fluids?

_____

If the patient receives 65 mL of the IV fluids, how many milligrams of LIDOCAINE would the patient receive? _____

12. A physician orders AMPICILLIN 2000 mcg/kg IV stat for a patient who weighs 165 lb. The medication is to be added to 50 mL of D-5-W to infuse for 20 minutes. The AMPICILLIN is reconstituted to 250 mg/5 mL.

What total strength in milligrams of AMPICILLIN should be added to the fluids?

_____

How many milliliters of AMPICILLIN should be added to the D-5-W?

_____

If the IV fluids are stopped at 15 minutes, how many milligrams of AMPICILLIN did the patient receive? _____

13. **EN DO** A physician orders METHYLPREDNISOLONE 125 mg IV in D-5-W 100 mL to run for an hour for a patient with asthma. The medication comes in a vial containing 250 mg/5 mL.

How many milliliters of METHYLPREDNISOLONE would be added to the fluids to complete the order? _____

If the patient receives the medication for 50 minutes, how many milligrams of METHYLPREDNISOLONE would the patient receive? _____

14. A 50 mL container of D-10-NS contains PENICILLIN 1.5 million units. These fluids are to be infused over 30 minutes.

How many grams of DEXTROSE are contained in the fluids? _____

If the patient receives the medication for 25 minutes, how many units of PENICILLIN did the patient receive? _____

15. A physician orders AMINOPHYLLINE as a loading dose of 5 mg/kg to be administered IVPB over 1 hour for a patient who weighs 154 lb. The available medication is AMINOPHYLLINE 250 mg/10 mL.

How many milligrams of medication should the patient receive?

_____

How many milligrams of medication should the patient receive each hour if the order is changed and the dose is to be infused over 2 hours? _____

The medication is to be administered at the prescribed mg/kg dose for 2 hours when added to 200 mL of IV fluids for infusion. If the infusion stops after 1½ hours, how many milligrams of medication would the patient receive? _____

16. A physician orders OXYTOCIN 2 units added to 1 L of D-5-W. The available medication is OXYTOCIN 10 units/mL.

How many units would be in 100 mL of solution? _____

If the patient receives 750 mL of the IV fluids, how much OXYTOCIN does the patient receive? _____

17. A physician orders MAGNESIUM SULFATE 10 g to be added to LACTATED RINGER'S solution 1 L. The available medication is 50% MAGNESIUM SULFATE.

What is the concentration of MAGNESIUM SULFATE in mg/mL?

_____

If this is to infuse over 5 hours, how many milligrams of MAGNESIUM SULFATE would the patient receive each hour? _____

18. A physician orders 1 L of D-10-½ NS to infuse over 10 hours.

How many grams of DEXTROSE would the patient receive per hour?

_____

*How many grams of SODIUM CHLORIDE would the patient receive per hour?

_____

19. A physician orders ERYTHROMYCIN 500 mg in 100 mL of NS for IVPB stat. The vial of medication contains 1 g of ERYTHROMYCIN to be diluted with 10 mL of sterile water and added to 100 mL NS.

How many milliliters of ERYTHROMYCIN should be added to the normal saline?

_____

If these IVPB fluids are to infuse for 2 hours, how many milligrams of ERYTHROMYCIN would the patient receive in 1 hour? _____

How many milligrams of ERYTHROMYCIN would the patient receive in 1 hour and 15 minutes? _____

20. EN DO A physician orders regular INSULIN 150 units to be added to 50 mL of NORMAL SALINE.

How many units of INSULIN are in each milliliter of fluids? _____

The fluids are to infuse over 20 minutes for the patient with severe hyperglycemia who is in a diabetic coma. The patient responds in 15 minutes, and the fluids are discontinued. How many units of INSULIN did the patient receive?

_____

CALCULATING INTRAVENOUS FLOW RATES IN DROPS PER MINUTE

In some medical instances fluids are infused without added medications, whereas in other circumstances medications are added for prophylactic or therapeutic reasons. The rate of administration varies depending on the patient's condition and the medications/fluids to be administered. The physician's order may state the number of milliliters per minute or per hour at which the fluids are to infuse, whereas in other circumstances the physician may state an amount of time for fluid infusion.

This section covers calculation of the drops or milliliters per minute (called **flow rate**). An IV infusion set (or equipment) includes the sealed container of sterile fluids and tubing connected to the needle for insertion into the vein for administration of the fluids. Equipment for IV infusions includes tubing for carrying fluid from the container to the person (Figure 12-1). The packaging for the tubing provides information on the number of drops per milliliter to be supplied. The rate of flow or the infusion rate in drops per minute is adjusted by the clamp on the tubing and the size of the drop from the drip chamber or the **drop factor** or by the use of infusion pump that calculates drops/minute based on the size of the drop.

For patient safety, the person preparing the fluids must ensure that the proper infusion set has been chosen to fill the physician's order. The size of the drop depends on the way the manufacturer designs the drop orifice. The larger the diameter of the drop orifice into the drip chamber, the larger the drop entering the chamber providing fewer drops

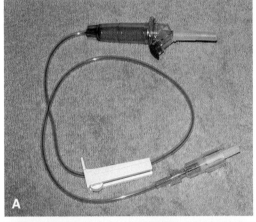
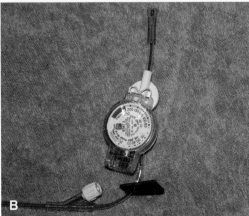
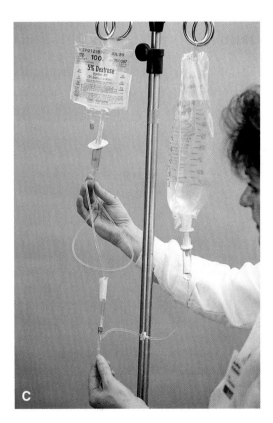

FIGURE 12-1 **A,** Primary infusion set showing drip chamber, tubing, and roller clamp. **B,** Primary infusion set for IVPB additions. **C,** IVPB being added to a primary line.

in 1 mL. Conversely, the smaller the opening into the drip chamber, the smaller the drops providing more drops per milliliter. The person preparing the fluids must be aware of the number of drops per milliliter (gtts/mL) or the drop factor to be used to complete a drop/minute (gtt/min) rate.

> **! TECH ALERT**
>
> The number of drops per milliliter for the infusion set is found on the box. Tubing is not interchangeable. This information is essential for proper fluid administration time and calculation of IV flow rates.

The most common drop factors for IV fluids are 10, 15, 20, and 60 gtts/mL (Figure 12-2, A). Drop factors that deliver fewer and larger drops per milliliter such as 10, 15, or 20 gtts/mL are called **macrodrip infusion sets**. Macrodrip sets are used when large volumes of fluids must be administered or if fluids must be administered at a rapid rate. Tubing that delivers 60 drops per milliliter is called a **microdrip infusion set**. These sets are used for slower delivery of fluids such as at rates of 50 mL per hour (see Figure 12-2, B).

The rate of infusion for IV fluids must be calculated to complete the physician's order, which provides type and amount of fluids and usually a desired infusion rate or infusion time. The proper infusion set must be chosen to supply the fluids as ordered. Therefore, the four factors to be considered with administration are as follows:

- The total amount of fluids to be administered in *milliliters (mL)*
- The calibration of the administration set in *drops/milliliter (gtts/mL)*
- The flow rate of the fluids in *drops/minute (gtts/min)*
- The time for the fluids to infuse in *minutes (min)*

Using the previous information, the formula for calculating the flow rate of IV fluids is as follows:

$$\text{Flow rate} = \frac{\text{Amount of fluid} \times \text{Calibration on administration set}}{\text{Time for infusion}}$$

OR

$$\text{Flow rate} = \frac{\text{mL ordered} \times \text{gtts/mL}}{\text{minutes for infusion}}$$

> **! TECH ALERT**
>
> 1 L of fluids is considered to be 1000 mL.

> **TECH NOTE**
>
> Be sure that all conversions within the formula are made before final calculations, such as hours to minutes or liters to milliliters.

EXAMPLE 12-3

A physician orders 1.5 L of LACTATED RINGER'S solution to be infused over 8 hours. The infusion administration set reads 20 gtts/mL.

> **TECH NOTE**
>
> In the following example calculation, 1.5 L has been converted to 1500 mL.

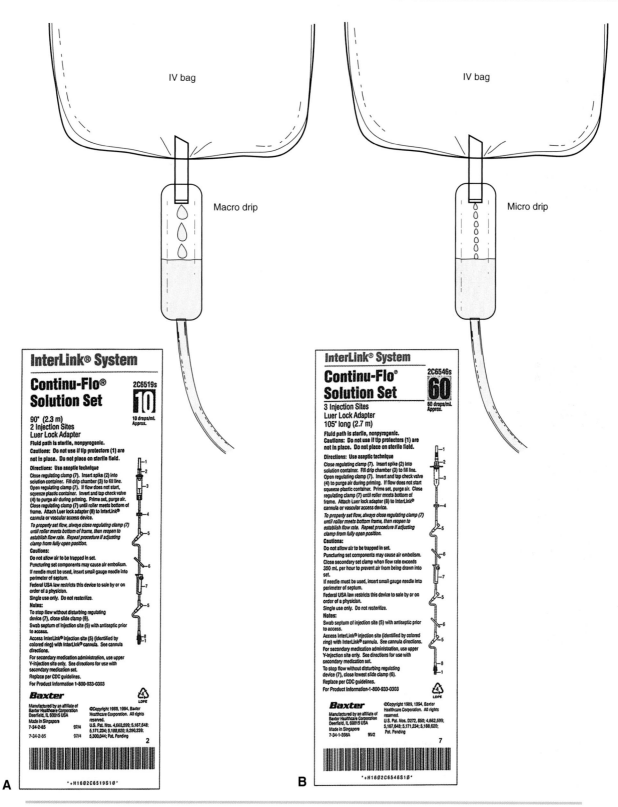

FIGURE 12-2 Infusion sets for administration of IV fluids. **A,** Macrodrip set shows 10 gtts/mL. **B,** Microdrip set shows 60 gtts/mL.

$$\text{Flow rate} = \frac{1500 \text{ mL} \times 20 \text{ gtts/mL}}{8 \text{ hr} \times 60 \text{ min/hr}}$$

$$\left.\text{Flow rate} = \frac{\dfrac{1500 \text{ mL}}{1} \times \dfrac{20 \text{ gtts}}{\text{mL}}}{\dfrac{8 \text{ hr}}{1} \times \dfrac{60 \text{ min}}{1 \text{ hr}}}\right\} \text{ Fractional units}$$

$$\left.\text{Flow rate} = \frac{\dfrac{1500 \text{ m\!L}}{1} \times \dfrac{20 \text{ gtts}}{\text{m\!L}}}{\dfrac{8 \text{ h\!r}}{1} \times \dfrac{60 \text{ min}}{1 \text{ h\!r}}}\right\} \text{ Fractional units}$$

$$\text{Flow rate} = \frac{1500 \times 20 \text{ gtts}}{8 \times 60 \text{ min}}$$

$$\text{Flow rate} = \frac{30,000 \text{ gtts}}{480 \text{ min}} \quad \text{or} \quad \frac{30000 \text{ gtts}}{480 \text{ min}}$$

$$\text{Flow rate} = 62.5 \text{ gtts/min} \quad \text{or} \quad 63 \text{ gtts/min}$$

Hint: Return to Chapter 2 if you need to review the rules for rounding decimals.
If it is easier for you to complete the infusion rate in two steps, the following two steps may be used.

EXAMPLE 12-4

A physician orders 1.5 L of LACTATED RINGER'S solution to be infused over 8 hours. The infusion administration set reads 20 gtts/mL.

Step 1: $\text{mL/hr} = \dfrac{\text{Total volume of fluids (TV)}}{\text{Total time in hours (TTH)}}$

$$\text{mL/hr} = \frac{1500 \text{ (TV)}}{8 \text{ h (TTH)}}$$

$\text{mL/hr} = 187.5 \quad \text{or} \quad 188$ milliliters per hour should be administered

Step 2: $\text{gtts/min} = \dfrac{\text{Drop factor (gtts/mL)}}{\text{Time in minutes (TM)}} \times \text{Total volume per 60 min}$

$$\text{gtts/min} = \frac{20 \text{ gtts/mL}}{60 \text{ min}} \times 188 \text{ mL/60 min}$$

$$\text{gtts/min} = \frac{20 \times 188}{60} \quad \text{or} \quad \frac{{}^{1}\!20 \times 188}{60_3}$$

$$\text{gtts/min} = \frac{188}{3}$$

$\text{gtts/min} = 62.7 \quad \text{or} \quad 63 \text{ gtts/min}$

If dimensional analysis is the preferred means of calculating dosage, see Example 12-5.

EXAMPLE 12-5

A physician orders 1.5 L of LACTATED RINGER'S solution to be infused over 8 hours. The infusion administration set reads 20 gtts/mL.

The following abbreviations will be used in the following formula:
D = Drop factor
CFV = **Conversion factor volume**
DV = **Dose volume**
DT = **Dose time**
CFT = **Conversion factor time**
FR = Flow rate in drops per minute

The necessary information for dimensional analysis with the preceding example is as follows:

Drop factor (DF) = 20 gtts/mL

Dose volume (DV) = 1.5 L

Dose time (DT) = 8 hr

Flow rate (FR) (flow rate in gtts/min) = x

Conversion factors: 1 L = 1000 mL (Conversion factor volume [CFV]); 1 hr = 60 minutes (Conversion factor time [CFT])

$$DF \times CFV \times DV \times DT \times CFT = FR \text{ (flow rate in gtts/min)}$$

$$\frac{20 \text{ gtts (DF)}}{1 \text{ mL}} \times \frac{1000 \text{ mL (CFV)}}{1 \text{ L}} \times \frac{1.5 \text{ L (DV)}}{\text{Dose}} \times \frac{\text{Dose}}{8 \text{ hr}} \times \frac{1 \text{ hr (CFT)}}{60 \text{ min}} = x \text{ (FR in gtts/min)}$$

$$\frac{20 \text{ gtts (DF)}}{1 \text{ mL}} \times \frac{1000 \text{ mL (CFV)}}{1 \text{ L}} \times \frac{1.5 \text{ L (DV)}}{\text{Dose}} \times \frac{\text{Dose}}{8 \text{ hr}} \times \frac{1 \text{ hr (CFT)}}{60 \text{ min}} = x \text{ (FR)}$$

$$\frac{20 \text{ gtts} \times 1000 \times 1.5 \times 1}{1 \times 1 \times 8 \times 60 \text{ min}} = x \text{ (FR)}$$

$$\frac{30,000 \text{ gtts}}{480 \text{ min}} = x \text{ (FR)}$$

$$\frac{30,000 \text{ gtts}}{480 \text{ min}} = x \text{ (FR)} \quad \text{or} \quad \frac{3000 \text{ gtts}}{48 \text{ min}} = x \text{ (FR)}$$

FR = 62.5   or   63 gtts/min should be administered

Remember that with dimensional analysis, you are completing the entire problem in one step.

Practice Problems B

Use the method that is most comfortable to calculate the flow rate in drops per minute of the following problems. Round all answers for medication weight/volume to the nearest tenth and for drops per minute to the nearest whole number. With this set of practice problems, the total volume of fluids for infusion is that given in the problem.

1. A physician orders 2 L of LACTATED RINGER'S solution over 12 hr. The drop factor is 20 gtts/mL.

    How many drops per minute would be infused? _____

2. A physician orders D-5-W 100 mL IV over 2 hours. The drop factor is 50 gtts/mL.

    How many drops per minute would be infused? _____

    How many milligrams of DEXTROSE are found in these fluids? _____

3. A physician orders 250 mL D-5-NS to be administered over 16 hours to keep a vein open. The drop factor is 60 gtts/mL.

    How many drops per minute would be administered? _____

    How many grams of DEXTROSE are in the fluids? _____

    How many grams of SODIUM CHLORIDE are in the fluids? _____

    How many milliliters will be administered per hour? _____

4. A physician orders 1000 mL D-10-1/2NS to be administered over 12 hours. The drop factor is 10 gtts/mL.

    How many drops per minute would be infused? _____

    How many grams of DEXTROSE are in these fluids? _____

    How many grams of SODIUM CHLORIDE are in these fluids? _____

5. A physician orders 150 mL of D-5-NS to be infused in 40 minutes. The drip factor is 15 gtts/mL.

    How many gtt(s)/min would be infused? _____

6. A physician orders a piggyback infusion containing AMPICILLIN 250 mg in 75 mL of NORMAL SALINE. The medication is to infuse over 1 hour using an infusion set labeled as 50 gtts/mL.

How many gtt(s)/min would be infused? _____

What weight (in mg) of AMPICILLIN is infused in 45 minutes? _____

7. A physician orders OXYTOCIN 10 units in 500 mL of NS to be infused over 30 minutes. The drop factor is 20 gtts/mL.

How many gtt(s)/min would be infused? _____

How many units of OXYTOCIN would the patient receive in 20 minutes?

_____

8. A physician orders ZANTAC 50 mg in 100 mL NS to infuse over 15 minutes. The drop factor is 15 gtts/mL.

How many gtt(s)/min would be infused? _____

How many milligrams of ZANTAC would the patient receive in 10 minutes?

_____

9. A physician orders METHYLPREDNISOLONE SODIUM SUCCINATE 500 mg in 150 mL NS to infuse over 2 hr. The drop factor is 20 gtts/mL.

How many gtt(s)/min would be infused? _____

How many grams of NaCl are found in the fluids? (Round to tenths.)

_____

If infused for 1 hour 15 minutes, how many grams of NaCl would be received by the patient? (Round to tenths) _____

How many milligrams of METHYLPREDNISOLONE SODIUM SUCCINATE would be administered to the patient in 1 hour 15 minutes? _____

10. A physician orders NAFCILLIN 1 g to be added to 100 mL D-5-W to run for 1 hour. The drop factor is 15 gtts/mL.

How many gtt(s)/min would be infused? _____

How many milligrams of NAFCILLIN would be infused in 50 minutes?

_____

11. A physician orders NOVOLIN R 60 units to infuse in 500 mL NS over 4½ hours. The drop factor is 15 gtts/mL.

How many gtt(s)/min would be infused? _____

How many units of INSULIN would be infused in 1 hour? _____

12. A physician orders TOBRAMYCIN 1 mg/kg in LR 50 mL IVPB to run for 50 minutes. The patient weighs 178 lb. The drop factor is 10 gtts/mL.

What dose (in mg) of TOBRAMYCIN should be prepared for the infusion?

_____

How many gtt(s)/min should be set for the infusion to meet the physician's order?

_____

How many milligrams of TOBRAMYCIN would be infused in 45 minutes?

_____

13. A physician orders CONJUGATED ESTROGENS 25 mg to be added to 50 mL D-2 1/2-W to run for 15 minutes. The drop factor is 15 gtts/mL.

How many gtt(s)/min should be infused? _____

How many milligrams of ESTROGEN would be infused in 6 minutes?

_____

14. A physician orders LIDOCAINE 300 mcg/kg IV for a heart patient who weighs 190 lb. The medication available is 4% LIDOCAINE solution.

How many milliliters of LIDOCAINE should be added to the desired fluids?

_____

The physician wants this medication added to 20 mL of D-5-W to run for 10 minutes. The drop factor is 10 gtts/mL. The infusion should be set for _____ gtt(s)/min.

How many total grams of DEXTROSE are in the fluids? _____

How many milligrams of LIDOCAINE would the patient receive in 4 minutes?

_____

15. A physician orders 2000 mL of 1/2 NS to run for 16 hours. The drop factor is 50 gtts/mL.

The infusion should be set for _____ gtt(s)/min.

How many total grams of NaCl would the patient receive? _____

16. A physician orders GENTAMICIN 0.02 g to be added to 50 mL NS for infusion over 45 minutes. The drop factor is 20 gtts/mL.

Set the infusion rate for _____ gtt(s)/min.

How many milligrams of GENTAMICIN would be added to the fluids?

_____

How many milligrams of NaCl would the patient receive in 30 minutes?

_____

How many milligrams of GENTAMICIN would the patient receive in 15 minutes?

_____

17. A physician orders FAMOTIDINE 20 mg in NS IV q12h to run over 25 minutes. The medication is available as FAMOTIDINE 10 mg/mL and a premixed IVPB of 20 mg/50 mL 0.9% NaCl.

Which available medication is most appropriate for use for this order?

_____

If medication from the available vial has to be added to 50 mL of NS, how many milliliters of FAMOTIDINE should be added? _____

Calculate the gtt(s)/min if the drop factor is 20 gtts/mL: _____

18. A physician orders CEFAZOLIN 1 g q4h to be mixed in 50 mL LACTATED RINGER'S solution and infused over 50 minutes. The medication available for reconstitution for this order is CEFAZOLIN 250 mg/vial.

How many vials of CEFAZOLIN would be necessary to complete this order?

_____

Because cefazolin is available as 1 g in 50 mL in NS premixed IVPB, could this be used for the order as written? _____

If the drop factor is 50 gtts/mL, how many gtt(s)/min would be administered?

_____

How many milliliters of NS would the patient receive in 20 minutes?

_____

How many milligrams of CEFAZOLIN would the patient receive in 30 minutes?

_____

19. A physician orders KETOROLAC 60 mg/day total dose IVPB to be divided and administered q6h over a 20-minute infusion time.

What dose of medication should be administered with each dose?

_____

The medication is added to D-5-W 25 mL. The tubing has a drop factor of 15 gtts/mL. How many gtt(s)/min would be administered? _____

How many milligrams of DEXTROSE would the patient receive per dose?

_____

20. A physician orders CLEOCIN 1.8 g/d to be administered in divided doses q8h to run over 45 minutes. CLEOCIN is available in vials of 300, 600, and 900 mg.

Which vial of medication would be used? _____

If this medication is added to 100 mL NS and the drip factor on the tubing is 15 gtts/mL, how would the infusion pump be set in gtt(s)/min? _____

How many milligrams of CLEOCIN would the patient receive in each dose? _____

How many milligrams of SODIUM CHLORIDE would the patient receive in each dose? _____

CALCULATING INTRAVENOUS INFUSION TIMES

In some instances the physician will provide an order for the amount of fluids to be infused and the milliliters per hour without providing the specific infusion time. The problem then becomes a decision on how long it will take for each volume of fluids to be infused using the rate ordered by the physician. As the pharmacy technician, you have a responsibility to be sure fluids are available at the necessary time for infusion and for the next dose as ordered. Therefore when the time is not designated for the fluids, but the amount of fluid is designated, the necessary calculation may include deciding how long the ordered fluids will infuse when the infusion rate and/or drop factor is provided.

TECH NOTE
  Remember that flow rate is indicated as drops/minute.

EXAMPLE 12-6

A physician orders 1000 mL D-5-NS to be administered at 20 gtts/min. The drop factor is 15 gtts/mL. What is the infusion time for these fluids?

Using the formula shown in the previous section and substituting information into the formula, the calculation can be made:

$$\text{Flow rate} = \frac{\text{mL ordered} \times \text{gtts/mL (drop factor)}}{\text{Minutes for infusion (TM)}}$$

Flow rate $= 20$ gtts/min

mL ordered $= 1000$ mL

gtts/mL $= 15$ gtts/mL

With these numbers, the equation would appear as follows:

$$20 \text{ gtts/min} = \frac{1000 \text{ mL} \times 15 \text{ gtts/mL}}{x}$$

20 gtts/min $x = 1000$ mL $\times 15$ gtts/mL

20 ~~gtts~~/min $x = 1000$ ~~mL~~ $\times 15$ ~~gtts/mL~~

$$20 \,(min)\, x = 15,000$$

$$x = \frac{15,000}{20 \text{ min}}$$

$$x = \frac{15,0\cancel{0}0}{2\cancel{0} \text{ min}}$$

$$x = 750 \text{ minutes} \quad \text{or} \quad 12.5 \text{ hours } (750 \text{ min} \div 60 \text{ min/hr})$$

TECH NOTE

Remember that when you cross the "=" sign while completing calculations, multiplication on the left side of the equation becomes division on the right side of the equation and vice versa.

EXAMPLE 12-7

A physician orders 1000 mL D-5-NS to be administered at 20 gtts/min. The drop factor is 15 gtts/mL. What is the total infusion time for the ordered fluids (using dimensional analysis)?

DF = Drop factor

CFV = Conversion factor volume

DV = Dose volume

DT = Dose time

CFT = Conversion factor time

FR = Flow rate in gtts/min

$$DF \times CFV \times DV \times FR = DT$$

Again, use substitution and complete the equation.

DF = 15 gtts/mL

DV = 1000 mL

DT = x

FR = 20 gtts/min

$$\frac{15 \text{ gtts (DF)}}{1 \text{ mL}} \times \frac{1000 \text{ mL (CFV)}}{1000 \text{ mL}} \times \frac{1000 \text{ mL (DV)}}{\text{Dose}} \times \frac{\text{Dose}}{20 \text{ gtts/min (FR)}} = DT$$

$$\frac{15 \cancel{\text{ gtts}} \text{ (DF)}}{1 \cancel{\text{ mL}}} \times \frac{1000 \cancel{\text{ mL}} \text{ (CFV)}}{1000 \cancel{\text{ mL}}} \times \frac{1000 \cancel{\text{ mL}} \text{ (DV)}}{\cancel{\text{Dose}}} \times \frac{\cancel{\text{Dose}}}{20 \cancel{\text{ gtts}}/\text{min (FR)}} = DT$$

$$\frac{15 \times 1 \times 1000}{1 \times 1 \times 20 \text{ min}} = DT$$

$$\frac{15,000}{20 \text{ min}} = DT$$

$$\frac{15,000}{20\ \text{min}} = \text{DT}$$

$$\frac{1500}{2\ \text{min}} = \text{DT}$$

DT = 750 minutes, then, convert minutes to hours = 12.5 hours (750 ÷ 60 min/hr)

Practice Problems C

Use either the formula method or dimensional analysis, whichever is more comfortable for you, to complete the following problems. Round time to the units of hours and minutes as indicated. Round drops to the nearest whole drop in the final answer. Drug weights/volumes and kilograms of body weight should be rounded to the nearest tenth, unless marked with an asterisk, and then round to the nearest hundredth. If asking for total hours, use tenths of hours; if asking for hours/minutes make the needed conversion. Show your work.

1. A physician orders 500 mL D-5-NS to be infused at 15 gtts/min. The drop factor is 10 gtts/mL.

   What time would be necessary to infuse these fluids? _____ min
   _____ hr

2. A physician orders 2500 mL D-5-½ NS to be infused at 30 gtts/min. The drop factor is 10 gtts/mL.

   How long would it take for these fluids to be infused? _____ min
   Hours and minutes _____?
   What is the metric weight of DEXTROSE in the entire order? _____
   What is the metric weight of SODIUM CHLORIDE in the entire order?

   _____

3. A physician orders AMIKIN 1 g in 100 mL D-5-W to infuse at 25 gtts/min using an infusion set calibrated to 60 gtts/mL.

   What is the running time for the infusion in minutes? _____ Hours? _____
   If the drug has a recommended infusion time of at least 1 hour, is this order safe for the patient? _____
   How many milligrams of AMIKIN would the patient receive in 10 minutes?

   _____

4. A physician orders MANNITOL 75 g IV for renal failure. The solution is provided in D-5-NS 50 mL. The infusion rate is 20 gtts/min with a drop factor of 50 gtts/mL.

What is the weight of MANNITOL in the solution? _____

How long would it take for the medication to infuse? _____

If the recommended time is 30 to 60 minutes, is the order correct for the patient?

_____

What is the metric weight of DEXTROSE in the fluids? _____

*What is the metric weight of SODIUM CHLORIDE in the fluids?

_____

5. A physician orders LR 250 mL to be infused at 50 gtts/min. The infusion set reads 10 gtts/mL.

What is the infusion time in minutes? _____

6. A physician orders 2 L of D-5-W to be infused at 25 gtts/min. The infusion set is 10 gtts/mL.

What time is necessary for infusion of these fluids in hours? _____

7. A physician orders GENTAMICIN 1.5 mg/kg/dose to be given q8h IVPB in 150 mL NS for a patient who weighs 148 lb. The infusion is to be infused at 25 gtts/min. The drop factor is 20 gtts/mL.

How many milligrams of GENTAMICIN should this patient receive?

_____

How long would it take for this medication to be infused in minutes?

_____

What total amount of GENTAMICIN would be infused daily? _____

How many milligrams would the patient receive in 45 minutes? _____

8. A physician orders OXACILLIN 12 g/day given in divided doses q3h IVPB.

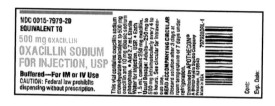

How many milligrams of OXACILLIN would be given to the patient with each dose?

_____

How many grams of OXACILLIN would be given to the patient with each dose?

_____

If this comes in an IV infusion prepared from the following label, how many vials of OXACILLIN would be necessary in 1 day? _____

What would be the volume of medication to be added to NS 100 mL of fluids to fill this order? _____

If the physician orders the medication to be given at 30 gtts/min, and the drop factor is 20 gtts/mL, how long would this infusion take for completion in hours and minutes? _____

9. A physician orders the solution shown in the following illustration to be administered at 30 gtts/min using a drop factor of 50 gtts/mL.

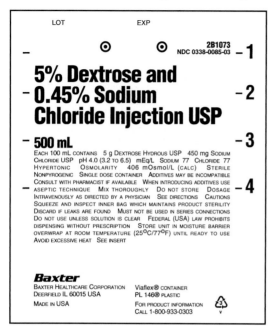

How long would it take for this infusion to occur in hours and minutes?

_____

How many grams of DEXTROSE are in these fluids? _____

*How many grams of SODIUM CHLORIDE are in these fluids? _____

10. A physician orders CEFOPERAZONE 2 g IV in LR 75 mL to be infused at 10 gtts/min. The drop factor is 25 gtts/mL.

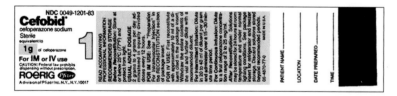

How long would it take for the medication to infuse in hours and minutes?

_____

Using the following label, how many vials of CEFOBID would be required for this physician's order? _____

After reconstitution, how many milliliters of CEFOBID should be added to the IV infusion? _____

How many milligrams of CEFOBID would be infused in 20 minutes?

_____

11.   A physician orders CEFTAZIDIME 750 mg IV in D-5-W 50 mL q12h for a severe case of pelvic inflammatory disease. The drop factor is 20 gtts/mL, and the fluids are to run at 2.5 mL/min. Using the following label, reconstitute the medication and prepare the fluids for infusion.

Hint: Be sure to include the correct volume for the added medication.

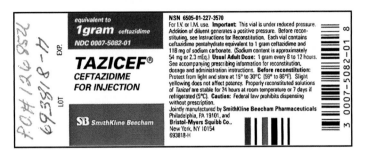

How many milliliters of sterile water would be added to the vial for reconstitution?

_____

How many milliliters in tenths of CEFTAZIDIME would be added to the fluids?

_____

What would be the total volume of fluids in the bag following the addition of medication? _____

How long would it take for the fluids to infuse? _____

What would be the powder displacement? _____

12.   A patient is to receive D-5-1/2 NS × 1.5 L at the rate of 100 gtts/min using an administration set of 10 gtts/mL.

What is the weight in milligrams of the DEXTROSE in the entire fluid order?

_____

What is the weight in milligrams of SODIUM CHLORIDE in the entire order?

_____

How long would it take for these fluids to infuse in minutes? _____

How long would it take in hours and minutes? _____

13. A physician orders AMPICILLIN 250 mg IVPB to be infused in 50 mL NS at 30 gtts/min. The drop factor is 10 gtts/mL.

Using ampicillin for injection 125 mg/vial, how many vials of medication would be necessary to complete this order? _____

If the volume of medication added to NS is 8 mL, how long would it take for the entire piggyback to infuse in minutes? _____

14. A physician orders AMINOPHYLLINE 750 mg IVPB to be added to 100 mL of fluids for a patient with severe asthma. The medication is available as AMINOPHYLLINE 500 mg/25 mL. The administration set is 60 gtts/mL, and the rate of infusion is 10 gtts/min.

How long in minutes would it take for the entire bottle of fluids to infuse?

_____

How long in hours and minutes would be needed to infuse the fluids?

_____

How many milliliters would be administered per minute? _____

15. A physician orders ERYTHROMYCIN 200 mg IVPB in 250 mL D-5-W. The medication is available as 400 mg/5 mL after reconstitution. The drop factor is 30 gtts/mL, and the rate of infusion is 20 gtts/min.

How many milliliters of ERYTHROMYCIN should be added to the bag of fluids?

_____

How many minutes would it take for the piggyback to infuse? _____

How many hours and minutes? _____

16. A physician orders 1000 mL LR + 20 mEq KCl per liter × 2 L. The drop factor is 10 gtts/mL. The infusion rate is 15 gtts/min.

How long would it take for this complete order to infuse in minutes?

_____ In hours and minutes? _____

17. A physician orders AMPHOTERICIN B 40 mg IVPB to be administered in D-5-W 250 mL to be infused at a rate of 20 gtts/min with a drop factor of 60 gtts/mL.

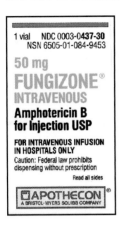

Using the following label, how many milliliters would be added to the fluids if the reconstituted AMPHOTERICIN B is 50 mg/10 mL? _____

How many minutes would the IV take to infuse? _____

How long in minutes would it take for AMPHOTERICIN 15 mg to infuse?

_____

18. A physician orders VANCOCIN 1 g in 100 mL D-5-W. The drop factor is 20 gtts/mL, and the infusion rate is 1.5 mL/min.

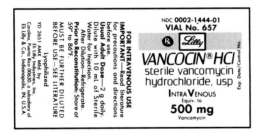

How long in minutes would it take for the VANCOMYCIN order to be infused?

_____

How many drops per minute would be infused? _____

Using the following label, how many vials of medication should be reconstituted to be added to the fluids? _____

What would be the time in hours and minutes for infusion? _____

What is the total volume of medication to be administered following the addition of VANCOCIN? _____

19. ⬤ A physician orders 150 mL D-5-W for a young child who is dehydrated. The drop factor is 60 gtts/mL, and the infusion rate is 0.5 mL/min.

How long in hours would it take for the fluids to be infused? _____

How many drops per minute would be infused? _____

20. 🧪 A physician orders HEPARIN SODIUM 3500 units to be added to 100 mL of NS for IV infusion. The drop factor is 60 gtts/mL, and the infusion rate is 20 gtts/min.

```
N 0469-1262-15    926201
HEPARIN SODIUM
INJECTION, USP
5,000 USP Units/mL
(Derived from Porcine
Intestinal Mucosa)
For IV or SC Use
1 mL Multiple Dose Vial
Usual Dosage: See insert.
▐◢ Fujisawa USA, Inc.
▐■ Deerfield, IL 60015-2548

          40213F

LOT
EXP
```

Using the following label, how many milliliters of HEPARIN should be added to the fluids? _____

How many minutes would it take for these fluids to infuse? _____

How many hours and minutes would it take for these fluids to infuse?

_____

REVIEW

Physicians order IV therapy for several reasons—maintenance, replacement, and restorative therapy. In some cases medications such as electrolytes and antibiotics may be added to the container of fluids for infusion over a period of time; such medications may be given by intermittent infusion over a short period of time (e.g., most by IVPB) or may be infused over long periods of time (e.g., continuous infusions or continuous IV fluid orders). To ensure that medications are supplied and infused as ordered by the physician, the pharmacy is responsible for providing the medications and fluids for the order. In some cases, the pharmacy may assist in providing the needed tubing with the correct drop factor for accurate administration.

After the correct fluids have been selected, as the pharmacy technician, you may be responsible for ensuring adequate amounts of fluids have been provided for the desired length of time. Furthermore, you may be asked to calculate the amount of time that a container of fluids will need for infusion, the necessary volume of fluids, or rate of infusion per minute or hour to provide the medication as ordered for the ordered time or the amount of medication that has been infused over a given period of time. Patient safety is ensured when the fluids are those ordered by the physician and are calculated for the correct infusion rate using formulas provided in this chapter. Because of the rapidity of administration of medications through an IV route, the pharmacy must take care with these calculations. As the pharmacy technician, you must be sure the correct fluids are chosen, along with the correct administration supplies. Rechecking calculations always enhances patient safety with intravenous medications.

Posttest

Before taking the Posttest, retake the Pretest to check your understanding of the materials presented in this chapter.

Calculate the following situations using the method most comfortable for you. Round to the nearest whole number for hours/minutes as appropriate. Round to the nearest tenth for weight/volume. If the question is marked with an asterisk, the answer should be rounded to the nearest hundredth. Round drops to whole numbers. Interpret each order for IV fluids and medications. Show your calculations.

1. A physician orders KEFUROX 1.5 g in D-5-NS 100 mL to be infused over 1 hr as IVPB. The drop factor is 20 gtts/mL. Use the following label for your calculation.

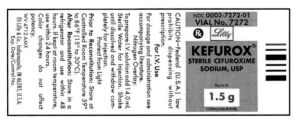

What is the necessary drip rate (gtt(s)/min) to fulfill this order? _____

If the patient received 80 mL of the IVPB, how many milligrams of KEFUROX would the patient receive? _____

If the patient received the IVPB for 35 minutes, how many milliliters of solution would the patient receive? _____

Continued

Posttest, cont.

2. A physician orders FUROSEMIDE 60 mg to be infused in D-5-W 500 mL. The drop factor is 20 gtts/mL, and the drop rate is 60 gtts/min. Use the following label for your calculations.

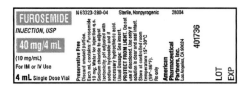

Calculate the amount of medication that must be added to the fluids.

_____

How long in minutes would the fluids infuse? _____

How many milligrams of FUROSEMIDE would the patient receive per minute?

_____

What are the total milligrams of DEXTROSE in the fluids? _____

3. A physician orders HUMULIN R 60 units added to D-2.5-½ NS 100 mL as an IVPB. The drop factor is 60 gtts/mL. The physician wants the INSULIN to infuse at 2.5 units/hr. Use the following label for your calculations.

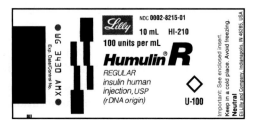

How many milliliters per hour would be infused to complete the order?

_____

How many milligrams of SODIUM CHLORIDE would be found in the fluids?

_____

How many milligrams of DEXTROSE would be found in these fluids?

_____

How long would the fluids need to infuse as ordered? _____

How many milliliters of INSULIN would be added to the fluids? _____

Posttest, cont.

4. A physician orders AMPICILLIN SODIUM 1 g to be added to LACTATED RINGER'S solution 100 mL. The drop factor is 60 gtts/mL. The medication must be given over a 2-hour time. Use the following label for calculations.

```
NDC 0015-7403-20
NSN 6505-00-946-4700
EQUIVALENT TO

500 mg AMPICILLIN

STERILE AMPICILLIN
SODIUM, USP
For IM or IV Use
CAUTION: Federal law prohibits
dispensing without prescription.
```

For IM use, add 1.8 mL diluent (read accompanying circular). Resulting solution contains 250 mg ampicillin per mL. Use solution within 1 hour. This vial contains ampicillin sodium equivalent to 500 mg ampicillin. Usual Dosage: Adults—250 to 500 mg IM q. 6h. READ ACCOMPANYING CIRCULAR for detailed indications, IM or IV dosage and precautions. APOTHECON® A Bristol-Myers Squibb Company Princeton, NJ 08540 USA   740320DRL-2

Cont:
Exp. Date:

How many vials of ampicillin would be added to the fluids? _____

What would be the flow rate (mL/min) for these fluids? _____

How many drops per minute would the patient receive? _____

If the order is repeated q6h, how many vials of medication would be necessary per day? _____

What would be the total dose of medication in milligrams given to the patient?

_____

How many milligrams of medication would be administered in 45 minutes?

_____

5. A physician orders NITROGLYCERIN IV 50 mg in D-5-W 250 mL to be infused at the rate of 50 mcg/min. The drop factor is 60 gtts/mL.

What is the amount of medication in micrograms per 1 mL of solution?

_____

*How many milliliters of solution would be necessary to fulfill the order for 50 mcg/min? _____

How long in minutes/hours would these fluids take to infuse? _____

How many milliliters would provide NITROGLYCERIN 5 mg? _____

Continued

Posttest, cont.

6. A physician orders D-5-NS 3000 mL to be infused over 24 hours. The drop factor is 15 gtts/mL.

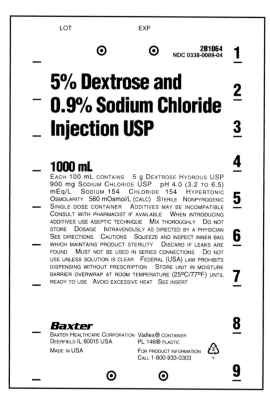

How many milliliters of fluids should be supplied for each 8-hour shift?

_____

Using the label, how many containers of solution should be provided for the physician's order? _____

How many milliliters per hour should be infused? _____

What would be the drip rate in mL/min? _____

If the physician stops the fluids after 5 hours of infusion, how many milliliters would the patient receive? _____

How many grams of DEXTROSE would the patient receive after 5 hours?

_____

Posttest, cont.

7. A physician orders AMIKIN 5 mg/kg q8h in 100 mL of fluids IVPB. The patient weighs 176 lb. The drop factor is 20 gtts/mL. The time of infusion is 2 hours.

How many milligrams of medication should be added to the fluids?

_____

If the medication is available as amikacin 50 mg/mL, how many milliliters should be added to fluids? _____

What would be the flow rate in drops per minute to ensure that the medication is given to physician's order? _____

Continued

Posttest, cont.

8. What is the time in minutes for infusion of the fluids shown in the following label if the drip rate is 3 mL/min, and the drop factor is 20 gtts/mL? _____

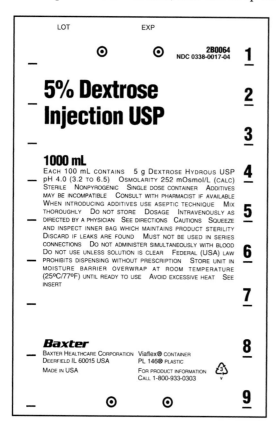

How many bags of fluids would be necessary if the physician orders the medications to run for 24 hours? _____

How many total milliliters of fluids are required in 24 hours? _____

How many grams of DEXTROSE would the patient receive with each container of fluids? _____

How many grams of DEXTROSE would the patient receive in a 24-hour period?

_____

Posttest, cont.

9. A physician orders 500 mL D-5-LR to be infused over 12 hours. The drop factor for the infusion set is 60 gtts/mL.

What would be the flow rate in mL/min? _____

How many milliliters of IV fluid would be infused in an hour? _____

How many gtt(s)/min should be infused? _____

10. A physician orders D-2.5 ½-NS 1000 mL for a child who is dehydrated. The physician wants the patient to receive 90 mL the first hour and the remainder over 12 hours. The drop factor is 60 gtts/mL.

What would be the flow rate in mL/min in the first hour? _____

What would be the flow rate in mL/min in the remaining hours? _____

If the patient receives only 6 hours of fluids, how many milliliters would the patient receive? _____

How many grams of DEXTROSE are in the fluids? _____

How many grams of SODIUM CHLORIDE are in the fluids? _____

11. A physician orders ROCEPHIN 25 mg/kg IVPB to run in 100 mL NS over 1 hour to be given q 12 h. The patient weighs 176 lb. The drop factor is 15 gtts/mL. The available medication is 2 g/vial.

How many grams of ROCEPHIN are administered to the patient every 12 hours?

_____

How many grams of medication would the patient receive in a day?

_____

How many vials of medication would be necessary to fulfill the order for a dose?

_____

What is the drip rate in mL/min to administer the medication as the physician ordered? _____

Continued

Posttest, cont.

12. A physician orders potassium chloride 30 mEq to be added to D-5-W 150 mL IVPB and infuse over 2½ hours. The drip factor is 20 gtts/mL.

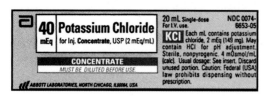

Using the label provided, how many milliliters of KCl should be added to the IVPB fluids to fulfill the physician's order? _____

How many milliliters of fluids should be infused in a minute? _____

How many milliliters of fluids should be infused in an hour? _____

How many grams of DEXTROSE should the patient receive? _____

How many gtt(s)/min should be infused? _____

13. A physician orders DOXYCYCLINE 150 mg IVPB in LR 85 mL to be administered over 1½ hours. The medication is available as DOXYCYCLINE 100 mg/10 mL. The drop factor is 20 gtts/mL.

How many vials of medication would be necessary for the physician's order?

_____

How many milliliters of DOXYCYCLINE should be added to the fluids?

_____

What would be the flow rate (mL/min) for this fluid order? _____

If the physician orders DOXYCYCLINE 75 mg IVPB for the next day and the medication is diluted in the same manner, how many milliliters of medication would be necessary for the order? _____

How many milliliters of LR would be necessary to provide a total of 100 mL when added to the medication on the second day? _____

What would be the rate of infusion in milliliters per minute if the physician wants these fluids to be infused over 1 hour? _____

Posttest, cont.

14. A physician orders RETROVIR (ZIDOVUDINE) 2 mg/kg IVPB to be administered to a patient who weighs 167 lb. The medication is to be infused in D-5-W 100 mL over a period of 1 hour. The drop factor is 15 gtts/mL. The order is to be repeated q4h × 24 hours.

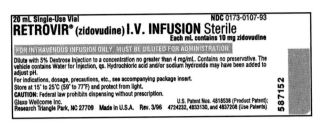

Using the label, how many milliliters of the medication should be added to the fluids for each dose? _____

What is the milliliter per minute rate that should be used to infuse this medication?

_____

How many mg of ZIDOVUDINE should the patient receive in a 24-hour period?

_____

How many gtt(s)/min should the patient receive with each dose? _____

Continued

Posttest, cont.

15. A physician orders AMPICILLIN 500 mg q6h in D-5-NS 50 mL to infuse over 15 min. The medication is available as shown in the following illustration. The drop factor for the infusion is 20 gtts/mL.

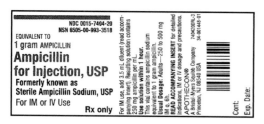

After reconstitution with sterile water the vial contains 9.5 mL, what volume of medication should be added to the vial? _____

What is the powder displacement with this medication on reconstitution?

_____

Hint: Remember to include the powder displacement as indicated in reconstitution for IM use.

How many vials of AMPICILLIN are necessary to fulfill this order for 24 hours?

_____

Hint: Read the label carefully.

What would be the milliliter per minute rate of infusion? _____

How soon ahead of the administration can this medication be prepared?

_____

How many gtt(s)/min would be infused? _____

Posttest, cont.

16. A physician orders HEPARIN SODIUM 20,000 units in NS 500 mL to run over 24 hours. The administration set is 60 gtts/mL. The medication available is shown on the following labels.

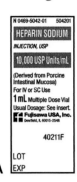 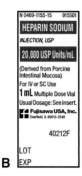

Which vial of HEPARIN should be used to add the medication to the fluids?

_____

How many milliliter of HEPARIN should be added to the fluids from that vial?

_____

What should be the flow rate in drops/min? _____

How many units of HEPARIN would the patient receive each hour?

_____

How many grams of NaCl would the patient receive with this infusion?

_____

17. A physician orders EPINEPHRINE 6 mg added to D-5-W 500 mL to be infused at 10 mL/hr. The drop factor is 60 gtts/mL.

*How many milligrams of EPINEPHRINE would the patient receive in an hour?

_____

How many mcg would the patient receive in a minute? _____

What volume would have infused in 24 hours? _____

How many gtt(s)/min should the patient receive? _____

Continued

Posttest, cont.

18. A physician orders LIDOCAINE 100 mg in D-5-W 250 mL to be infused over an hour. The lidocaine is available in 10 mg/mL. The drop factor is 40 gtts/mL.

What volume of LIDOCAINE should be added to the fluids? _____

What is the flow rate in milliliters per minute that the patient would receive?

_____

How many gtt(s)/min should be administered to the patient? _____

How many milligrams of LIDOCAINE per minute would the patient receive?

_____

How many milliliters should be administered in 25 minutes? _____

19. A physician orders EPINEPHRINE 50 mcg/min to be administered from fluids that contain epinephrine 5 mg in D-5-LR 500 mL. The drop factor is 20 gtts/mL.

What is the rate of infusion in gtt(s)/min? _____

What would be the flow rate in milliliters per hour? _____

How long would it take in minutes and hours for these fluids to infuse?

_____

If the patient receives 300 mL, how many milligrams of EPINEPHRINE should the patient receive? _____

20. A physician orders AMPHOTERICIN B 200 mg IVPB to be added to D-5-W 500 mL to infuse over 6 hours. The medication is available in a 100-mg/20-mL vial. The drop factor is 15 gtts/mL.

How many milliliters of amphotericin must be added to the fluids?

_____

How many vials of medication would be necessary to complete the order?

_____

How many drops per minute would be necessary to complete this order?

_____

If the fluids infuse for 4 hours, how many milligrams of amphotericin B should the patient receive? _____

How many milliliters per hour should be infused? _____

REVIEW OF RULES

Interpreting the Amounts of Solutes in Intravenous Fluids

- Remember that 1 mL of water equals 1 g in weight.

- Percentage is based on 100, so 5% indicates that 5 g solute is found in 100 mL of solvent.

- The easiest method for calculating weight of solute by ratio and proportion is as follows:

  Known solute : Known volume :: Desired-to-know solute : Desired-to-know volume

Calculating Intravenous Flow Rates in Drops per Minute

- Tubing used for the IV infusion set provides information for the number of drops per milliliter to be supplied to the patient.

- The drop factor is found on the packaging for the infusion set and may be either microdrops or macrodrops.

- To calculate the flow rate, consider the following factors:

  The total amount of fluid to be administered in milliliters

  The calibration of the administration set in drops/milliliter

  The flow rate of the fluid in drops/minute

  The time for the fluid to infuse in minutes

- The flow rate of IV fluids may be calculated using the following formula:

  $$\text{Flow rate} = \frac{\text{Amount of fluid (mL)} \times \text{Calibration on administration set (gtts/mL)}}{\text{Time for infusion (min)}}$$

  OR

  $$\text{Flow rate} = \frac{\text{mL ordered} \times \text{gtts/mL}}{\text{minutes for infusion}}$$

- This calculation may also be accomplished using two steps:

  Step 1:

  $$\text{mL/hr} = \frac{\text{Total volume of fluids (TV)}}{\text{Total time in hours (TTH)}}$$

  Step 2:

  $$\text{gtts/min} = \frac{\text{Drop factor (gtts/60 min)}}{\text{Time in minutes (TM)}} \times \text{Total volume (mL)}$$

- If dimensional analysis is used, the formula is based on the following: DF = Drip factor; CFV = Conversion factor volume; DV = Dose volume; DT = Dose time; CFT = Conversion factor time; FR = Flow rate in gtts/min.

  $$\text{DF} \times \text{CFV} \times \text{DV} \times \text{DT} \times \text{CFT} = \text{FR}$$

Calculating Intravenous Infusion Times

- If a physician orders fluids without a specific running time, the problem is to decide the total time of the infusion. This calculation provides availability of fluids for follow-up infusions at the appropriate time to meet physician's order.

- The formula for calculating the infusion time is as follows:

$$\text{Flow rate} = \frac{\text{mL ordered} \times \text{gtts/mL (Drop factor)}}{\text{minutes for infusion}}$$

- In this case the minutes for infusion becomes x, and the given amounts are placed in the equation.

- If using dimensional analysis, use the same abbreviations found earlier. The formula is as follows:

$$DT = DF \times CFV \times DV \times FR$$

CHAPTER 13

Calculation of Mixtures from Stock Medications

OBJECTIVES

- Interpret labels for the weight/volume of solute in solvent
- Dilute stock medications to the required strength using strengths expressed as percentages, fractions, and ratios
- Calculate the weight/volume of active ingredient in a substance
- Using alligation, calculate the weight/volume of stock medications needed to prepare a desired compound

KEY WORDS

Alligation Mathematical method for determining amount of two solutes of different percentage strengths necessary to prepare a compound to a required percentage strength

Alligation medial Calculation method by which the weighted average percentage strength of a mixture of two or more substances of known quantity and concentration may be determined

Dilution Process of making a more concentrated solution less concentrated

Medication strength Concentration of active ingredient in a medication

Ratio strength Strength of weak solutions or liquid preparations expressed in ratio terms; because all ratios may be stated as parts of 100, same as expressing percentage strength

Stock medication Medication kept on hand for use in preparing prescriptions; medication of a higher percentage of active ingredient that is used to prepare a medication of a lower percentage

Pretest

Interpret the following labels to show the weight/volume of solute in the solvent. In those instances in which the solvent is unknown, state as the drug "in the solvent." Round answers to tenths. Show all calculations.

1. A label for isopropyl alcohol reads 70% isopropyl alcohol.

Interpret the label in the metric system using ratio strength. _____

2. A label reads Zephiran chloride 0.2%.

Interpret the label in the metric system using ratio. _____

Continued

515

Pretest, cont.

3. A label reads sodium hypochlorite 10%.

   Interpret the label in the metric system using ratio strength. _____

4. A label reads epinephrine 2.25% nebulizer.

   Interpret the amount of epinephrine on the label in the metric system using ratio strength. _____

5. The label on isopropyl alcohol reads 1:2.

   How many parts of alcohol are in the solution? _____

   How many parts of solvent are in the solution? _____

6. The label on a 25 mL saline vial shows a 1:25 solution.

   What is the metric weight of NaCl in the solution? _____

7. A Burrow's solution 100-mL label reads 1:7.5.

   What is the metric volume of Burrow's solution in the total volume?

   _____

   What is the volume of solvent in the mixture? _____

8. A physician orders 1 L of a 10% boric acid solution to be used for compresses.

   How many grams of boric acid should be added to the solvent for this order?

   _____

Pretest, cont.

9. A physician orders 65 mL of a 1:15 sodium hypochlorite solution to be used in the office.

   How many milliliters of sodium hypochlorite should be used to prepare the solution?

   _____

   How many milliliters of solvent would be necessary? _____

   If the physician changes the order to 130 mL of 1:15 sodium hypochlorite solution, how many milliliters of the solute would be needed? _____

   Now, how many milliliters of solvent would be needed? _____

10. An order is to supply 10 mL of a drug at 50 mg/mL. The stock supply is 2.5 g/10 mL.

    How many milliliters of stock supply would be necessary? _____

    How many milliliters of diluent would be necessary? _____

11. A physician asks that 500 mL of a 10% solution of a medication be prepared. The stock supply of the solution is 75%.

    Note this calculation is completed using a formula.

    How many milliliters of diluent would be necessary? _____

    How many milliliters of the medication stock solution would be necessary?

    _____

12. A physician asks that 325 mL of a 1% sodium bicarbonate solution be prepared. The stock medication is 650 mg/tab.

    How many tablet(s) would be necessary to prepare the solution? _____

    How many milliliters of solution would be necessary? _____

Continued

Pretest, cont.

13. A physician asks the pharmacy to prepare 1 L of a 1:2000 silver nitrate solution to be used for an irrigation solution. The stock solution is 1% silver nitrate solution.

How many milliliters of silver nitrate stock solution would be necessary to prepare the solution? _____

How many milliliters of solvent would be necessary? _____

14. Prepare 250 mL of a 0.02% benzalkonium chloride solution to be used for cleansing skin before surgery. Stock strength of the solute is 1%.

How many milliliters of solute would be necessary? _____

How many milliliters of solvent would be necessary? _____

How many milliliters of solute would be needed for 500 mL of solution?

_____

How many milliliters of solvent would be needed for 500 mL of solution?

_____

15. A physician desires 3 L of a 15% Neomycin solution to use for irrigation of a wound. The available Neomycin is found in 0.5 g tablets.

How many grams of Neomycin would be added to fulfill the order?

_____

How many tablets of Neomycin would be added to each liter of the product?

_____

16. A physician wants a patient to receive epinephrine 4 mg. The available medication is 1:1000 injectable. The medication is to be added to 500 mL of D-5-W.

How many milliliters of epinephrine would be added to the fluids for injection?

_____

How many milliliters of epinephrine would be needed to be added to 1000 mL to provide the ordered strength of medication shown above? _____

If the physician wanted the patient to receive epinephrine 3 mg in the 500 mL of D-5-W to follow the 1000 mL, how many milliliters of the medication would be added to the fluids for injection? _____

Pretest, cont.

17. A physician orders calcium gluconate 0.5 g to be used to prepare 1 L IV fluids. The medication is available in a vial marked calcium gluconate 1:2000 injectable.

How many milliliters of calcium gluconate would be added to the fluids?

_____

How many milliliters of IV fluids would be used? _____

18. A medical office needs 0.25 L of a 10% Lysol solution for disinfecting the office.

How many milliliters of the 25% Lysol would be necessary to prepare the solution?

_____

How many milliliters of solvent are needed for the solution? _____

19. A physician desires 100 mL of a 50% creosol solution to be prepared from a 1:2 creosol solution.

How many milliliters of the 1:2 creosol solution should be obtained to prepare this order? _____

How many milliliters of solvent should be added for the order as above?

_____

20. A stock bottle of sodium perborate 1:50 solution is available. The dentist asks that 200 mL of solution be prepared.

How many grams of sodium perborate would be found in the 200 mL of solution?

_____

INTRODUCTION

Special populations such as geriatric or pediatric patients often require an adjustment of **medication strength** found in **stock medications** supplied by manufacturers. Stock solutions may also be stored in concentrated amounts, to save space and for economic reasons, for **dilution** later. Stock supplies are usually found in commonly used solution strengths. By diluting the stock medication, the amount of medication necessary may be placed in a volume that is more easily measured or in a volume that may meet the needs of the physician's prescription or order. The pharmacy is responsible for preparing weaker solutions to meet physicians' orders or to make the administration of the correct amount of medication more accurate.

Remember from previous chapters that a solution is made of the solute (the drug to be dissolved) and the solvent (the liquid in which the solute will be dissolved). First, the amount of solute in a solution must be understood before dilution may occur. Using a process of dilution called **alligation**, the medication strength may be changed to meet the required strength. Dilution means to make a strong concentration of medication weaker or to add more solvent to the solute. Alligation is the mathematical calculation that determines the necessary amount of two different concentrations required to prepare the desired concentration for the medication order.

INTERPRETING SOLUTION LABELS AND CALCULATING SOLUTIONS IN PERCENTAGES

A solution is a mixture of two or more substances with a percentage of weight/volume being greater than the other. These substances are present as a gas/liquid, liquid/liquid, or solid/liquid. The solution may be prepared by mixing two liquids, as in mixing chocolate syrup with milk to make chocolate milk; mixing a gas with a liquid, as in adding carbon dioxide to water to prepare carbonated water for a fountain soda; or mixing a solid with a liquid, such as adding water to powdered instant tea. The material with the highest percentage of weight/volume to be mixed in the solid or gas form is considered a solute, whereas the substance with the lower percentage of weight/volume is a solvent. But what if both substances are liquids? In this case the liquid in the smaller amount is considered the solute or concentrate, and the greater amount of liquid is considered the solvent or the diluent. When the solute is shown as part of the solvent, the resultant solution may be expressed as a **ratio strength** or percentage strength.

As a review of previous chapters, percentage means that there are so many parts per 100. So 25% is 25 parts of solute in 100 parts of total solution or the parts of the percentage represent 1 g of solute in 100 mL of solvent. Percentages may be expressed as weight in weight (w/w) showing the number of grams of a solute in 100 g of total solvent. Percent of weight in volume (w/v) is the number of grams of solute in 100 mL of solvent. Finally, percentage may be expressed as volume in volume (v/v) or the number of milliliters of solute in 100 mL of total solvent. Weight in weight is found with semi solid or solid preparations, whereas weight in volume and volume in volume are found with liquid preparations.

With percentage preparations, the easiest method for calculation is the ratio and proportion method. If a review of the ratio and proportion method is necessary, see Chapter 2.

Calculating Weight-in-Weight Solutions

With weight-in-weight percentage calculations, the solutes and solvents will be expressed in weights such as grams, milligrams, grains, pounds, and other weights. Therefore the percentage will measure the total weight of one substance in the total weight of the final compound. With the solute being a solid weight and the solvent being a solid or semi-solid weight, the final product will be either a solid or a semi-solid preparation such as powder, cream, or ointment. Remember that the units used in the equation for ratio and proportion must be in the same measurements such as grams and milligrams.

EXAMPLE 13-1

A physician asks that you prepare 100 grams of 2.5% hydrocortisone cream from available hydrocortisone cream 10%.

What is the weight of hydrocortisone in the stock medication? _____

What is the weight of hydrocortisone in each 100 g of base to complete this order?

_____

What weight of the 10% stock medication is needed to prepare the 2.5% cream?

_____

How many grams of hydrocortisone would be needed to prepare 5 g of the 2.5% cream?

_____

What is the weight of hydrocortisone in stock medication?

The label interpretation of 10% is 10 g in 100 g of stock medication.

What is the weight of hydrocortisone in each 100 g of base to complete this order?

_____

The desired weight of hydrocortisone in the order is 2.5 grams.

What weight of the 10% stock medication is needed to prepare the 2.5% cream?

$$2.5 \text{ g} : x = 10 \text{ g} : 100 \text{ g base}$$

$$2.5 \text{ g} : x = 10 \text{ g} : 100 \text{ g}$$

$$10 \text{ g } x = 2.5 \text{ g} \times 100 \text{ g}$$

$$10 \text{ g } x = 2.5 \text{ g} \times 100 \text{ g}$$

$$10x = 250 \text{ g}$$

$$x = \frac{250}{10} \text{ or 25 g of 10% hydrocortisone to prepare a 2.5% hydrocortisone cream}$$

How many grams of hydrocortisone are needed to prepare 5 g of the 2.5% cream?

$$2.5 \text{ g} : 100 \text{ g base} :: x : 5 \text{ g of base}$$

$$100 \text{ g } x = 2.5 \text{ g} \times 5 \text{ g}$$

$$100x = 12.5 \text{ g}$$

$$x = \frac{12.5}{100} \text{ or 0.125 g of hydrocortisone per 5 g of cream}$$

Calculating Weight-in-Volume Solutions

Calculations for weight-in-volume percentages will show a strength or weight such as grams, milligrams, and other weights of medication in a volume such as liters, milliliters, drams, pints, or other liquid measures of solvent. A weight-in-volume is similar to a weight-in-weight because in a 1% solution, 1 g of solute is found in 100 mL of the solvent if the solvent has the same specific gravity of water. Again, the ratio and proportion method is preferred for calculating these solutions. With weight-in-volume, the numerator or solute is measured in grams, whereas the denominator or solvent is measured in milliliters.

TECH NOTE
Remember that 1 g of water is equivalent to 1 mL of water, or 1 mL of water weighs 1 g.

EXAMPLE 13-2

 How many milliliters of a 10% boric acid solution can be made from 20 g of boric acid?

10 g : 100 mL :: 20 g : x

$10x = 100$ mL $\times 20$ (Notice that the grams have been canceled.)

$10x = 2000$

$x = 200$ mL

Calculate Volume-in-Volume Solutions

Again using ratio and proportion, the amount of liquid solute in liquid solvent can be calculated. The percentage indicates the weight of solute in the solvent in a volume measurement.

EXAMPLE 13-3

A physician orders 15 mL of a 10 mcg/mL dilution of a drug for a child. The stock medication is 40 mcg/mL.

How many micrograms of the drug will be needed to prepare the order?

10 mcg : 1 mL :: x : 15 mL

$x = 10 \times 15$ mcg or 150 mcg of the medication is necessary

How many milliliters of the stock medication are necessary?

40 mcg : 1 mL :: 150 mcg : x

$40\,x = 150$ mL

$x = \dfrac{150}{40}$ or $\dfrac{15}{4}$ (Notice that the zeros are canceled.)

$x = 3.75$ mL of stock solution are necessary

How many milliliters of diluent are necessary?

15 mL Total volume of solution – 3.75 mL volume of stock solution
  = 11.25 mL volume of diluent necessary

Calculate the Amount of Drug and Solvent

In some cases the calculation of the quantity of the pure drug, either liquid or solid, must be determined to prepare a solution of a certain strength. The amount of solvent is the amount of diluent added to the solute to make the required volume of the necessary solution. The final volume of solution will contain the amount of stock medication required for the physician's order.

The following formula will allow the calculation of these solutions:

Strength of solution available   **Desired or new volume of solution**

$$\frac{\text{Amount or volume of solute}}{\text{Total volume of solution}} = \frac{\text{Amount of desired or new solute}}{\text{Volume of desired solution}}$$

The first step is to write the percentage strength as a ratio and then write the desired solution as a ratio. Then solve for x.

EXAMPLE 13-4

 A physician desires a 1% lidocaine preparation in hand lotion for itching. How many grams of lidocaine would be necessary to prepare 50 mL of this solution?

First interpret that 1% is 1 g/100 mL.

Strength of solution   **Desired amount of solution**

$$\frac{1\text{ g (Amount of solute)}}{100\text{ mL (Total volume of solution)}} = \frac{x\text{ (Amount of desired solute)}}{50\text{ mL (Volume of desired solution)}}$$

$$\frac{1\text{ g}}{100\text{ mL}} = \frac{x}{50\text{ mL}}$$

$$100\text{ mL} \times x = 50\text{ mL} \times 1\text{ g}$$

$$100\text{ m\cancel{L}} \times x = 50\text{ m\cancel{L}} \times 1\text{ g}$$

$$100\,x = 50\text{ g}$$

$$x = 50\text{ g} \div 100$$

$$x = 0.5\text{ g of lidocaine is necessary to prepare this solution}$$

If the medication available is lidocaine 5%, what volume of lidocaine is necessary for this order?

$$5\text{ g} : 100\text{ mL} :: 0.5\text{ g} : x$$

$$5\text{ g} \times x = 0.5\text{ g} \times 100\text{ mL}$$

$$5\text{ \cancel{g}} \times x = 0.5\text{ \cancel{g}} \times 100\text{ mL}$$

$$5\,x = 50\text{ mL}$$

$$x = 10\text{ mL}$$

To calculate volume of solvent in volume of solution, use the following:

Volume of solvent = Volume of finished solution − Volume of solute

What is the amount of hand lotion that should be used to prepare this solution?

Volume of solvent = 50 mL (finished solution) − 10 mL (Volume of solute)

Amount of solvent (hand lotion) = 50 mL − 10 mL or 40 mL

Reducing and Enlarging Ordered Preparations

When a volume of a known solution requires reducing or enlarging to meet a physician's order, the original strength of the preparation may be used for the calculation of the new volume or weight of the preparation. For example, using the above calculations in Example 13-4, if the physician desires 100 mL, the answer can be figured using ratio and proportion.

10 mL (solute) : 50 mL (prepared medication) :: x : 100 mL (prepared medication)

50 mL (prepared medication) $x = 10$ mL (solute) $\times 100$ mL (prepared medication)

$50 x = 1000$ mL (solute)

$x = 20$ mL of solute is needed to prepare 100 mL of ordered medication

40 mL (solvent) : 50 mL (prepared medication) :: x : 100 mL (prepared medication)

50 mL (prepared medication) $x = 40$ mL (solvent) $\times 100$ mL (prepared medication)

50 mL (solvent) $x = 4000$

$x = 80$ mL of solvent to prepare 100 mL of ordered medication

The volume of solute to solvent for 100 mL of ordered medication would be 20 mL solute to 80 mL of solvent.

Practice Problems A

Calculate the following problems. Round all answers to tenths. Show all your calculations.

1. How many grams of sucrose must be dissolved in 500 mL of water to make a 75% solution? _____

   How many grams of sucrose would be needed to make 1000 mL of 75% solution?
   _____750_____

   How many grams of sucrose would be needed for 250 mL of 75% solution?
   _____187.5_____

2. How many milliliters of 10% solution can be made from 750 g of a chemical?
   _____7,500_____

3. A stock lotion contains 10% methyl salicylate.

How many milliliters of 10% methyl salicylate would be necessary to prepare 3 pints of 4% lotion?

Hint: Remember that the units must be in the same measurements.

_____576_____

4. If 15 mL of peppermint oil is in 500 mL of a solution, what is the percentage strength of the fluids? _____3_____

5. Epinephrine is available in 5% solution.

How many milliliters would be necessary to prepare 10 mL of a 2.5% solution of epinephrine? _____5 ML_____

6. A 20-mL vial of medication contains 50 mg/mL.

What is the total weight of the medication in the vial? _____1,000 Mg_____

What is the percentage strength of the medication? _____5%_____

7. How many grams of boric acid would be necessary to prepare 60 mL of a 5% solution? _____3_____

8. On hand is a 15% solution of sodium hypochlorite. The physician wants 1 L of a 0.15% solution.

How many milliliters of sodium hypochlorite would be necessary?

_____

How many milliliters of solvent should be added? _____

9. A stock liter contains 50% sodium bicarbonate. A physician desires 2 L of 6% solution.

How many milliliters of 50% sodium bicarbonate would be necessary to fill this order? _____

How many milliliters of solvent would be necessary for this solution?

_____

10. A physician desires 100 mL of a 15% iodine preparation. Ten mL of solution is to be added to 1 pt of water as a soak.

How many grams of iodine would be in the stock solution? _____

What would be the percentage strength of the iodine after it has been diluted?

_____

11. A physician orders a 2% vinegar solution as a douche. A patient asks how much vinegar should be put in each pint of water. (Round to the whole number.)

What would be the answer for this patient? ___10 ML_____

How could the patient measure this in household utensils? ___2 tsp_____

12. How many milliliters of a 50% dextrose solution would be administered to a patient in hypoglycemia to provide 150 mg of dextrose? ___0.3 uL_____

How many milliliters of the 50% dextrose would be needed to provide 300 mg of dextrose? ___2.6_____

How many milliliters of dextrose 50% would be needed to provide 375 mg? (Round to hundredths.) ___0.75_____

13. How many milliliters of sterile water should be added to 75 g of sucrose to make a 2.5% solution? ___3,000 mL___

14. How many grams of dextrose are necessary to prepare 3000 mL of a 10% solution? ___300 g___

15. A prescription is written to prepare a mouthwash containing tetracycline 1 g, nystatin suspension 60 mL, Benadryl 60 mL and qs to 240 mL with dexamethasone.

What is the percentage of tetracycline in the final compound? _____

What is the percentage (v/v) of nystatin suspension in the final mixture?

___5%___

What volume of dexamethasone is needed to prepare the desired volume?

___120 ML___

16. A prescription is written to prepare a lotion using Aristocort Lotion 1% to be mixed with 60 mL of hand lotion to make a 0.5% lotion.

What is the weight of Aristocort 1% in the prepared lotion? ___60 g___

17. A dentist sends a prescription for a mouth swish for pain.

Lidocaine 0.5%

Benadryl

Maalox

Sig: a̅a̅qs 120 mL

What volume of each medication would be necessary to prepare this prescription?

Lidocaine ___40 ML___

Benadryl ___40 ML___

Maalox ___40 ML___

What would be the percentage (v/v) strength of each?

Lidocaine ___33.3%___

Benadryl ___33.3%___

Maalox ___33.3%___

18. A physician orders a 30% solution of dextrose in 500 mL.

How many grams of dextrose would be necessary to make this solution?

___150___

19. How many grams of 100% zinc oxide would be necessary to prepare 4 oz of a 10% ointment?

Hint: Be sure to calculate ounces to the metric system before any other calculations.

(Round to hundredths.) ___12___

20. A dermatologist writes a prescription for 0.25% menthol and 0.5% phenol in Vaseline to make 1 g of ointment.

How many milligrams of menthol would be necessary to prepare this hand preparation? ___2.5 mg___

How many milligrams of phenol would be necessary to prepare this hand preparation? ___5 mg___

INTERPRETING SOLUTION LABELS AND CALCULATING MEDICATION IN RATIO DOSAGES

Weak solutions are often expressed in terms of ratio strength such as $1:10$, which is merely another way to express percentage strength. The $1:10$ ratio means that 1 part of solute is found in 10 parts of total solution, or 10 parts of solute are found in 100 parts of total solution, or a 10% compound. If the $1:10$ ratio were a weight (solid) solute found in a volume (liquid) of solvent, 1 g of solute would be found in 10 mL of total solution. If both the solute and solvent were in liquid form, 1 mL of solute would be found in 10 mL of total solution. Finally, if both the solvent and solute are solid (weight), 1 g of solute would be found in 10 g of total compound. To calculate the ratio strengths in a solution or mixture, you may use the ratio and proportion method.

> **TECH NOTE**
>
> Remember that 1 mL of liquid is equal to 1 g of solid in weight.

EXAMPLE 13-5

A medication with ratio strength of $1:500$ has what percentage strength?

1 part : 500 parts :: x : 100%

$500x = 100$

$x = 100 \div 500$ or $x = 1\emptyset\emptyset \div 5\emptyset\emptyset$

$x = 0.2\%$

EXAMPLE 13-6

A medication contains 4 mg/mL of solution. What is the ratio strength of the solution?

Remember that the ratio strength is expressed in grams per 100 mL, so a conversion from milligrams to grams must first be calculated.

4 mg = 0.004 g

0.004 g : 1 mL :: 1 g : x

$0.004 \text{ g} \times x = 1 \text{ mL} \times 1 \text{ g}$

$0.004\,\cancel{g} \times x = 1 \text{ mL} \times 1\,\cancel{g}$

$0.004x = 1 \text{ mL}$

$x = 250 \text{ mL}$

Ratio strength $= 1 : 250$

EXAMPLE 13-7

What ratio strength of a solution can be made by dissolving Benadryl 50 mg in a lotion to make 150 mL?

Again, change 50 mg to grams to get 0.05 g.

0.05 g : 150 mL :: 1 g : x mL

$0.05 \text{ g} \times x = 150 \text{ mL} \times 1 \text{ g}$

$0.05\,\cancel{g} \times x = 150 \text{ mL} \times 1\,\cancel{g}$

$$0.05x = 150$$

$$x = 3000 \text{ mL}$$

Ratio strength $= 1 : 3000$

Practice Problems B

Calculate the following problems for medications in ratio dosage. Round answers to hundredths unless otherwise indicated. Show all your calculations.

1. Prepare 500 mL of a $1 : 200$ vinegar solution to be used as a douche.

   What is the percentage strength of the solution? ___0.5%___

2. Prepare 1000 mL of a $1 : 25,000$ silver nitrate solution to be used by a urologist.

   What is the percentage strength of silver nitrate? (Round to thousandths.)
   ___0.04%___

3. How many milligrams of a drug are in 1.5 mL of a $1 : 5000$ solution?
   ___0.03___

4. How many milligrams of a drug are found in 1500 mL of a $1 : 750$ solution?
   ___2 grams___

5. How many grams of NaCl would be necessary to make 500 mL of a $1 : 5000$ solution?
   ___0.1 g___

6. How many fluid ounces of water should be added to 4 mL of a $1 : 4$ concentration to make a $1 : 6$ concentration? ___0.07 ounces___

   How many mL would be added? ___2 ML___

7. If a medication is available in 1:500 concentration, how many milliliters would be necessary to provide 750 mg? _____375 ML_____

8. A boric acid solution is 1:10 strength. How many milliliters of 1:10 boric acid solution would be necessary to prepare 100 mL of a 5% solution?
_____50 ML_____

9. An order is written for 1500 mL of a 1:10 antiseptic solution. The stock solution is 1:5.

How many milliliters of the stock solution would be necessary to complete this order? _____150_____

How many milliliters of solvent would be necessary to complete this order?
_____150_____

10. Epinephrine is available in a 1:10,000 solution for the treatment of asthma.

How many milliliters of this medication should be supplied to provide the patient with 2.5 mg? _____25_____

11. A physician orders a 4% solution of potassium permanganate.

How many grams of potassium permanganate would be necessary to prepare 500 mL? _____20_____

12. Tylenol with codeine elixir is 25% codeine.

What is the ratio strength? _____1:4_____

13. A physician orders 1 L solution of sodium chloride 1:200.

   How many grams of sodium chloride would be necessary to complete this order?

   _____ 5 g _____

14. A physician orders a 10% dextrose solution.

   How many grams of dextrose would be necessary to make 0.5 L?

   _____ 50 g _____

15. [icon] A dentist desires an antiseptic mouthwash of sodium bicarbonate 1:40.

   How many grams of sodium bicarbonate would be necessary to make 6 oz?

   _____ 4.5 g _____

16. [icon] A floor order is received for epinephrine 0.5 mg to be administered IM stat. The supply of epinephrine is 1:1000 solution in a 1-mL vial.

   What is the milligram strength of the vial of epinephrine? _____ 1 mg : 1 ML _____
   How many vials of 1:1000 epinephrine would be necessary to fill the order?

   _____ 1 _____

   How many vials of epinephrine should be supplied to the floor? _____ 1 _____
   What volume should be administered? _____ 0.5 _____
   What syringe should be supplied for administration of the dose? _____ ML _____

17. [icon] A physician orders Prostigmin 0.4 mg IM stat. The available medication is Prostigmin 1:2000 in a 1-ml vial.

   What is the milligram strength of the available Prostigmin? _____ 0.5 mg _____
   How many milliliters of medication should be administered to the patient?

   _____ 0.8 ML _____

18.   A physician desires a solution of 500 mL of isopropyl alcohol 30%. The available alcohol is isopropyl alcohol 7:10.

How much sterile water should be added to prepare the necessary solution?

_____285.7_____

How much stock alcohol should be used to prepare the 30% solution?

_____214.3_____

19.   A physician orders desoximetasone cream 0.25% 5 g to be used for a patient with allergic dermatitis. The available medication is desoximetasone cream 1:2.

What is the weight in grams of stock 1:2 desoximetasone that should be used to prepare the cream? (Round to hundredths.) _____0.025 g_____

20.   A physician asks that 0.4 g of potassium permanganate be dissolved to prepare a finished pint of solution. (Round to hundredths.)

What is the percentage strength of the solution? _____0.08%_____

What is the ratio strength of the solution? _____1:1250_____

CALCULATING THE DILUTION OF STOCK SOLUTIONS

Diluting stock solutions may be necessary to prepare a solution ordered by the physician. The ability to prepare these solutions from stock medication is also a way in controlling the numbers of medications that are kept in stock. Stock medications are generally more potent or concentrated than the usual desired solution for prescriptions; therefore this medication must be diluted or compounded to a weaker strength. Using stock solutions that are purer and stronger forms of the drug, larger volumes of medications may be prepared from small medication quantities, and space in the pharmacy is saved. Stock solutions have the strength written on the label, and a diluent is added to prepare the compound as ordered. When diluting compounds, the amount of active ingredient or solute remains the same and the solvent amount is increased, reducing the percentage or dilution of the stock solution. Remember from earlier in this chapter that the solvent and solute may be in solid forms, as well as liquid.

Two rules are important in simplifying this process:

Rule 1—When ratio strengths are given, convert these to percentage strengths using ratio and proportion. It is much easier to calculate in a percentage than in the fraction equivalent found with ratio strengths, such as 1:20, which would become 5%.

Rule 2—Reduce proportional parts to the lowest terms if these must be used, such as 75 parts : 50 parts becomes 3:2.

TECH NOTE

Remember that when calculating these problems, as with all math calculations for medication administration, you must use the parts or units in the equivalent measurement system.

Two formulas are available for diluting medications. Either may be used, so the choice depends on what is most comfortable for the person doing the calculation.

EXAMPLE 13-8

A physician orders 1 L of 10% boric acid solution to be prepared from 40% boric acid solution.

FORMULA 1

$$\text{Amount of stock solution necessary} = \frac{\text{Amount of solution prescribed} \times \text{Strength prescribed}}{\text{Strength of stock solution}}$$

$$\text{Step 1—}x \text{ (Amount of stock solution necessary)} = \frac{1000 \text{ mL (amount of solution desired)} \times 10\% \text{ (strength desired)}}{40\% \text{ (Strength of stock solution)}}$$

$$x = \frac{1000 \text{ mL} \times 10\%}{40\%}$$

$$x = \frac{1000 \text{ mL} \times 10\%}{40\%}$$

$$x = \frac{1000 \text{ mL} \times 10}{40} \quad \text{or} \quad \frac{10,000 \text{ mL}}{40}$$

$$x = 250 \text{ mL of boric acid solution}$$

Step 2—To complete this calculation, take the amount of solute (250 mL) and subtract it from the final amount of the solution (1000 mL).

1000 mL (total amount of solution ordered) – 250 mL of boric acid solution (amount of solute necessary) = 750 mL (Amount of solvent necessary to prepare the amount of fluid to the physician's order)

FORMULA 2

$$\text{SV (Stock volume)} \times \text{S\% (Stock percentage)} = \text{DV (Desired volume)} \times \text{D\% (Desired percentage)}$$

$$\text{Step 1—}x \text{ (SV)} \times 40\% = 1000 \text{ mL} \times 10\%$$

$$40\% \times x = 10\% \times 1000 \text{ mL}$$

$$40\% \times x = 10\% \times 1000 \text{ mL}$$

$$40\,x = 10,000 \text{ mL}$$

$$x = 10,000 \text{ mL} \div 40 \text{ (or } 1000 \text{ mL} \div 4 \text{ after cancelling zeros)}$$

$$x = 250 \text{ mL of boric acid}$$

Step 2—To complete this calculation, you must take the amount of solute (250 mL) and subtract this from the final amount of the solution (1000 mL).

1000 mL (Total amount of solution necessary) – 250 mL (Amount of solute necessary) = 750 mL (Amount of solvent necessary to prepare the amount of fluid to the physician's order)

Practice Problems C

Calculate the following problems using either formula described earlier. Round to tenths as appropriate and to other decimal places as indicated. Show your calculations.

1. Prepare 1 L of Lysol 3% from a stock solution of Lysol 10%.

   How many milliliters of stock solution are necessary for this preparation?

   _____

   How many milliliters of solvent are necessary for this preparation?

   _____

2. Prepare 500 mL 5% creosol solution from a stock solution of creosol 1:10.

   Hint: Remember to change ratio to percentage.

   How many milliliters of stock solution are necessary? _____

   How many milliliters of solvent are necessary? _____

3. How many milliliters of sterile water are necessary to prepare 8 oz of 40% solution of isopropyl alcohol from a 70% stock solution? _____

   How many milliliters of stock solution are necessary? _____

4. Prepare 1.5 L of creosol 1:200 from a 2% stock solution.

   How many milliliters of stock solution are necessary? _____

   How many milliliters of solvent are necessary? _____

5. Prepare 1 oz of a 0.002% solution of Merthiolate from a 1% stock solution. (Round to hundredths.)

Hint: Be sure the measurements are in the same measurement system.

How many milliliters of stock solution are necessary? _____

How many milliliters of solvent are necessary? _____

6. A physician orders glycerin solution 15% 250 mL to be used as an enema. The available stock solution is glycerin 25%.

How many milliliters of stock solution would be necessary? _____

How many milliliters of solvent would be necessary? _____

7. A physician orders 1 pint of 7.5% dextrose in water. The stock solution of dextrose is 50%.

How many milliliters of stock solution would be necessary? _____

How many milliliters of solvent would be necessary? _____

8. How many milliliters of 20% Zephiran chloride are necessary to prepare 8 ounces of a 7.5% solution?

How many milliliters of stock solution are necessary? _____

How many milliliters of solvent are necessary? _____

9. A physician desires 1.5 L of potassium chloride 15% from a stock solution that is 20% potassium chloride.

How many milliliters of stock solution would be necessary? _____

How many milliliters of solvent would be necessary? _____

10. A medical office needs 3 L of a 1:10 solution of hypochlorous acid. The stock solution is Clorox 25%.

How many milliliters of stock solution would be necessary? _____

How many milliliters of solvent would be necessary? _____

11. A physician desires 8 oz of Betadine solution 2%. The stock solution is Betadine 10%.

How many milliliters of stock solution would be necessary? _____

How many milliliters of solvent would be necessary? _____

12. Prepare 3 L of hydrogen peroxide 1:40. The stock solution is hydrogen peroxide 5%.

How many milliliters of stock solution are necessary? _____

How many milliliters of solvent are necessary? _____

13. Prepare 600 mL of a 2.5% solution from a 10% hydrogen peroxide solution.

How many milliliters of stock solution are necessary? _____

How many milliliters of solvent are necessary? _____

14. Prepare 4 L of a 1:50 solution of potassium permanganate from a 5% potassium permanganate stock solution.

How many milliliters of stock solution are necessary? _____

How many milliliters of solvent are necessary? _____

15. Prepare 10 mL of 0.01% adrenaline solution for injection from a 2% adrenaline ampule. (Round to hundredths.)

How many milliliters of stock solution are necessary? _____

How many milliliters of solvent are necessary? _____

16. A physician desires 500 mL of 2% calcium chloride solution to be given IV. The stock solution is calcium chloride 10%.

How many milliliters of stock solution would be necessary? _____

How many milliliters of solvent would be necessary? _____

If the calcium chloride is available in 5-mL ampules, how many ampules would be necessary to prepare the solution? _____

17. How many fluid ounces of a 6% solution can be made from 30 mL of a 36% solution?

Hint: Insert the knowns and unknowns in the proper places in the formulas.

_____

18. A stock solution of 1:50 of mercuric chloride is available to prepare 250 mL of 0.02% solution. How many milliliters of stock solution are necessary?

_____

How many milliliters of solvent are necessary? _____

19. Prepare 500 mL of 10% disinfectant from a 50% stock solution.

How many milliliters of stock solution would be necessary? _____

How many milliliters of solvent would be necessary? _____

20. 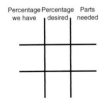 A physician orders 1 pint of 10% ethyl alcohol. The stock solution is 100 mL of 95% ethyl alcohol.

How many milliliters of stock solution would be necessary? _____

How many milliliters of solvent would be necessary? _____

How many total milliliters of 10% ethyl alcohol can be prepared from the available stock solution? _____

CALCULATING MEDICATION DILUTIONS USING ALLIGATION

Alligation is a mathematical method of solving calculations involving the mixing of solutions or compounds possessing different percentage strengths. Alligation alternate is a method of calculating the number of parts of two components of a given strength that are mixed to prepare a mixture of the desired strength. A final proportional calculation permits the translation of relative parts found by alligation to the desired specific amount.

! TECH ALERT

Alligation indicates the parts of two given stock medications needed to prepare the desired compound strength.

! TECH ALERT

Preparation of diluted compounds from stock medications to meet a prescription ordered compounds is actually accomplished in two distinct steps. The first calculation is to find the parts of each stock medication needed for the compound (Steps 1-7 below). The second calculation is to find the volume/weight of each stock medication needed to prepare the ordered strength (Step 8 below).

The final strength of the mixture must lie somewhere between the strengths of the component parts. This means that the prepared mixture must be stronger than its weakest part and weaker than the strongest component. Therefore the strength of the prepared mixture is "weighted" by the relative amounts of the components involved. If the mixture contains more of the weaker component, the prepared mixture will lie closer to the weaker component. If the mixture contains more of the stronger component, the mixture will be closer to that side of the equation.

To begin alligation alternate, think of preparing a box for playing tic-tac-toe to allow the numbers to be placed in the four corners and in the center box.

Percentage   Percentage   Parts
we have   desired   needed

Step 1—Prepare the graph.
Step 2—Place the strength to be calculated in the center box.
Step 3—Place the highest percentage concentration in the left upper corner.
Step 4—Place the lowest percentage concentration in the lower left corner.
Step 5—Subtract the center square from the left upper square and place in the lower right square to reveal the parts of the lowest percentage concentration to be used in the new mixture.

Step 6—Subtract the lower left square from the center box and place in the upper right corner to reveal the parts of the highest percentage concentration to be used in the new mixture.

Step 7—Add the calculated parts together to find the total parts of the two ingredients in the compound.

Step 8—When the total quantity of the mixture is included in the prescription, then the parts of the mixture are placed into two ratio and proportion equations to calculate the exact amount of each ingredient to use. The total number of calculated parts is placed in the first ratio with the total amount of compound. The second ratio set in the proportion is the calculated number of parts of the stock ingredients to the unknown total compound amount. This step must be calculated for each part of the compound.

EXAMPLE 13-9

Prepare 1 L solution of 70% alcohol from 50% alcohol and 95% alcohol.

Step 1—Draw the graph for calculating alligation.

Percentage Percentage Parts
we have   desired needed

Step 2—Place the strength to be calculated in the center box.

Percentage Percentage Parts
we have   desired needed

70%

Step 3—Place the highest percentage concentration in the left upper corner.

Percentage Percentage Parts
we have   desired needed

95%

70%

Step 4—Place the lowest percentage concentration in the lower left corner.

Percentage Percentage Parts
we have   desired needed

95%

70%

50%

Step 5—Subtract the center square from the left upper square and place in the lower right square to reveal the parts of the lowest percentage concentration to be used in the new mixture.

 TECH ALERT

Notice that the answers are now in parts, not unit values.

Step 6—Subtract the lower left square from the center box and place in the upper right corner to reveal the parts of the highest percentage concentration to be used in the new mixture.

Step 7—Add the parts of the concentration to find the total parts in the compound.

To prepare this solution, mix 20 parts of 95% alcohol with 25 parts of 50% alcohol.

Remember, this is a proportional amount that must be used to find the exact part amounts when the total weight or volume of the compound is indicated.

Step 8—Using the previous example, the total amount of the solution is 1 L of 70% alcohol.

The total number of compound parts as calculated using the alligation graph is 45 parts in 1000 mL (1 L) of solution.

First, calculate the number of milliliters of 95% alcohol (stock solution).

$$45 \text{ parts} : 1000 \text{ mL} :: 20 \text{ parts} : x$$

$$45 \text{ parts} \times x = 20 \text{ parts} \times 1000 \text{ mL}$$

$$45 \text{ parts} \times x = 20 \text{ parts} \times 1000 \text{ mL}$$

$$45x = 20{,}000 \text{ mL}$$

$$x = 444.4 \text{ mL of } 95\% \text{ alcohol} \quad \text{or} \quad 444 \text{ mL of } 95\% \text{ alcohol}$$

Second, calculate the total number of milliliters of 50% alcohol (stock solution).

$$45 \text{ parts} : 1000 \text{ mL} :: 25 \text{ parts} : x$$

$$45 \text{ parts} \times x = 1000 \text{ mL} \times 25 \text{ parts}$$

$$45 \text{ parts} \times x = 1000 \text{ mL} \times 25 \text{ parts}$$

$$45x = 25{,}000 \text{ mL}$$

$$x = 555.6 \text{ mL of } 50\% \text{ alcohol} \quad \text{or} \quad 556 \text{ mL or } 50\% \text{ alcohol}$$

Now check your calculations:

444 mL of 95% alcohol + 556 mL of 50% alcohol = 1000 mL of 70% alcohol

Therefore the calculations are correct.

DILUTING STOCK MEDICATIONS USING STRENGTHS IN PERCENTAGE, FRACTIONS, AND RATIOS

Alligation medial is a method of calculation that may be used to define the weighted average percentage strength of a mixture of two or more substances with known quantities and strengths. When two or more solutes must be added to one compound, this method allows rapid calculation. The percentage strength must be expressed as a whole number for each component. The quantities must be expressed in common measurements such as same weight or same volume indicators. If a percentage of the solvent is not provided, in most cases it may be considered to be 0%.

Alligation medial, another means of checking for accuracy, involves multiplying the percentage as a decimal by the total number of milliliters in the preparation to obtain the total number of grams in the compound. Then multiply the components by the same formula and add the total grams together to check for calculation accuracy.

EXAMPLE 13-10

Following is the calculation of the previous solution using alligation medial to prove the calculation was made correctly.

Amount desired (milliliters, etc.) × Percent (in a decimal) = Grams

Prepare 1 L solution of 70% alcohol from 50% alcohol and 95% alcohol

$$1000 \text{ mL} \times 0.7 \ (70\%) = 700 \text{ g}$$
$$556 \text{ mL} \times 0.5 \ (50\%) = 278 \text{ g}$$
$$444 \text{ mL} \times 0.95 \ (95\%) = 422 \text{ g}$$
$$278 \text{ g} + 422 \text{ g} = 700 \text{ g}$$

This calculation shows that the calculations using alligation alternate are correct.

Practice Problems D

Complete these problems using alligation and calculation of the necessary amounts of each component to prepare the amount of compound ordered. Round to tenths unless otherwise indicated. Verify calculations for accuracy using alligation medial. Indicate the calculation of weight/volume of the solute/solvent on each line by indicating the solute/solvent with the answer, such as _____ of (15%). Show your work.

1. On hand is a 6% solution of sodium hypochlorite and a 15% solution of sodium hypochlorite. Prepare 500 mL of a 10% solution of sodium hypochlorite.

   _____

   _____

2. Available are two ointment strengths containing 5% boric acid and 20% boric acid. Prepare 1 g of a 12.5% ointment.

   _____

   _____

3. A physician orders 20 g of a 15% tannic acid ointment. Available are two tannic acid ointments in 12% and 25%.

   _____

   _____

4. Prepare 500 mL of 15% potassium chloride solution using 20% potassium chloride and 5% potassium chloride solution.

   _____

   _____

5. Prepare 500 mL of 0.9% sodium chloride solution from a 10% sodium chloride solution.

Hint: The diluent of sterile water necessary for this calculation has 0% sodium chloride.

_____

_____

6. Prepare 750 mL of 3% sodium bicarbonate solution from a 15% solution and 1% solution.

_____

_____

7. Prepare 200 mL of 10% dextrose solution using 5% dextrose solution and 50% dextrose solution.

_____

_____

8. Prepare 3 L of 3% Lysol solution using 1.5% Lysol and 5% Lysol solutions.

_____

_____

9. A physician desires 50 g of a 7.5% ointment. The available ointments are 2.5% and 15%.

_____

_____

10. Prepare 2 L of 40% alcohol from 10% alcohol and 55% alcohol.

_____

_____

11. Prepare 500 mL of 4% potassium permanganate solution using 1:10 potassium permanganate solution and 1:50 potassium permanganate solution.

Hint: Remember to change ratio to percentage strength.

_____

_____

12. Prepare 250 mL of 8% dextrose solution. The available dextrose solutions are D-5-W and D-10-W.

_____

_____

13. A physician orders 50 mL dextrose 7.5% to be administered IV stat. The available dextrose is D-5-W and dextrose 50% solution.

_____

_____

14. Prepare 200 mL of 5% potassium chloride. The available potassium chloride is 20%.

Hint: Remember that sterile water is 0%.

_____

_____

15. Prepare 50 mL of 1.8% sodium chloride solution. The available sodium chloride solutions are 0.9% and 5%. (Round answers to hundredths.)

_____

_____

16. Prepare 2.5 g of hydrocortisone ointment 7.6%. The available hydrocortisone ointments are in strengths of 2.5% and 10%.

_____

_____

17. A physician orders 1.5 L of a 12% Burrow's solution. The available Burrow's solutions are 5% and 25%.

_____

_____

18. Prepare 75 mL 9% solution of dextrose in water. The available medications are D-5-W and dextrose 25% solution.

_____

_____

19. A patient needs epinephrine for an acute asthma attack. The physician orders 100 mL of epinephrine 4%. The available epinephrine is 1:10 and 1:100.

_____

_____

20. [PA IN] A physician orders 8 oz of 3% lidocaine solution. The available lidocaine is 1% and 4%.

_____

_____

REVIEW

Stock supplies are often used to prepare compounds that are less concentrated in weight/ volume than the stock medications. Stock supplies are often found in commonly used strengths. To obtain the correct amount of medication for the physician's order or for administering a dose of medication more accurately, the stock medication may need dilution. The processes of dilution or alligation may be used for these purposes. Dilution is the adding of more solvent to the solute to prepare the weaker solution. This can be accomplished using ratio and proportion. If the medication is in two different concentrations, alligation is the method for preparing the medication. However, if the "weighted average" percentage strength is necessary for mixture of two or more substances with a known quantity and concentration, alligation medial may be used for the calculation. As the pharmacy technician, you must know how to calculate the strength and must also know the correct method for calculation on the basis of the information given.

Posttest

Before taking the Posttest, retake the Pretest to check your understanding of the materials presented in this chapter.

Calculate the following problems using the appropriate method for each. As previously, show all of your work. Round to tenths, unless otherwise indicated.

1. How many grams of dextrose must be dissolved in sterile water to prepare 100 mL of a 60% solution? _____

2. If 15 mg of amoxicillin is added to 100 mL of sterile water, what is the percentage strength of the total volume of prepared medication? (Round to thousandths.)

_____

Continued

Posttest, cont.

3. A physician orders 5 mL of epinephrine 1% added to 45 mL of sterile water to prepare 50 mL of solution.

   What is the weight in milligrams of the epinephrine that has been added?

   _____

4. A lotion of 5% methyl salicylate is to be prepared for a patient with allergic dermatitis.

   What amount of a 10% methyl salicylate lotion would be necessary to prepare 8 oz?

   _____

5. A lotion of 250 mL of 3% calamine lotion is to be prepared from a 7.5% calamine lotion.

   What amount of 7.5% calamine lotion would be necessary to prepare this lotion?

   _____

   How much solvent would be necessary for this prescription? _____

6. A stock pint of sodium bicarbonate contains 60% solution. The physician prescribes 1.5 L of 15% sodium bicarbonate solution.

   What volume of stock solution would be necessary to prepare the solution?

   _____

   What volume of solvent should be added to the stock supply to complete the order?

   _____

7. Prepare 250 mL of a 1:500 silver nitrate solution.

   What is the percentage strength of this solution? _____

   How many milligrams of silver nitrate are necessary to prepare this solution?

   _____

Posttest, cont.

8. A liquid stock is available in a 1:350 concentration. You are asked to prepare a pint of 1:500 solution.

How many milliliters of stock solution are necessary? _____

How many milliliters of solvent are necessary? _____

9. A boric acid solution of 1:5 is available as a stock solution. A physician asks that you prepare 10 oz of 15% solution.

How many milliliters of boric acid are necessary to prepare the 15% solution?

_____

How many milliliters of solvent are necessary? _____

If the physician had written for a 2% solution, how many milliliters of boric acid would be necessary? _____

How many milliliters of solvent would be necessary for the 2% solution?

_____

10. A physician orders 250 mL 0.05% epinephrine solution. The available epinephrine is 1:500 in 10 mL vials.

How many milliliters of 1:500 epinephrine would be necessary to prepare the solution? _____

How many milliliters of sterile water would be necessary as a solvent?

_____

How many vials of medication would be necessary to complete the order?

_____

11. Prepare 500 mL of creosol 1:150 from a stock solution of creosol solution 2.5%.

How many milliliters of 2.5% creosol are necessary to prepare this compound?

_____

How many milliliters of solvent are necessary? _____

Continued

Continued

Posttest, cont.

12. A physician orders 250 mL of 15% dextrose in water. The stock solution is 50% dextrose in 10-mL ampules.

How many milliliters of stock solution would be necessary for this order?

_____

How many milliliters of sterile water would be necessary to complete the order?

_____

How many ampules of dextrose would be necessary to complete the order?

_____

13. A physician orders 6 oz of glycerin solution 7.5% to be used as a retention enema. The available stock glycerin solution is 25%.

How many milliliters of 25% glycerin should be used to prepare the enema?

_____

How many milliliters of solvent would be necessary? _____

14. Prepare 250 mL of a 3% hydrogen peroxide solution from a 12% hydrogen peroxide solution.

How many milliliters of 12% hydrogen peroxide would be necessary?

_____

How many milliliters of solvent would be necessary? _____

15. Prepare a 2.5% solution from a 1-pt stock hydrogen peroxide 15% solution.

How many milliliters of 2.5% solution can be prepared from the entire stock bottle?

_____

Posttest, cont.

16. On hand is a 5% sodium hypochlorite solution and a 20% sodium hypochlorite solution. Prepare 1 L sodium hypochlorite 12% solution. Check your calculations by alligation medial.

   _____

   _____

17. Prepare 500 mL of a 12.5% dextrose solution. Available is D-5-W and dextrose 50%. Check your calculations by alligation medial.

   _____

   _____

18. Prepare 2.5 L of 6% Lysol solution using 5% Lysol and 8% Lysol. Check your calculations using alligation medial.

   _____

   _____

19. Prepare 750 mL of 0.75% sodium chloride solution from 0.9% NaCl and 0.45% NaCl solutions. Verify your calculations using alligation medial.

   _____

   _____

20. Prepare 2 L of 12.5% KCl solution using 20% KCl and 10% KCl. Verify the calculations using alligation medial.

   If this order is prepared in 1-L sterile solutions for IV infusion, how many milliliters of each percentage of KCl would be combined for each container of fluids?

   _____

   _____

REVIEW OF RULES

Interpreting Solution Labels

- A solute expressed as a percentage shows the number of grams of solute in 100 mL of solvent or the parts of the solute/100 parts of solvent.

Calculating the Amount of Solute and Solvent

- To calculate the amount of solute and solvent, use the following formula:

$$\frac{\textbf{Strength of solution available}}{\begin{array}{c}\text{Amount or volume of solute}\\\hline\text{Total volume of solution}\end{array}} = \frac{\textbf{Desired or new volume of solution}}{\begin{array}{c}\text{Amount of desired solute}\\\hline\text{Volume of desired solution}\end{array}}$$

The first step is to write the percentage strength as a ratio and then write the desired solution as a ratio. Finally, solve for x.

- To calculate volume of solvent in volume of solution, use the following equation:

Volume of solvent = Volume of finished solution − Volume of solute

- To calculate the ratio strengths in a solution or mixture, you may use the ratio and proportion method.

Calculating the Dilution of Stock Solutions

- Rule 1—When ratio strengths are given, convert these to percentage strengths using ratio and proportion.
- Rule 2—Reduce proportional parts to the lowest terms.

FORMULA 1

$$\begin{array}{c}\text{Amount of stock}\\\text{solution necessary}\end{array} = \frac{\text{Amount of solution prescribed} \times \text{Strength prescribed}}{\text{Strength of stock solution}}$$

FORMULA 2

SV (Stock volume) × S% (Stock percentage) = DV (Desired volume) × D% (Desired percentage)

- To complete the calculation using either of these formulas, you must take the amount of solute and subtract it from the final amount of the solution ordered.

Calculating Medication Dilutions Using Alligation

Step 1—Prepare the graph.

Step 2—Place the strength to be calculated in the center box.

Step 3—Place the highest percentage concentration in the upper left corner.

Step 4—Place the lowest percentage concentration in the lower left corner.

Step 5—Subtract the center square from the upper left square and place in the lower right square to reveal the parts of the lowest percentage concentration to be used in the new mixture. Notice that the answers are now in parts and not in unit values.

Step 6—Subtract the lower left square from the center box and place in the upper right corner to reveal the parts of the highest percentage concentration to be used in the new mixture.

Step 7—Add the calculated parts together to find the total parts of the two ingredients in the compound.

Step 8—When the total quantity of the mixture is included in the prescription, the parts of the mixture are placed into ratio and proportion to calculate the exact amount of each compound to use. The total number of parts is placed in ratio with the total amount of compound. The second ratio is the calculated number of parts to the unknown. This formula must be calculated for each part of the mixture.

- Alligation medial is another means of checking calculations for accuracy, using the following formula:

  Amount desired (milliliters, etc.) $\times$ Percent (in a decimal) = Grams

- Alligation medial may be used when two or more substances are to be mixed. The quantities to be mixed must be in a common denomination whether in weight or in volume.

Interpreting Physicians' Orders for Dosages

OBJECTIVES

- Calculate total dosage of medication when quantity is unknown
- Calculate number of doses of medication from total dosage presented on a prescription
- Calculate the number of doses in a prescription if medication is taken according to a physician's order, including duration in days
- Read and interpret prescriptions to calculate doses and dosages

Pretest

Using the information provided, calculate the doses or dosages for the prescriptions as appropriate. Note that all doses will be administered on the first day as ordered unless otherwise stated. Note that a month means 30 days unless otherwise stated. Round answers to measurable doses depending on the utensil to be used or the available form of medication. Show your work.

1. A physician prescribes amoxicillin suspension 250 mg/5 mL 150 mL to be taken 1 teaspoonful three times a day until the entire amount has been taken. A dosespoon is to be included with the prescription.

   How many days would the medication last? _____

   What total volume of amoxicillin would be administered daily? _____

   How many milligrams of antibiotic would the child receive daily? _____

   Indicate label directions using a dosespoon. _____

   What dose of medication would the person receive with each administration?

   _____

2. A physician prescribes furosemide 20 mg po daily × 1 mo c̄ refills × 2. The available medication is furosemide 40 mg/tablet.

   How many tablets would the patient take daily from the available stock medication?

   _____

   How many tablets would be provided for a month's supply to the patient from the stock bottle? _____

   Indicate prescription label directions. _____

Pretest, cont.

3. Using the provided prescription, how many tablets are necessary to fill the prescription? _____

Interpret the prescription. _____

Indicate prescription label directions. _____

Lawrence Merry, M.D.
4th Street and Jones Ave.
Holly, GA 00111
phone# - 001-555-2176

Patient Name_____ Date _____
Address_____ Age _____

℞ Topamax 25mg

4V tabs Bid x 1 month

_____ Refill _____

DEA#_____

What medication has been ordered? _____

4. A physician prescribes NPH insulin 80 units qam. The vial contains 10 ml of NPH insulin U-100. Indicate the amount of medication on the syringe so that you can supply patient instruction for self-administration.

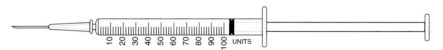

How many days would this vial of medication last? _____

If the patient needs the insulin for 1 month, how many vials of medication would be necessary? _____

Continued

Pretest, cont.

5. An order is written for the preparation of CEFTIZOXIME 500 mg in 50 mL of D-5-W to be infused at the rate of 50 mg/kg per day. CEFTIZOXIME is available for dilution at 1 g/10 mL of sterile water.

   How many milliliters of infusion would a patient weighing 88 lb receive per day?

   _____

   If this is to be administered in divided doses q6h, how many milliliters would the patient receive with each dose? _____

   How many milligrams would the patient receive per day? _____

   How many milligrams would the patient receive with each dose? _____

6. A physician prescribes Vibramycin 100 mg po tab ii stat and repeat in 12 hours. The prescription then reads to provide the patient with 100 mg/d for one week.

   How many Vibramycin 100 mg tabs would be supplied to fill the prescription?

   _____

   How many milligrams would the patient receive with the first dose? _____

   Indicate prescription label directions. _____

7. A physician orders AMPICILLIN 0.2 g/kg/d IV in divided doses q6h. The physician wants AMPICILLIN 500 mg to be added to each 100 mL of D-5-W. AMPICILLIN is available in 500 mg vials for reconstitution with 1.2 mL of diluent. The patient weighs 110 lb.

   How many milliliters of D-5-W would be necessary for the addition for each dose of the AMPICILLIN according to physician orders for dilution? _____

   How many milligrams would the patient receive with each dose? _____

   How many grams of AMPICILLIN would the patient receive daily? _____

   How many total milliliters of fluids would the patient receive daily? _____

Pretest, cont.

8. Use the prescription provided to make the necessary calculations. The tablet is available as Toprol-XL 25 mg.

How many tablets would be necessary to fill the prescription for a month's supply?
_____

What metric weight of drug would the patient receive with each dose? _____

Interpret the prescription as written. _____

Indicate prescription label directions. _____

Lawrence Merry, M.D.
4th Street and Jones Ave.
Holly, GA 00111
phone# - 001-555-2176

Patient Name_____ Date _____
Address_____ Age _____

℞   Toprol XL 25

½ P.O.   Q Day

_____ Refill _____
DEA#_____

9. A patient weighing 198 lb is to receive chloramphenicol 50 mg/kg/d in divided doses q4h to be administered in D-5-NS 500 mL for a *Salmonella typhi* infection. The available medication is in 1-g vials at 100 mg/mL.

Hint: Only full vials are available for use.

How many milliliters of chloramphenicol are in a full vial? _____

How many milliliters of chloramphenicol would be added to each container of fluids

for the ordered dose? _____

How many vials of chloramphenicol would be necessary to supply the daily

chloramphenicol for the physician's order? _____

Explain your answer. _____

Continued

Pretest, cont.

10. A child has a streptococcal infection of the throat. The child weighs 66 lb. The physician tells the pharmacist to supply the accurate amount of medication so that the child receives erythromycin 40 mg/kg/day in divided doses to be administered q6h for 10 days. The medication is available as erythromycin 200 mg chewable tablets.

What would the prescription label read for the prescription with the medication shown as available? _____

If the parent states that the child will not chew the tablet but will take oral liquids, after obtaining the physician's permission, what volume of medication would be supplied to the child with each dose if the erythromycin is available as 400 mg/5 mL? _____

How would the label read in household measurements? _____

How many tablets would be necessary to complete the order if chewable tablets are used? _____

How many milliliters of medication would be used to prepare the prescription?

_____

Using a choice of utensils for dispensing with the medication, what utensil should be chosen for more exact administration of the medication at home? _____

Hint: Go back to Chapter 7 to see available utensils.

11. The patient presents the provided prescription for preparation. The patient has no drug insurance coverage and wants 2 months' supply. The prescription has prn refills for one year. The medication is available in 40-mg capsules.

How many capsules would be prepared for the amount of medication requested?

_____

Interpret the prescription as written. _____

Indicate prescription label directions. _____

```
+-------------------------------------------------+
|              Lawrence Merry, M.D.               |
|             4th Street and Jones Ave.           |
|                  Holly, GA 00111                |
|              phone# - 001-555-2176              |
|                                                 |
|   Patient Name_____  Date _____   |
|   Address_____   Age _____   |
|        R    Strattera 40mg                      |
|             TT PO Quening                       |
|   _____  Refill prn x 1 yr        |
|   DEA#_____                           |
+-------------------------------------------------+
```

What is the medication ordered? _____

Pretest, cont.

 12. A physician prescribes amoxicillin 62.5 mg po tid for 10 days for a child weighing 44 lb. Available is amoxicillin 125 mg/5 mL in 100-mL and 150-mL containers.

Which container of amoxicillin would be provided for the prescription? _____

What quantity of the medication would the parents give to provide the correct dose?

_____

How much medication would be discarded if the orders are followed correctly?

_____

Indicate prescription label directions for the prescription using household measurements. _____

 13. A physician writes a prescription for Humulin N 65 units subcutaneously qam and qpm. The prescription also contains an order for Humulin R 25 units subcutaneously with the afternoon dose.

How many 10-mL vials of Humulin N (100 units/mL) are necessary for a month's supply? _____

How many 10-mL vials of Humulin R (100 units/mL) are necessary for a month's supply? _____

What size insulin syringes should be supplied to administer both injections?

_____

Indicate the volume of medication to be administered in AM and in PM on the appropriate syringe. Label the time for the appropriate syringe.

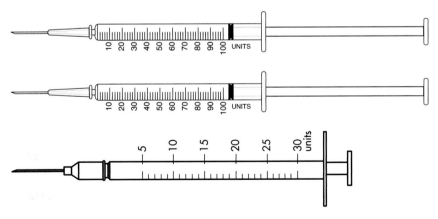

Continued

Pretest, cont.

14. A physician prescribes atenolol 75 mg po qam and 25 mg po at bedtime. The available stock medication is atenolol 50 mg.

How many tablets would be necessary for a 30-day supply? _____

Indicate prescription label directions. _____

15. A physician prescribes ibuprofen liquid 10 mg/kg to be administered po qid prn for pain for a child who weighs 66 lb. The available medication is 100 mg/5 mL. The volume of medication to be dispensed is 8 ounces.

How many milliliters of medication would be needed for one day? _____

How many milliliters of medication would be administered to the child with each dose? _____

How many doses of medication are available in this prescription? _____

Indicate the prescription label directions. _____

INTRODUCTION

This chapter's objective is to bring together mathematical skills learned in previous chapters so you, as the pharmacy technician, can accurately prepare a medication for dispensing given the information provided on a prescription. In some instances the medical professional accidentally omits the number of doses of medication necessary or omits the dose to be given from a total dosage. In many instances, because only one element is missing, pharmacy staff may be able to make the necessary calculation from the prescription without an inquiry to the physician. Therefore this chapter provides the knowledge base needed for making accurate decisions for doses and dosages to ensure patient safety.

PREPARING MEDICATIONS WHEN THE QUANTITY FOR DISPENSING IS UNKNOWN

In some cases physicians may accidentally write orders for the dispensing of medications and do not include the amount of medication that should be dispensed. In those cases the pharmacy staff is responsible for ensuring that the patient has sufficient medication to complete the desired medication cycle. The formula for calculating the total dose quantity required follows:

Total dosage required = Number of doses per day × Total number of days

EXAMPLE 14-1

A physician prescribes digoxin 0.125 mg tab ii stat then tab i daily. How many tablets would be necessary for a 30-day supply if the available medication is that seen on the following label?

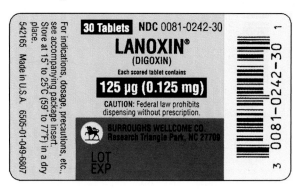

Total dosage necessary = 2 tablets now and 1 tablet daily for 29 days

Total dosage necessary = 2 tablets + 29 tablets

Total dosage necessary = 31 tablets

Prescription label directions: Take two tablets now then one tablet daily

Practice Problems A

Calculate the following problems, showing all calculations. Note that a month means 30 days unless otherwise stated.

1. A physician prescribes phenobarbital gr i$\overline{\text{ss}}$ po q6h for epilepsy. The order is to provide a month's supply with each prescription refill.

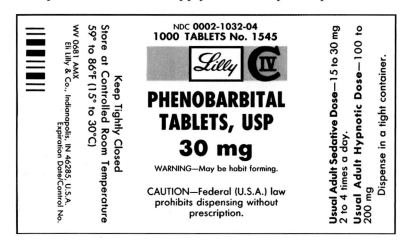

Using the provided label, how many tablets would be provided for the patient?

_____

What is the dose q6h in tablets? _____

What is the dose in milligrams? _____

Indicate prescription label directions. _____

2. A physician prescribes Voltaren 50 mg po tid with meals or snack. How many tablets are necessary to fill this prescription for a month? ___90___

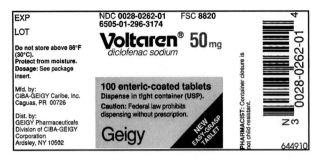

Indicate prescription label directions. _____

3. A physician prescribes cephalexin oral suspension 62.5 mg po q6h × 10 days. Indicate the dose on the available utensil below.

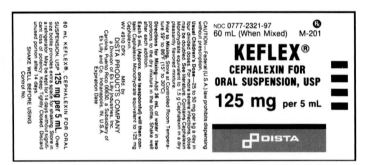

What volume of medication would be administered with each dose? _____

Would the label shown provide adequate medication to fulfill the prescription? ___yes___

If this is adequate, what volume of medication would be discarded? _____

If the amount is inadequate, how many more milliliters of medication would be necessary for the prescription? _____

What would be the dose in household measurements? _____

Indicate prescription label directions using an oral dose syringe. _____

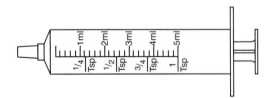

4.   A physician prescribes Macrodantin 0.1 g to be given po qid for a month for a severe urinary tract infection.

NDC 0149-0008-05
LIST 70805

50 mg

Macrodantin
(nitrofurantoin
macrocrystals)

Avoid excessive heat (over 104°F or 40°C).
THIS IS A BULK CONTAINER AND
NOT INTENDED FOR DISPENSING.
Dispense in a tight container.

**URINARY TRACT
ANTIBACTERIAL**

100 Capsules

CAUTION: Federal law
prohibits dispensing
without prescription.

DOSAGE: Adults: 50 to 100 mg
q.i.d. with food.
See package insert for indications,
precautions, and dosage.

Manufactured by Eaton Laboratories, Inc.
Manati, Puerto Rico 00701
Distributed by
Norwich Eaton Pharmaceuticals, Inc.
A Procter & Gamble Company   © 1984 NEPI
Norwich, New York 13815   00805-L5

Norwich Eaton

Using the provided label, how many capsules would be necessary to complete the order? _____

Indicate the prescription label directions. _____

5. Using the provided prescription, how many tablets would be necessary to fill the prescription? _____

Interpret the prescription. _____

Indicate prescription label directions. _____

Lawrence Merry, M.D.
4th Street and Jones Ave.
Holly, GA 00111
phone# - 001-555-2176

Patient Name_____ Date _____
Address_____ Age _____

℞   Trilephl (150 g/tab)
      ⁓ī⁓ī⁓ī po bid
      # 1 month supply

_____ Refill _____
DEA#_____

6. Using the provided prescription, what volume of medication must be supplied to fill the order? _____

Interpret the prescription. _____

The medication is available in 80 mL, 100 mL, and 150 mL containers. Which container should be chosen to prepare the medication? _____

What volume of medication should be discarded by the patient if the medication is taken correctly? _____

Indicate prescription label directions using household measurements. _____

```
                     Lawrence Merry, M.D.
                   4th Street and Jones Ave.
                        Holly, GA 00111
                   phone# - 001-555-2176

    Patient Name_____  Date _____
    Address_____  Age _____

        ℞   Keflex  250mg/5mL
                7 days
                5mL po qid

        _____  Refill _____
        DEA#_____
```

7. During a severe influenza epidemic, the physician writes the provided prescription as a prophylactic in an older adult with COPD. The only amoxicillin in stock is amoxicillin 250 mg/capsule.

How many capsules should be given to the patient to complete this order? _____

Interpret the prescription. _____

Indicate the prescription directions that would be on the label. _____

```
                     Lawrence Merry, M.D.
                   4th Street and Jones Ave.
                        Holly, GA 00111
                   phone# - 001-555-2176

    Patient Name_____  Date _____
    Address_____  Age _____

        ℞   Amoxicillin 500 mg bid
                  × 10 days.

        _____  Refill _____
        DEA#_____
```

8. Using the provided prescription, what volume of medication must be provided to fulfill this order? _____

Interpret the prescription. _____

Indicate the prescription label directions. _____

```
            Lawrence Merry, M.D.
          4th Street and Jones Ave.
               Holly, GA 00111
            phone# - 001-555-2176

  Patient Name_____    Date _____
  Address_____      Age _____

  Rx   Ceftin  125mg/tsp
          ½ tsp po Bid
                 x 7 days

  _____    Refill _____
  DEA#_____
```

9. A patient presents the provided prescription for preparation. _____

How many patches does the patient need for a month's supply? _____

Interpret the prescription. _____

Indicate the prescription label directions. _____

```
            Lawrence Merry, M.D.
          4th Street and Jones Ave.
               Holly, GA 00111
            phone# - 001-555-2176

  Patient Name_____    Date _____
  Address_____      Age _____

  Rx   Oxytrol 3.9mg/d
        Apply q3d @ 9A

  _____    Refill _____
  DEA#_____
```

10. On Friday a nurse orders medication to be sent to the floor for the weekend using the provided medication label. The patient is to receive cimetidine 300 mg IM q6h.

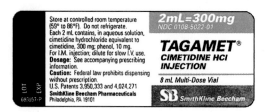

How many vials of medication would be sent to the floor for Friday noon through the weekend with sufficient amount to provide the medication on Monday 6 am?

_____

11. A physician orders Solu-Cortef 150 mg IM q8h for a patient with severe allergic dermatitis.

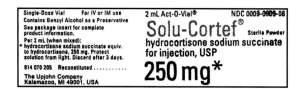

How many vials of medication would be sent to the floor for administration in 1 day using the provided label? _____

12. A physician prescribes cyanocobalamin 1.5 mg subcutaneously for administration twice a week for a month. Use 4 weeks for a month with this calculation.

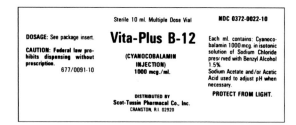

Using the provided label, how many vials of cyanocobalamin would be provided to the patient for this order? _____

What syringe should be provided with the prescription to meet this prescription?

_____

Indicate the amount of medication that should be shown as patient education on the appropriate syringe.

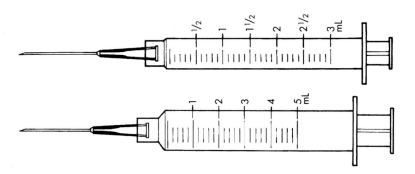

13. A physician prescribes Keflex 500 mg to be given po qid.

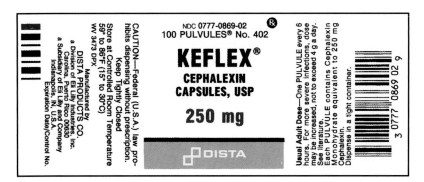

Using the provided label for available medication, how many capsules would be supplied for 2 weeks? _____

Interpret the prescription. _____

Indicate the prescription label directions. _____

14. How many tablets would be necessary to supply this medication for 2 weeks?
_____

Interpret the prescription. _____

Indicate the prescription label directions. _____

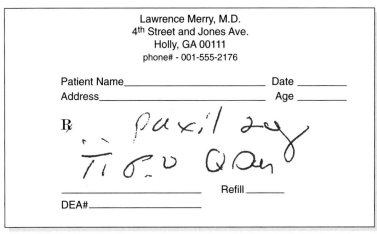

15. **EN DO** How many tablets are necessary for a month's supply of the provided prescription? _____

If each refill is for a month's supply, how many total tablets would the patient receive over the period of the prescription for 3 months? _____

Interpret the order. _____

Indicate the prescription label directions. _____

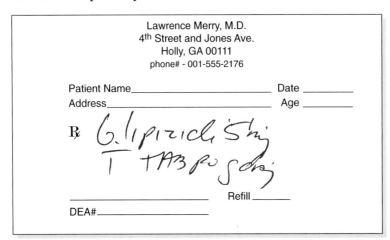

16. The physician orders phenobarbital gr 1/4 po q8h for seizures.

How many tablets would be provided for one week's supply? _____

Indicate prescription label directions. _____

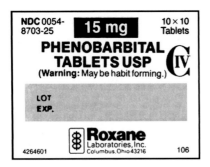

17. Four prescriptions are written as shown in the provided illustration. Determine how many tablets of each medication would be necessary for the prescription as written.

```
┌─────────────────────────────────────────────────────┐
│              Lawrence Merry, M.D.                      │
│              4th Street and Jones Ave.                 │
│                  Holly, GA 00111                       │
│               phone# - 001-555-2176                    │
│                                                        │
│    Patient Name_____  Date _____│
│    Address_____   Age _____ │
│                                                        │
│    R   Depakote ←(1 month)→ Xanax ½ mg                 │
│     x  Sig: 1000mg PO q HS *   Sig: 3½ mg PO q AM      │
│                                                        │
│        Desyrel ←(1 month)→ Zoloft                      │
│        Sig: 150mg PO q HS *   Sig: 250mg PO            │
│                                          q D           │
│    _____  Refill _____         │
│    DEA#_____                            │
└─────────────────────────────────────────────────────┘
```

Depakote 500-mg tablet is available.

Depakote to be supplied: _____

Interpret the order for this medication. _____

Indicate label directions. _____

Desyrel 50-mg tablet is available.

Desyrel to be supplied: _____

Interpret the order for this medication. _____

Indicate label directions. _____

Xanax 0.5-mg tablet is available.

Xanax to be supplied: _____

Interpret the order for this medication. _____

Indicate label directions. _____

Zoloft 100-mg tablet is available.

Zoloft to be supplied: _____

Interpret the order for this medication. _____

Indicate label directions. _____

*These abbreviations are found on the TJC Do Not Use List and ISMP's List of Error-Prone Abbreviations, Symbols, and Dose Designations due to medication safety issues. They should not be used. You are being tested on them here because these abbreviations may still appear in the pharmacy setting.

18. ♥ A physician prescribes Cardizem 120 mg qid.

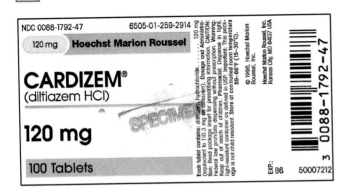

Using the provided label, how many tablets are necessary to fill the order for 5 days? _____

Indicate the prescription label directions. _____

19. 👤 A patient who has difficulty swallowing tablets is to receive Mellaril 45 mg bid.

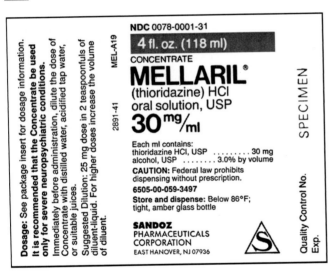

How many milliliters of medication are necessary for a month's supply using 30 days as a month? _____

How many milliliters are necessary for a week's supply? _____

What size medication bottle in ounces would be necessary to hold the month's supply? _____

What is the daily AM dose in household measurements using a medicine dropper calibrated in ¼ tsp increments? _____

20. 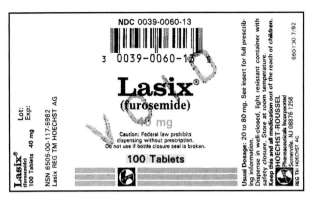 A physician prescribes Lasix 80 mg po stat, then Lasix 40 mg po daily thereafter.

How many tablets would be necessary for the first month's supply? _____

Indicate prescription label directions. _____

CALCULATING THE NUMBER OF MEDICATION DOSES IN A GIVEN CONTAINER

Some physicians write prescriptions to last a specified amount of time. If the size of the dose and the amount of medication in a container is known, the number of doses in the container can be calculated to ensure the patient has a sufficient amount of medication for the expected time for administration. To calculate this information, the following formula should be used:

$$\text{Number of doses in a container} = \frac{\text{Total amount of medication in container}}{\text{Dose size}}$$

TECH NOTE

Calculations of doses of medication must have the same measurement system in the numerator and denominator.

EXAMPLE 14-2

A physician orders a dose for 1 tsp of an antibiotic from a bottle containing 120 mL.

Notice that a teaspoon is in the household measurement system and milliliter is in the metric system, so a conversion to a common measurement system must be performed. The first step is to convert the 1 tsp to 5 mL. Now you can do the necessary calculation.

$$\text{The number of doses in the container} = \frac{120 \text{ mL (Total amount of medication)}}{5 \text{ mL (Amount of medication per dose)}}$$

$$\text{The number of doses in the container} = \frac{120 \text{ mL (Total amount of medication)}}{5 \text{ mL (Amount of medication per dose)}}$$

$$\text{The number of doses in the container} = 120 \div 5$$

$$\text{Number of doses} = 24$$

Does the container of medication contain adequate doses for 10 days if the medication is given tid?

The amount of medication per day is 15 mL or 3 doses. To last 10 days, there must be 30 doses, so the amount of medication provided is not adequate for the ordered amount because 24 doses are available and 30 doses are needed.

Practice Problems B

In the following problems, determine the number of doses in the container. Note that a month means 30 days unless otherwise stated. Show your work.

1. 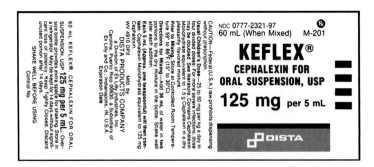 How many full doses are available with this prescription? _____

   Interpret the prescription. _____

   Indicate prescription label directions. _____

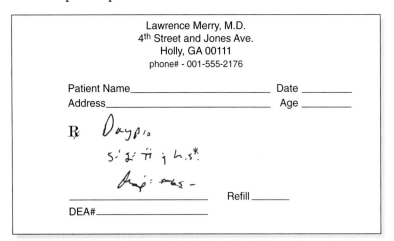

```
                    Lawrence Merry, M.D.
                   4th Street and Jones Ave.
                        Holly, GA 00111
                    phone# - 001-555-2176

   Patient Name_____  Date _____
   Address_____   Age _____

   R̶x    Daypro

         5' 2' Ti ᵢ h.s.*

         Amp̶: tabs -

   _____   Refill _____
   DEA#_____
```

2. A physician prescribes Keflex Suspension 125 mg q6h for 10 days.

```
NDC 0777-2321-97                          ℞
60 mL (When Mixed)      M-201

KEFLEX®
CEPHALEXIN FOR
ORAL SUSPENSION, USP

125 mg   per 5 mL

⊡ DISTA
```

   Using the label supplied, how many doses are in the container? _____

   Will one container be sufficient for the prescription? _____

*These abbreviations are found on the TJC Do Not Use List and ISMP's List of Error-Prone Abbreviations, Symbols, and Dose Designations due to medication safety issues. They should not be used. You are being tested on them here because these abbreviations may still appear in the pharmacy setting.

If not, how many containers would be needed if the medication provided on the label is the available medication? _____

Indicate the prescription label directions in household measurements. _____

_____

3. 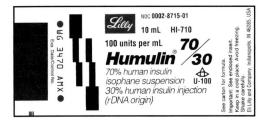 A patient is to take furosemide 80 mg po daily.

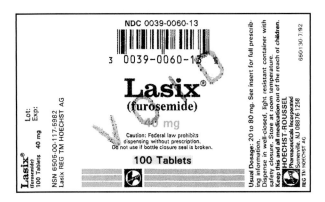

How many doses are in the provided container? _____

Indicate the prescription label directions. _____

4. **EN DO** A physician orders Humulin 70/30 63 units subcutaneously daily.

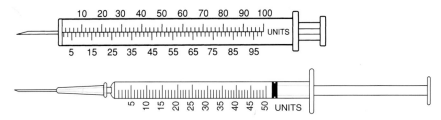

How many doses are in the provided vial? _____

How many vials would be necessary for a month's supply? _____

How many packages of insulin syringes would be necessary per month if each package contains 10 syringes? _____

Indicate the prescription label directions. _____

Indicate the volume of medication to be administered on the correct syringe.

5. 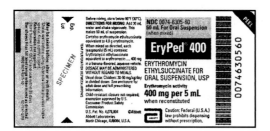 A physician orders EryPed 200 mg qid for a child with acute bronchitis.

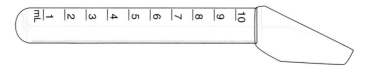

How many doses are in the provided container? _____

How many days would this container provide the necessary medication? _____

If this is the size of container of medication available, how many containers would be necessary for 2 weeks? _____

Indicate prescription label directions. _____

Indicate the approximate volume of medication to be administered on the dosespoon below.

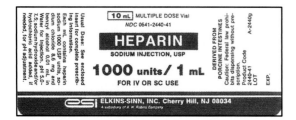

6. A physician desires that a patient receive heparin 2500 units IV q8h. The vial of medication available is shown as follows.

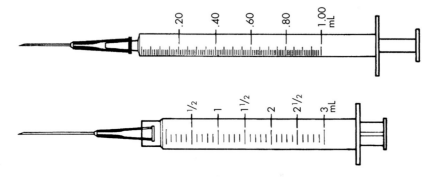

How many doses of heparin are in this vial? _____

How many vials would be necessary for a 3-day supply? _____

Indicate the prescribed amount on the correct syringe.

7. How many doses of medication are in this prescription? _____

What metric strength of Omnicef is the patient receiving with each dose? _____

Indicate the prescription label directions using an oral dose syringe. _____

_____

Lawrence Merry, M.D.
4th Street and Jones Ave.
Holly, GA 00111
phone# - 001-555-2176

Patient Name_____ Date _____
Address_____ Age _____

Rx   Omnicef 125mg/5cc   60cc*

4cc* PO BID

_____   Refill _____

DEA#_____

8. A physician prescribes Halcion 0.25 mg hs prn sleep.

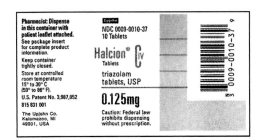

Pharmacist: Dispense in this container with patient leaflet attached.	Upjohn NDC 0009-0010-37 10 Tablets
See package insert for complete product information.	
Keep container tightly closed.	Halcion® C IV Tablets
Store at controlled room temperature 15° to 30° C (59° to 86° F).	triazolam tablets, USP
U.S. Patent No. 3,987,052 815 831 001	0.125mg
The Upjohn Co. Kalamazoo, MI 49001, USA	Caution: Federal law prohibits dispensing without prescription.

How many doses are in the container shown? _____

If the patient has taken Halcion 125 mcg for 3 doses, how many full doses are left in the prescription? _____

Indicate prescription label directions. _____

*Per ISMP's List of Error-Prone Abbreviations, Symbols, and Dose Designations, the abbreviation "cc" should not be used. It is included here because it may still be seen in a pharmacy setting.

9. A physician prescribes rifampin 600 mg daily 1 hr ac for tuberculosis.

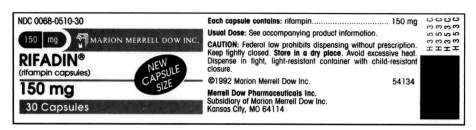

How many full doses of medication are found in the container with the provided label? _____

How many containers would be necessary for a month's supply? _____

Indicate the prescription label directions. _____

10. A physician orders digoxin 0.25 mg stat and in AM and then digoxin 125 mcg daily.

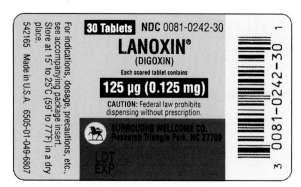

How many daily doses of 0.125 mg are in the provided container? _____

Indicate the prescription label directions. _____

11. A physician orders Procanbid 1 g stat and repeat in 30 min. Then give Procanbid 500 mg q12h as a maintenance dose to control atrial fibrillation.

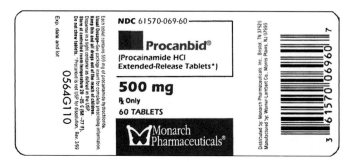

How many total doses are available of Procanbid in the container following the administration of the two initial doses? _____

The physician prescribes the stock bottle with the label shown for the patient to take with the orders for the daily dose as given previously. Ten days after starting the medication, the physician changes the dose to be Procanbid 1 g qam and 0.5 g qpm. How long in days would the prescription last until needing to be refilled?

_____

How many stock containers of medication would be needed to be sure the patient has sufficient medication for 90 days using the last order for the medication?

_____

12.   A physician orders Lopid 600 mg qam and 300 mg qpm.

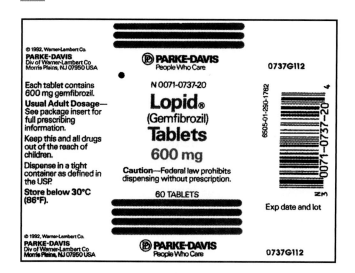

How many days can the patient expect the prescription to last using the provided label? _____

Indicate the prescription label directions. _____

13.   A vial of Compazine with the provided label has been provided to the medical floor for a patient with postoperative emesis.

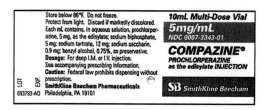

How many doses of Compazine 10 mg can be obtained from this vial? _____

14. Using the provided prescription, the pharmacist supplies 50 mL of the medication on the prescription. The dropper holds 1 mL. Round to whole doses.

> Lawrence Merry, M.D.
> 4th Street and Jones Ave.
> Holly, GA 00111
> phone# - 001-555-2176
>
> Patient Name_____   Date _____
> Address_____   Age _____
>
> R
>
> _____   Refill _____
> DEA#_____

How many doses of medication are in the 50-mL container? _____

Interpret the prescription. _____

Indicate the prescription label directions. _____

15. As the pharmacy technician, you are checking the floor narcotics for the amount of meperidine that has been administered. Meperidine 50 mg has been given to four patients over the past 24 hours. The floor stocks a box of 75 mg/mL ampules in a floor locked cabinet, as labeled below.

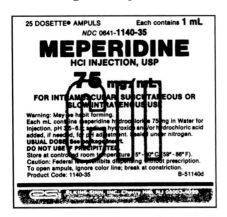

How many ampules should be left in the 75 mg/mL ampule box if the floor stock supply had not been used except for these injections? _____

Explain your answer. _____

16. Using the provided prescription, how many doses of Brovex would be supplied to the patient? _____

Interpret the prescription. _____

Indicate the prescription label directions. _____

Lawrence Merry, M.D.
4th Street and Jones Ave.
Holly, GA 00111
phone# - 001-555-2176

Patient Name_____ Date _____
Address_____ Age _____

R̶x   Brovex
Sig   1 tsp p bid p cm
802
_____ Refill _____
DEA#_____

17. How many doses of amoxicillin are found with this prescription? _____

How many milligrams of amoxicillin is the patient receiving with each dose?

_____

Interpret the prescription. _____

Indicate the prescription label directions using household utensils. _____

Lawrence Merry, M.D.
4th Street and Jones Ave.
Holly, GA 00111
phone# - 001-555-2176

Patient Name_____ Date _____
Address_____ Age _____

R̶x   Amoxicillin 20/5
Disp 150ml
Sig 7.5ml po BID
_____ Refill _____
DEA#_____

18. 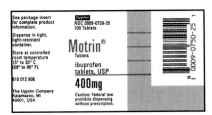 The physician prescribes ibuprofen 0.8 g tid pc for a patient with osteoarthritis.

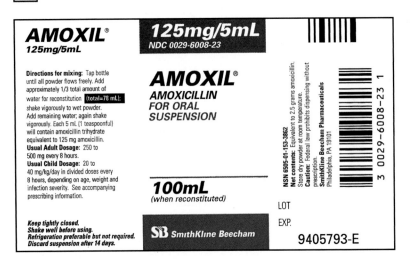

How many doses are in the bottle shown with the provided label? _____

Indicate the prescription label directions. _____

19. A physician prescribes amoxicillin 250 mg to be taken tid.

How many doses are available using the provided label? _____

If the medication is available as amoxicillin 250 mg/5 mL in a 150-mL bottle, how many doses would be available? _____

Indicate prescription label directions using a dose syringe. _____

20.   A physician orders Lincocin 0.6 g IM q12h.

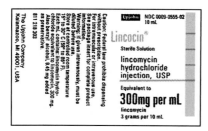

How many doses of medication are found in the vial with the provided label?

_____

DETERMINING THE LENGTH OF TIME A PRESCRIPTION WILL LAST

In some cases it is important to calculate how long the medication prescription will last if taken appropriately. In today's market, where insurance claims may be submitted only after a specified period of time following the last prescription dispensing, the pharmacist or pharmacy technician needs to know if the medication has been taken properly or if the medication should be refilled at the specific time.

 TECH ALERT

If the proper length of time between prescription refills is inappropriate, the pharmacist should be notified that the prescription cannot be refilled. The pharmacist then notifies the physician for further directions and so patient education can occur by both the pharmacist and physician to be sure medications are being administered as ordered.

The time that the prescription should last may be determined using the following equation:

$$\text{Total dose administration time} = \frac{\text{Total amount of medication}}{\text{Number of doses to be administered in a specific time}}$$

EXAMPLE 14-3

A physician orders 60 tablets of antibiotic to be administered qid. How many days will the prescription last if taken properly?

$$\text{Total dose administration time} = \frac{\text{Total amount of medication}}{\text{Number of doses to be administered in a specific time}}$$

$$\text{Total dose administration time} = \frac{60 \text{ tablets}}{4 \text{ tablets/day}}$$

$$\text{Total dose administration time} = \frac{60 \text{ tablets}}{4 \text{ tablets/day}}$$

$$\text{Total dose administration time} = 15 \text{ days}$$

TECH NOTE

Again, be sure the medication measurements in the numerator and denominator are the same. If not, make the needed conversion calculations.

Practice Problems C

Complete the following problems, showing all calculations. Note that a month means 30 days unless otherwise stated. Calculate as full days unless otherwise stated.

1. ♥ How long would the provided prescription last? _____

Interpret the prescription. _____

Indicate prescription label directions. _____

```
            Lawrence Merry, M.D.
          4th Street and Jones Ave.
               Holly, GA 00111
            phone# - 001-555-2176

   Patient Name_____      Date _____
   Address_____        Age _____

   R   ZAmorrs 2.5
        T po 賁 q3d

        R 30
   _____    Refill _____
   DEA#_____
```

2. 🫁 How long would the medication in the provided prescription last? _____

Interpret the prescription. _____

Indicate prescription label directions. _____

```
            Lawrence Merry, M.D.
          4th Street and Jones Ave.
               Holly, GA 00111
            phone# - 001-555-2176

   Patient Name_____      Date _____
   Address_____        Age _____

   R

   AllegraD ɿ bid # 30

   _____    Refill _____
   DEA#_____
```

3. 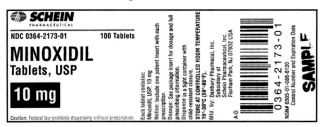 A physician writes a prescription for minoxidil 0.04 g to be administered po daily. The pharmacist fills the prescription with 40 tablets of the medication shown on the provided label.

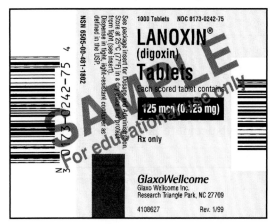

How many days would this prescription last? _____

How many tablets would be necessary for a month's supply? _____

Indicate prescription label directions. _____

4. 🤍 A physician writes a prescription for Lanoxin 0.125 mg tablets #40. The patient is to take Lanoxin 0. 5 mg stat and 0.375 mg in am and then to take tab i daily.

How long would this prescription last after the two initial doses? _____

Indicate prescription label directions. _____

5. 🦠 Using the provided prescription, how long would the medication last? _____

Interpret the prescription. _____

Indicate prescription label directions. _____

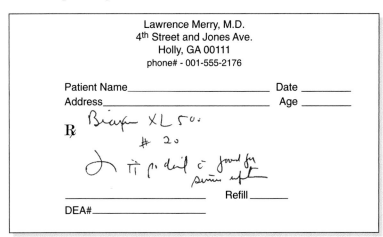

6. How long would the medication in the provided prescription last if taken appropriately? _____

Interpret the prescription. _____

Indicate prescription label directions. _____

Lawrence Merry, M.D.
4th Street and Jones Ave.
Holly, GA 00111
phone# - 001-555-2176

Patient Name_____ Date _____
Address_____ Age _____

R̸ _Altace 5ɣ_
H 62

ᴈ T b.d BP

_____ Refill _____
DEA#_____

7. A physician prescribes erythromycin ethylsuccinate 200 mg tid using the label provided.

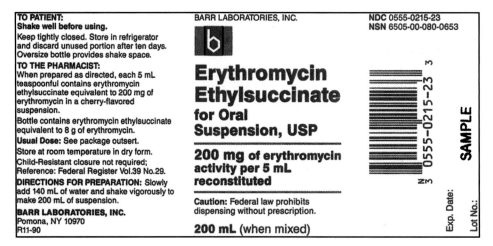

TO PATIENT:
Shake well before using.
Keep tightly closed. Store in refrigerator and discard unused portion after ten days. Oversize bottle provides shake space.
TO THE PHARMACIST:
When prepared as directed, each 5 mL teaspoonful contains erythromycin ethylsuccinate equivalent to 200 mg of erythromycin in a cherry-flavored suspension.
Bottle contains erythromycin ethylsuccinate equivalent to 8 g of erythromycin.
Usual Dose: See package outsert.
Store at room temperature in dry form.
Child-Resistant closure not required; Reference: Federal Register Vol.39 No.29.
DIRECTIONS FOR PREPARATION: Slowly add 140 mL of water and shake vigorously to make 200 mL of suspension.
BARR LABORATORIES, INC.
Pomona, NY 10970
R11-90

BARR LABORATORIES, INC.

Erythromycin Ethylsuccinate
for Oral Suspension, USP

200 mg of erythromycin activity per 5 mL reconstituted

Caution: Federal law prohibits dispensing without prescription.

200 mL (when mixed)

NDC 0555-0215-23
NSN 6505-00-080-0653

0555-0215-23   NM3   SAMPLE

Exp. Date:
Lot No.:

How many days would the medication last if taken as ordered? _____

How many doses of medication are available in the container? _____

Indicate prescription label directions using household utensils. _____

8. How long would the provided prescription last if taken appropriately?

_____

Interpret the prescription. _____

Indicate prescription label directions. _____

```
            Lawrence Merry, M.D.
           4th Street and Jones Ave.
              Holly, GA 00111
            phone# - 001-555-2176

    Patient Name_____  Date _____
    Address_____  Age _____

                      □250mg
    ℞ Levaquin® ☑500mg   begin day
       # 4                before BX
         SIG:  ī  PO  QD

    _____    Refill _____
    DEA#_____
```

9. How long would the provided prescription last if taken appropriately?

_____

Interpret the prescription. _____

Indicate prescription label directions. _____

```
            Lawrence Merry, M.D.
           4th Street and Jones Ave.
              Holly, GA 00111
            phone# - 001-555-2176

    Patient Name_____  Date _____
    Address_____  Age _____

    ℞      Pepcid 20mg
          Sig: ī po BID
          Disp! # 20

    _____    Refill _____
    DEA#_____
```

10. How long would this medication last if taken as specified on the provided prescription? _____

Interpret the prescription. _____

Should this prescription be refilled? _____ Explain your answer _____

Indicate the prescription label directions. _____

Lawrence Merry, M.D.
4th Street and Jones Ave.
Holly, GA 00111
phone# - 001-555-2176

Patient Name_____ Date _____
Address_____ Age _____

R Pen VK   500 mg
   Disp: 28
   Sig : c̄ tab qid until gone

_____ Refill _____

DEA#_____

11. How long would the provided prescription last if taken appropriately?
_____

Interpret the prescription. _____

Indicate the prescription label directions. _____

Lawrence Merry, M.D.
4th Street and Jones Ave.
Holly, GA 00111
phone# - 001-555-2176

Patient Name_____ Date _____
Address_____ Age _____

R Urocit. K   10 mEq
   #540   (1080 mg)
   Sig: ī po TID

_____ Refill _____

DEA#_____

12. 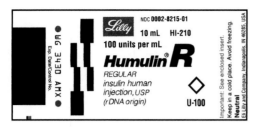 A physician prescribes Humulin R 50 units subcutaneously at breakfast and 40 units subcutaneously before the evening meal.

How long would the vial last? _____

How many vials of Humulin R would be necessary for a month's supply for this patient if injected according to physician's order? _____

Select the correct syringe for each dose and label AM and PM as appropriate. Show the amount on selected syringes.

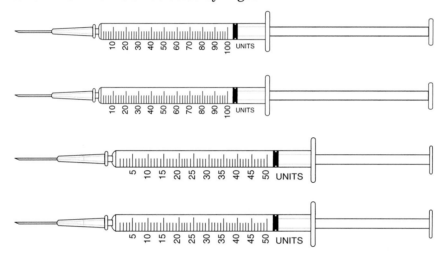

13. 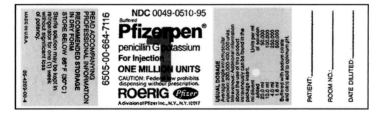 A physician prescribes penicillin G potassium 200,000 units bid. The medication has been diluted with 1.6 mL of diluent.

How many doses can be obtained from this vial of medication? _____

How many vials of medication would be provided for a 24-hour supply? _____

What is the powder volume of the container? _____

What volume of medication should be given for each dose? _____

14. A physician prescribes 200 mg of Lorabid po bid.

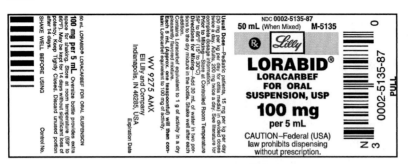

How many days would the container with the provided label last? _____

How many containers of Lorabid would be dispensed for a 10-day supply? _____

What is the powder volume of this container? _____

Indicate the prescription label directions in household measurements. _____

15. A physician prescribes Dilantin 0.3 g to be taken po each am and Dilantin 100 mg to be taken po at bedtime for epilepsy.

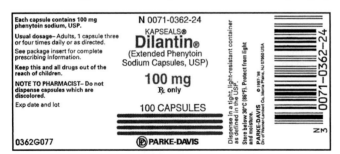

Using the provided label, how many days would that container of medication last? _____

How many extra capsules would be necessary for a month's supply if the medication is taken as ordered? _____

Indicate the prescription label directions. _____

16. A physician prescribes Prozac Liquid 40 mg po qam.

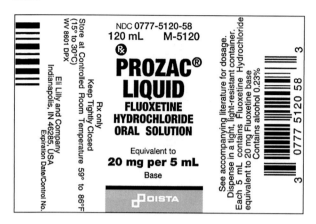

How many days would the medication shown on the provided label last if it is taken appropriately? _____

Indicate the prescription label directions using household utensils. _____

_____

17. A physician prescribes Benadryl elixir 18.75 mg po tid.

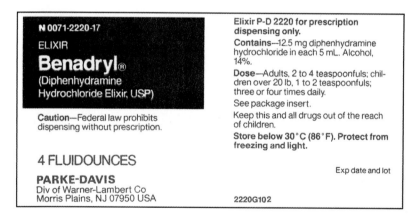

Using the label provided, how many doses of medication are available if the patient takes the medication as ordered? _____

Indicate the label directions using a dose syringe. _____

Indicate the prescription label directions using household utensils. _____

_____

18. A physician prescribes Biaxin 500 mg po bid. The available medication is shown on the provided label.

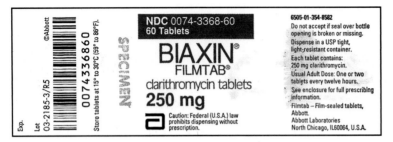

How long would the container of medication last if taken as ordered? _____

Indicate the prescription label directions. _____

19. The physician prescribes KCl 80 mEq po qam. The medication is supplied in the container with the provided label.

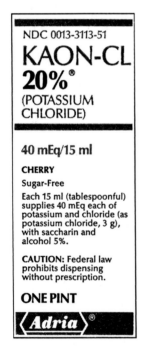

How many days would the medication last if the patient takes the medication as ordered? _____

How many containers of medication would be needed for a 90-day supply?

_____

Indicate the prescription label directions in household measurements. _____

20. **EN DO** A patient is to take Lantus insulin 35 units qam. Using the syringes below, show the amount of Lantus to be administered on the correct syringe for the order.

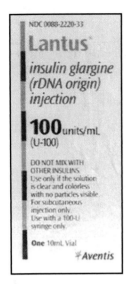

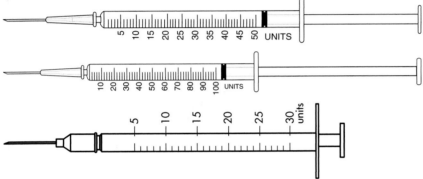

How long would the vial seen here last? _____

How many vials of Lantus would be necessary to provide a month's supply?

_____

Hint: Be sure that you calculate full doses for each day and 1 month is 30 days for this calculation.

How many vials of medication would be needed for a 90-day supply? _____

REVIEW

In some cases, pharmacists may be asked to calculate the amount of medication to be dispensed when the number of doses per day and the number of days for treatment is known. On other occasions, the calculation of the number of doses of medications in a container may be necessary to ensure the patient has adequate medication to complete the prescription or physician's order. Finally, for refills and occasionally when insurance companies have restrictions on the amount of medication that can be dispensed at a given time, you may be required to determine just how long the medication will last. All of these tasks may be necessary to accurately dispense medications and calculations of the time must be accomplished.

Posttest

Before taking the Posttest, retake the Pretest to check your understanding of the materials presented in this chapter.

Use the correct technique to complete the following calculations. A month is 30 days unless otherwise stated. As always, show your calculations. All calculations should be for full days.

1. Determine the number of tablets necessary to fill this prescription. _____

   Interpret the prescription. _____

   Lawrence Merry, M.D.
   4th Street and Jones Ave.
   Holly, GA 00111
   phone# - 001-555-2176

   Patient Name_____ Date _____
   Address_____ Age _____

   ℞   Trazodone 100mg
        1 no >gg'g
        1/2 tab po gam
        1/2 tab g pm
        1 1/2 po g hs*

   _____ Refill _____
   DEA#_____

   Indicate the prescription label directions. _____

2. Determine the number of tablets necessary to complete the provided prescription for 30 days. _____

   Interpret the prescription. _____

   Indicate prescription label directions. _____

   Lawrence Merry, M.D.
   4th Street and Jones Ave.
   Holly, GA 00111
   phone# - 001-555-2176

   Patient Name_____ Date _____
   Address_____ Age _____

   ℞   Nepranta · 300mg
        #
        gg 1 tab po daily
        X 3 days then
        1 tab bid X 3 day
        then 1 tab po tid
        thereafter

   _____ Refill _____
   DEA#_____

   ---

*These abbreviations are found on the TJC Do Not Use List and ISMP's List of Error-Prone Abbreviations, Symbols, and Dose Designations due to medication safety issues. They should not be used. You are being tested on them here because these abbreviations may still appear in the pharmacy setting.

Posttest, cont.

3. How many Alora patches are necessary for a 30-day supply? _____

Indicate the prescription label directions. _____

Lawrence Merry, M.D.
4ᵗʰ Street and Jones Ave.
Holly, GA 00111
phone# - 001-555-2176

Patient Name_____   Date _____
Address_____   Age _____

℞ *Alora Oil*

     #

     S. ÷ Twice weekly
       i

_____   Refill _____

DEA#_____

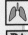

4. A physician writes a prescription for a 1:1:1 proportion of the following:

Benadryl

Lidocaine 1% viscous

Maalox

What is the amount of each component necessary to make 6 oz? _____

How many doses of medication are available if the patient swishes and spits 1 tsp q4h? _____

What percentage of the mouthwash is lidocaine? _____

Indicate the prescription label directions using household utensils. _____

Continued

Posttest, cont.

5. A physician writes a prescription for Decadron as shown on the provided label on a sliding scale of tabs 1 qid × 2 days, tid × 2 days, bid × 2 days, and daily × 4 days.

```
This Package Not For          NDC 0054-      100 Tablets    EXP. LOT
Household Use                 4179-25
See Package Insert for            0.5 mg
Complete Prescribing Information.
Store at Controlled          DEXAMETHASONE            S
Room Temperature                Tablets USP
15°-30°C (59°-86°F)
                                GLUTEN-FREE
PROTECT FROM MOISTURE          Each tablet contains
Dispense in a well-closed,    Dexamethasone 0.5 mg
light-resistant container     Caution: Federal law prohibits
as defined in the USP/NF.     dispensing without prescription.

                                                   4155001
TABLETS IDENTIFIED            Roxane                 034
   54 299                     Laboratories, Inc.   © RLI, 1994
                             Columbus, Ohio 43215
```

How many tablets are necessary to fill this prescription? _____

How many milligrams of dexamethasone would the patient receive on each day of the sliding scale? _____ Days 1 and 2: _____ Days 3 and 4: _____ Days 5 and 6: _____ Days 7 to 10: _____

Indicate the prescription label directions. _____

6. How many days would the provided prescription last if the medication is taken as written? _____

Interpret the prescription. _____

Indicate the prescription label directions. _____

```
                    Lawrence Merry, M.D.
                   4th Street and Jones Ave.
                       Holly, GA 00111
                    phone# - 001-555-2176

   Patient Name_____  Date _____
   Address_____  Age _____

   R     Atend-l  50mg

         1.5  MB  sd*

         H  60

   _____   Refill _____
   DEA#_____
```

*Per ISMP's List of Error-Prone Abbreviations, Symbols, and Dose Designations, "qd" should not be used. It is used here because it may still be seen in the pharmacy setting.

Posttest, cont.

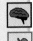

7. How long would the prescription for Gabitril last if taken appropriately? _____

How long would the prescription for Colace last if taken as a daily dose as prescribed prn? _____

Interpret both prescriptions. _____ _____

Indicate the prescription label directions for each medication. _____ _____

```
            Lawrence Merry, M.D.
           4th Street and Jones Ave.
               Holly, GA 00111
            phone# - 001-555-2176

   Patient Name_____  Date _____
   Address_____  Age _____
            Gabitril 4mg PO Q8°
   R̈           #90

            Colace 100mg PO Q12° PRN
                 #60
   _____  Refill _____
   DEA#_____
```

8. How long would the provided prescription last if taken as ordered? _____

Interpret the prescription. _____

Indicate the prescription label directions. _____

```
            Lawrence Merry, M.D.
           4th Street and Jones Ave.
               Holly, GA 00111
            phone# - 001-555-2176

   Patient Name_____  Date _____
   Address_____  Age _____
   R̈   Cipro    5w
              2u
            ⅰ BId
   _____  Refill _____
   DEA#_____
```

Continued

Posttest, cont.

9. A physician orders erythromycin ethylsuccinate 300 mg po tid for 10 days.

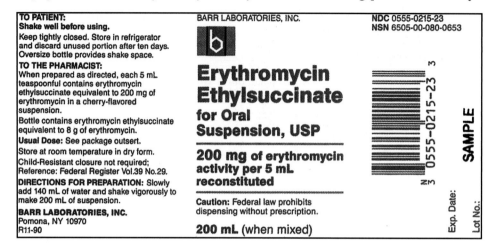

TO PATIENT:
Shake well before using.
Keep tightly closed. Store in refrigerator and discard unused portion after ten days. Oversize bottle provides shake space.
TO THE PHARMACIST:
When prepared as directed, each 5 mL teaspoonful contains erythromycin ethylsuccinate equivalent to 200 mg of erythromycin in a cherry-flavored suspension.
Bottle contains erythromycin ethylsuccinate equivalent to 8 g of erythromycin.
Usual Dose: See package outsert.
Store at room temperature in dry form.
Child-Resistant closure not required; Reference: Federal Register Vol.39 No.29.
DIRECTIONS FOR PREPARATION: Slowly add 140 mL of water and shake vigorously to make 200 mL of suspension.
BARR LABORATORIES, INC.
Pomona, NY 10970
R11-90

BARR LABORATORIES, INC.

Erythromycin Ethylsuccinate
for Oral Suspension, USP

200 mg of erythromycin activity per 5 mL reconstituted

Caution: Federal law prohibits dispensing without prescription.

200 mL (when mixed)

NDC 0555-0215-23
NSN 6505-00-080-0653

0555-0215-23   SAMPLE

Exp. Date: Lot No.:

How many milliliters of medication would be necessary for each dose? _____

What total metric strength of erythromycin would be given each day? _____

What total volume of medication would be necessary for the prescription as ordered? _____

Is there sufficient medication in the container as shown on the label given?

_____

How should the dose ordered be indicated on an oral dose syringe? _____

Indicate the prescription label directions using an oral dose syringe. _____

_____

Indicate the prescribed amount on the syringe below.

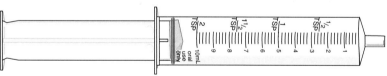

Posttest, cont.

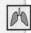

10. A physician writes an order for Voltaren 50 mg bid with food for 7 days and decrease to daily for a 30 day supply.

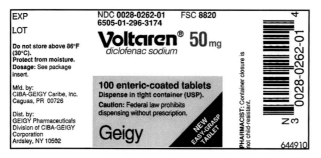

How many Voltaren tablets would be necessary for this prescription? _____

If the person takes the medication at home, what would the label directions be?

_____

11. If the patient uses the albuterol as ordered on a regular basis and does not skip a dose, how long would the provided medication last? _____

Indicate the prescription label directions. _____

Lawrence Merry, M.D.
4th Street and Jones Ave.
Holly, GA 00111
phone# - 001-555-2176

Patient Name_____ Date _____
Address_____ Age _____

℞ Albuterol Unit Dose 25/3ml

Disp 25

Sb Use in Jet Neb Q8°
in cap

_____ Refill _____

DEA#_____

Continued

Posttest, cont.

12. How many capsules would be necessary to provide a 3-month supply? _____

After the first month the physician increases the HCTZ to bid. How much longer will the original amount of medication last? _____

Interpret the order as written. _____

Indicate the prescription label directions. _____

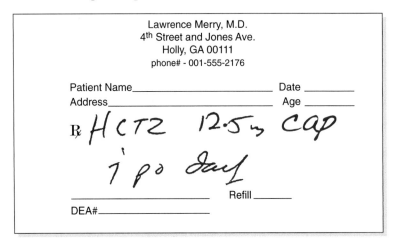

Lawrence Merry, M.D.
4th Street and Jones Ave.
Holly, GA 00111
phone# - 001-555-2176

Patient Name_____ Date _____
Address_____ Age _____

℞ HCTZ 12.5 ₃ Cap

i po day

_____ Refill _____
DEA#_____

13. A physician orders Coumadin 5 mg po on Sunday, Tuesday, Wednesday, Friday, and Saturday and Coumadin 7½ mg po on the other days of the week.

COUMADIN®   2½ mg
(Warfarin Sodium Tablets, USP)
Crystalline
DuPont Pharma
Wilmington, Delaware 19880
LOT JJ275A
EXP

COUMADIN®   5 mg
(Warfarin Sodium Tablets, USP)
Crystalline
DuPont Pharma
Wilmington, Delaware 19880
LOT KA009A
EXP

How many tablets would be necessary for a week's supply? _____

What amount of Coumadin in milligrams would be taken in a week? _____

How many tablets would be necessary for a month's supply? _____

Using the provided labels, which Coumadin provides the least number of tablets and still allows patient safety with administration? _____

Indicate prescription label directions. _____

Posttest, cont.

 14. If the patient takes the medication as ordered at one tablet q4h, as well as before an appointment, how many days would this medication last? _____

Interpret the prescription. _____

Indicate the prescription label directions. _____

Lawrence Merry, M.D.
4th Street and Jones Ave.
Holly, GA 00111
phone# - 001-555-2176

Patient Name_____ Date _____
Address_____ Age _____

℞ *[handwritten] Talwin 50mg*

_____ Refill _____

DEA#_____

---

15. How many days would the provided prescription last if taken as written? _____

Interpret the prescription. _____

Indicate the prescription label directions. _____

Lawrence Merry, M.D.
4th Street and Jones Ave.
Holly, GA 00111
phone# - 001-555-2176

Patient Name_____ Date _____
Address_____ Age _____

℞ *[handwritten] Amoxicillan 500mg #30 BID for infection*

_____ Refill _____

DEA#_____

Continued

Posttest, cont.

16. The medication as prescribed is available in a 5-mL container.

> Lawrence Merry, M.D.
> 4th Street and Jones Ave.
> Holly, GA 00111
> phone# - 001-555-2176
>
> Patient Name_____ Date _____
> Address_____ Age _____
>
> R͟ *Acular Ophthalmic, 0.5%*
>   *1 drop left eye tid*
>
> _____ Refill _____
> DEA#_____

If no medication were wasted, how many days would this medication last? _____

Interpret the prescription. _____

Indicate the prescription label directions. _____

17. How many doses of the medication are found in the provided prescription as ordered? _____

What weight of Motrin is the patient receiving with each dose? _____

Interpret the prescription. _____

Indicate the prescription label directions. _____

> Lawrence Merry, M.D.
> 4th Street and Jones Ave.
> Holly, GA 00111
> phone# - 001-555-2176
>
> Patient Name_____ Date _____
> Address_____ Age _____
>
> R͟ *Motrin 100m/5L   4oz*
>   *6 cc PO Q8° PRN*
>
> _____ Refill _____
> DEA#_____

Posttest, cont.

18. A physician prescribes Dilantin 200 mg po bid for 14 days.

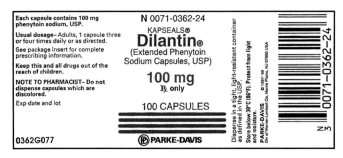

Using the provided label, how many tablets would be provided to fill the prescription? _____

Indicate the prescription label directions. _____

19. A physician writes for Thorazine 50 mg po qam and 75 mg po at bedtime.

How many tablets would be necessary for a 21-day supply? _____

What is the total dosage per day of the medication? _____

Indicate the prescription label directions. _____

Continued

Posttest, cont.

20. How long would the provided medication last if taken as ordered? _____

Interpret the prescription. _____

Interpret the prescription label directions. _____

> Lawrence Merry, M.D.
> 4th Street and Jones Ave.
> Holly, GA 00111
> phone# - 001-555-2176
>
> Patient Name_____ Date _____
> Address_____ Age _____
>
> ℞ Cuftin 250 tabs
>   #20
>   Tabobid
> _____ Refill _____
> DEA#_____

REVIEW OF RULES

Preparing Medications When the Quantity for Dispensing Is Unknown

Total dosage necessary = Number of doses per day × Total number of days

Calculating the Number of Medication Doses in a Given Container

$$\text{The number of doses in a container} = \frac{\text{Total amount of medication in container}}{\text{Dose size}}$$

Determining the Length of Time a Prescription Will Last

$$\text{Length of time for administration} = \frac{\text{Total amount of medication}}{\text{Number of doses to be administered in a specific time}}$$

Posttest, cont.

6. A medication has an AWP of $75.60 for 50 tablets. The contract with the third-party payer is AWP + 15% + $7.85 filling fee for the prescription for 50 tablets.

   What would the total be that should be billed to the insurance company?

   _____

   If the store bought 100 tablets of the medication for $152.50 with a 15% discount for payment made within 10 days, what would be the profit for the store for the above prescription? _____

   If the store had no discount on the medication, what would be basic cost per tablet if 50 tablets of the medication cost as shown above? _____

7. A pharmacy has a capitation contract with an insurance company to pay the pharmacy $250 a month for an elderly patient who takes multiple medications. The patient takes prescriptions costing the pharmacy $7.68, $15.98, $46.32, and $48.21.

   If these were the only prescriptions obtained in a month, what would be the profit from the prescriptions for this patient? _____

   If the patient adds prescriptions costing $24.89, $50.65, and $12.50 to be taken on a regular basis for the next 4 months, and the contract will not be recalculated during this time, what would be the profit or loss per month to the store during the next 4 months? _____

   What would be the total profit or loss during the 6 months? _____

8. The par level for reorder of Enablex is 500 tablets. The pharmacy technician takes an inventory on Monday for reorder on Tuesday. The count on the tablets is 150. The medication is available in containers of 250 tablets.

   How many containers of the tablets should be reordered for a week's supply?

   _____

   However, on Monday evening the technician assists in filling prescriptions for 90 tablets each for two patients prior to the reorder. Could the prescriptions for both patients be filled as ordered with the inventory available? _____
   Explain your answer. _____

   How many containers should be ordered with the filled prescriptions taken into account? _____

Continued

Posttest, cont.

9. Joseph is on an insurance plan that pays AWP plus 12.5% and a filling fee of $12.75. He brings prescriptions to the pharmacy for medications with an AWP of $34.50, $12.35, and $5.35.

What would be the amount that should be charged to the third-party payer for the prescription with AWP of $34.50? _____

What would the profit be on this prescription if the prescription costs the pharmacy $29.50? _____

What would be the amount to be charged for the prescription with an AWP of $12.35? _____

What would be the profit if this prescription costs the pharmacy $15.45?

_____

What would be the amount to be charged for the prescription with an AWP of $5.35? _____

What would be the profit on this prescription if the medication costs the pharmacy $5.69? _____

Which prescription would provide the highest gross profit? _____

10. A pharmacy has depreciation of $4325/month, inventory costs of $2678.36 an average week, utilities of $1025.25 per month, telephone of $568 per month, and salaries of $4500 a week for the pharmacist and $1500 a week for two pharmacy technicians. The income for the month is $65,342.

What would be the total overhead expense for the month? _____

What would be the net profit or loss for the month? _____

If the pharmacist gives a 5% discount on all merchandise for a week during the month, what would be the average total of the discount for a week based on the inventory costs? _____

If the pharmacy has a basic 20% markup on all inventory, what would be the discount based on average sales after markup for the week? _____

Using the figures given above, what would be the overhead spent in a day?

_____

What would be the daily gross profit, using the above figures to calculate a daily profit? _____

What would be the net profit for the day? _____

What would the 5% discount cost the pharmacy per day based on a 7-day week and the price after markup? _____

REVIEW OF RULES

Calculation of Annual Depreciation

- Annual depreciation is used to indicate the loss of asset value over a years time.

  Annual depreciation = Cost ÷ Estimated time of use

Overhead Expenses

- Overhead expenses are all of the expenses required to do business except the cost of merchanise.

  Overhead = Total of all business expenses

Markup of Prescriptions

- The markup amount is the difference in the purchase cost of the drug and the selling price of the same drug.

  Markup (or gross margin) = Selling price – purchase cost

Percentage of Markup

- Percentage of markup provides the calculation of which prescription medications have the greatest percentage of profit.

  Markup percentage = (Gross margin ÷ Cost) × 100

Profit or Loss

- The gross profit is the difference between the sales price and the cost of the inventory.

  Gross profit (or Loss) = Sales – Cost of inventory
- Net income is difference between selling price and costs related to the business.

  Net income = Sales – (Inventory + Overhead)
- Markup rate is the difference between selling price and purchase price.

  Markup rate = Selling price – Purchase price

  Markup Rate Percentage = (Gross profit ÷ Purchase price) × 100

Discounts

- Discounts are given for multiple reasons and reduce the selling price for the item. These include calculating the discount amount and then subtracting this amount from the selling price. Discounts may also be given when using manufacturers' coupons. The amount of the coupon should be subtracted from the selling price and the coupon placed in the cash drawer.

  Discount amount = Selling price × Discount percentage

  AND

  Discounted price = Selling price – Discount amount

Insurance Reimbursements

- The third-party price for a prescription may be computed using AWP or the average wholesale price nationally.

  Reimbursement of prescription = AWP ± Percentage of AWP allowed +
  Dispensing fee (if applicable)

- The pharmacy needs to know if the reimbursement provides a profit or loss using the reimbursement fee less the cost of preparing the prescription.

  Profit (or Loss) for prescription = Reimbursement fee – Cost

- Capitation fees are a set reimbursement fee usually paid to the pharmacy per month by the third-party insurance carrier.

  Profit (or Loss) of prescription = Capitation fee – Medication costs

- A minimal/reorder level is predetermined by sales history or human input and is used to maintain the drug flow and minimize the need for extra shelf space while replacing medications as needed to maintain business efficiency. This predetermined point is called the par level.

  Needed available inventory = Par or reorder level – Amount dispensed

- Inventory turnover rate is the frequency at which medications sell over a specified time. This calculation is used to control the amount of cash that is tied up in inventory.

  Inventory turnover rate = Total purchases for a given time ÷ Inventory value

Daily Cash Report

- The daily cash report checks payments received during a day to show the cash received balances with the amount of money in the cash drawer at the time of preparation of the report.

  Cash in drawer = Opening cash balance + Sales for day – Credit card
  payments – Checks – Miscellaneous disbursements

Chapter 1

Pretest

3. nothing by mouth
6. four times a day
9. bedtime
12. microgram
15. grain
18. do not repeat
21. every 2 hours
24. intravenous
27. three times a day
30. sufficient quantity
33. ointment
36. suppository
39. ounce
42. teaspoon
45. before
48. every 12 hours
51. telephone order
54. with

Basic Math Skills Proficiency Self-Test

3. 1.59
6. 13.11
9. 8 5/8
12. XXX
15. 2 2/9
18. 2/5
21. 5 1/12
24. 1/150
27. 3.5
30. 3 7/8
33. 10 mL
36. 60
39. 5500 mg
42. 24.2
45. 20
48. $26.10

Chapter 2

Pretest

3. 94
6. 3626
9. 816.789
12. 11/24
15. 2 1/2
18. 81
21. 11 19/24
24. 2/3
27. 16 1/8
30. 2
33. 75
36. 126.44
39. 1.75
42. 34 : 68 = 1 : 2

45. 1.5
48. 0.8
51. milliliter
54. gram
57. tablespoon
60. pint

Practice Problems A

3. 1599
6. 373 lb
9. 22
12. 75 mL
15. 35 mL
18. 251 kg

Practice Problems B

3. 8700
6. 24,150
9. 23,530
12. 21
15. 10
18. 23
21. 1100 mL
24. 12,000 kg
27. 1666.67 units
30. 2500 mg
33. three times

Practice Problems C

3. 7; 15

Practice Problems D

3. 8 3/4
6. 3
9. 1 1/2 L
12. 1 ¼ c
15. 23/8
18. 33/7
21. 9/2 tab
24. gr 11/8
27. 4 5/6
30. 3
33.

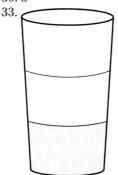

Practice Problems E

3. 2/3
6. ¼

9. 5/4; 1 1/4
12. 16/8; 2
15. 16/10; 1 3/5
18. 14/6 c; 2 1/3 c

Practice Problems F

3. 5/7
6. 4/8 = ½
9. 1/7
12. 5/8 c
15. ¾ oz
18. 3 9/16
21. 3 19/24
24. 2 ¾ qt
27. 8 5/8 c
30. 3 1/8
33. 2 1/16
36. 4 11/16 qt
39. 1 15/16 lb
42. ¼ gal
45. 1 9/16 oz

Practice Problems G

3. 3/8
6. 4/15
9. gr 1/8
12. 1 ¼ qt
15. 8 13/15
18. 10 61/72
21. 15 1/8 c
24. 7 3/16 oz
27. 2 ¼
30. 1/12
33. gr ½
36. 5 1/3
39. 48/61
42. gr 1/2
45. 9 c
48. three tablets; nine tablets; 270 tablets

Practice Problems H

3. six and seven hundred fifty thousandths
6. thirty-five ten thousandths
9. seven hundred and eighty thousandths

Practice Problems I

3. 33/100
6. 5/100
9. 1244/10,000

Practice Problems J

3. 36.45
6. 8.24
9. 3.5
12. 12.1

635

15. 1.5 mg
18. 10
21. 2 mg
24. 1 mg

Practice Problems K

3. 1363.08
6. 12.43
9. $153.59
12. 2.81
15. 13.44
18. $12.44
21. 49.5 mg
24. 212.75 mg; 287.25 mg

Practice Problems L

3. 42.5
6. 8.25
9. 2379.41
12. 75 mL
15. 277.5 mg
18. 25 mg

Practice Problems M

3. 5
6. 35.59
9. $61.70
12. 1.2 mg
15. 0.25 g
18. 3.56 L

Practice Problems N

3. 2.5
6. 556
9. 1040
12. 1300
15. 2150
18. 467

Practice Problems O

3. 0.78
6. 3.25
9. 0.32
12. 12.45
15. 0.146
18. 0.035

Practice Problems P

3. 0.0075
6. 0.0125
9. 0.0213
12. 0.0014
15. 0.0383
18. 0.0183

Practice Problems Q

3. 40
6. 22.73

9. 680
12. 37.5
15. 167
18. 612.5

Practice Problems R

3. 1/80
6. 33/100
9. 21/2000
12. 1/200
15. 33/5000
18. 1/3

Practice Problems S

3. 5 : 25 = 1 : 5
6. 19 : 20
9. 3 : 5
12. 2 : 25
15. 1 : 10
18. 0.75 lb : 2 lb or 3 oz : 8 oz
21. $0.10 : $1.10 or
     $0.01 : $0.11
24. 1 ml : 25 ml

Practice Problems T

3. yes
6. yes
9. no

Practice Problems U

3. 40
6. 25
9. 4.4
12. 3 g
15. 8 lb
18. 16 qt
21. 0.06 g
24. 25 mg
27. two tab/dose; six tab/day
30. 30 mL/day

Practice Problems V

3. 45
6. 2%
9. 11%
12. 5.12 oz
15. 0.12 mg
18. 12 oz
21. 25%
24. 7.2 oz

Posttest

3. 154.449; 154.45
6. 100.00; 100
9. 1 5/8
12. 5/6
15. 3 31/44
18. 1 2/5

21. 0.56
24. 5.93
27. 1 16/25
30. 10 4/5
33. 2 : 1
36. 375 tab
39. 240 tab
42. 42 tab
45. 9 tab
48. 6.25 mL

Chapter 3

Pretest

3. liv
6. xcv
9. 8
12. 97
15. 37 ½
18. 44 ½
21. 0730
24. 1159
27. 2042
30. 5:20 AM
33. 12:01 AM
36. 12:35 PM
39. 37° C
42. 85.3° F
45. 5.4° C
48. 50° F
51. 35.3° C
54. 100° C

Practice Problems A

3. xxi
6. ix
9. lxxv
12. xxxv
15. xxxiii ss
18. cxxvi

Practice Problems B

3. 19
6. 66
9. 95
12. 37 ½
15. 99
18. 20 ½

Practice Problems C

3. 0615
6. 0345
9. 0655
12. 2020
15. 2100
18. 1804
21. 11:30 AM
24. 12:30 AM

27. 8:30 AM
30. 9:45 PM
33. 10:20 AM
36. 10:44 PM
39. 2:02 AM

Practice Problems D

3. 1.7° C
6. 93.2° F
9. 37° C
12. 37.9° C
15. 118.8° F
18. yes; 37.9° C is the temperature in the conversion

Posttest

3. 93 1/2
6. xxxvi ss
9. lxxv
12. 125
15. clxv
18. 4:25 PM
21. 12:45 AM
24. 1210
27. 1526
30. 6:35 AM
33. 97.7° F
36. 37.6° C
39. 82.2° C
42. 212° F
45. 35.6° F
48. 101.5° F; yes
51. 90 tablets
54. 0600; 1200; 1800; 2400
57. 1630
60. –2.8° C or roughly –3° C

Chapter 4

Pretest

3. gram
6. inch
9. milliequivalent
12. teaspoon
15. ¼
18. 0.001
21. 32
24. 0.25
27. 5600
30. 5
33. 704
36. 0.0025
39. 48

Practice Problems A

3. ½
6. 40

9. 1 ½
12. 1 ¼
15. 56
18. 90
21. 180
24. 3

Practice Problems B

3. 2 teaspoons

Practice Problems C

3. 4000
6. 500
9. 0.05
12. 25
15. 0.025
18. 0.5
21. 300
24. 0.51
27. 0.25 gm
30. 175 mcg

Practice Problems D

3. 1/15
6. xl (40)
9. 3/4

Posttest

3. 180
6. 1 1/4
9. 0.01
12. ½
15. ½
18. 1,300,000
21. ii
24. 40,500
27. 0.25
30. 0.25
33. 4
36. 1200
39. 28
42. 0.01
45. x
48. 50
51. 125 mcg
54. 75 mg
57. 2 tbsp
60. 10 mg

Chapter 5

Pretest

3. 7 ½
6. 1
9. 6
12. ii
15. 15 (15 gtts/mL)

18. 900
21. 32
24. 4 1/5
27. 0.5 mg
30. 5
33. 20
36. 30
39. 12

Practice Problems A

3. 16 (1 gtt = ℳ i)
6. 24 (1 gtt = ℳ i)
9. 1 ½
12. 25 (1 gtt = ℳ i)
15. 3
18. 5
21. 6 (℥ i = ʒ viii)
24. 5
27. 3 tablespoons; every 3 to 4 hours as needed
30. approximately ½ teaspoon (60 gtts = 1 tsp)

Practice Problems B

3. 17.6
6. 12.7
9. 2
12. 10
15. 2.1/2
18. 3/4
21. 1/2
24. 3 1/4
27. 15.9 kg
30. 1 mL

Practice Problems C

3. 1
6. 1 ½
9. 80 (75)
12. 25
15. 30
18. 0.75 (30 mL = ℥ i)
21. 4 (4 mL = ʒ i)
24. 0.1
27. 30 (15 minims = 1 mL)
30. no, this prescription would be 15 mg

Posttest

3. 45
6. 1/100
9. 40 (16 gtts = 1 mL)
12. 5.05
15. 5
18. 40.64
21. 5.5
24. 9 (5 mL = 1 tsp)
27. 2.5

30. 127.56
33. 176 (16 minims = 1 mL)
36. 2.78
39. 3
42. 5.21
45. 1 ½ teaspoons
    (5 mL = 1 tsp)
48. 40.94 in

Chapter 6

Pretest

3. chlorothiazide 0.25 g one tablet by mouth every morning as needed for swelling; Take one tablet by mouth every morning as needed for swelling
6. Premarin 1.25 mg tablet by mouth daily for 21 days; Take one tablet by mouth daily for 21 days
9. Zithromax 250 mg two tablets by mouth now, then one tablet by mouth daily on days 2 through 5; Take two tablets by mouth now and then one tablet by mouth daily on days 2 through 5
12. Thorazine 100 mg, 100 tablets, one tablet by mouth three times a day; Take one tablet by mouth three times a day
15. lovastatin 10 mg, 30 tablets, one tablet by mouth daily with evening meal or bedtime with a snack for hyperlipidemia; Take one tablet by mouth daily with evening meal or at bedtime with a snack for hyperlipidemia
18. diazepam 10 mg, 30 tablets, one half to one tablet by mouth every 4 to 6 hours as needed for anxiety or muscle spasms; Take one half to one tablet by mouth every 4 to 6 hours as needed for anxiety or muscle spasms

Practice Problems A

3. Premarin 0.625 mg, 30 tablets, one tablet by mouth daily at

approximately the same hour every day; Take one tablet by mouth daily at approximately the same hour each day
6. Allegra 180 mg, 30 tablets, one tablet by mouth daily; Take one tablet by mouth every day
9. furosemide 40 mg, 30 tablets, one tablet by mouth daily at 10 AM; Take one tablet by mouth daily at 10 AM
12. Neurontin 600 mg, 50 tablets, one tablet by mouth daily for 5 days, one tablet by mouth twice a day for 5 days, then one tablet by mouth three times a day; Take one tablet by mouth daily for 5 days, then take one tablet by mouth twice a day for 5 days, then take one tablet by mouth three times a day
15. Prilosec 40 mg, 30 tablets, one capsule by mouth daily in the morning; Take one capsule by mouth daily in the morning

Practice Problems B

3. cephalexin 500 mg by mouth every 8 hours for 3 days
6. discontinue Septra; start Cipro 500 mg by mouth twice a day for 2 days
9. K-Dur 20 mg by mouth three times daily for 2 days, then twice daily
12. Elavil 25 mg by mouth at bedtime
15. Advair Diskus 250/50, inhale one puff twice daily
18. Flonase one spray in each nostril twice a day

Practice Problems C

3. 500 mg; 500; Bristol-Myers Squibb Co.; Glucophage; metformin hydrochloride; light-resistant container
6. chewable tablets; tight container, protect from moisture; Tegretol (carbamazepine) 100 mg;

100; Geigy; Tegretol; Carbamazepine; protect from moisture
9. Liquid; Adria; 1 tablespoonful; milliequivalent; yes/ medication is sugar free; 1 pt; potassium and chloride; registered trademark; 15 mL

Practice Problems D

3. Lilly; 100 units per mL; 10 mL; Regular
6. isophane insulin suspension; NPH Iletin I; 100 units; injection SC; Lilly; 10 mL
9. 10 mL; 3,000,000 units; 300,000 units; store below 46° F or 8° C; penicillin G procaine suspension, USP

Posttest

3. Mycostatin Oral Suspension, 60 mL, shake then swish and swallow with 5 mL every 4 to 6 hours; Shake medication and use one teaspoon to swish and swallow every 4 to 6 hours
6. amlodipine 5 mg, 30 tablets, one tablet by mouth daily at 10 AM; Take one tablet by mouth daily at 10 AM
9. Ocuflox ophthalmic solution, 5 mL, one drop in each eye four times a day for 5 days; Instill one drop in each eye four times a day for 5 days
12. Septra 2 teaspoons by mouth every 4 hours until all medication is taken
15. Tagamet 300 mg intramuscularly now
18. digoxin 250 mcg by mouth every morning with pulse over 60
21. furosemide; Hoechst-Roussel; 0039-0060-13; 100 tablets; 40 mg/tablet; 20 to 80 mg daily
24. 324 mg/tablet; 5 grains; iron deficiency in hypochromic anemias;

tablet; one or two tablets three times daily after meals; keep all medication out of reach of children; 100 tablets

27. 105 mL; 150 mL; 250 mg/5 mL; 20 mg/kg/day in divided doses every 8 hours; 250 mg every 8 hours; amoxicillin; 14 days; No store below 30° C

Chapter 7

Pretest

3. 1 tablet
6. 2 tablets
9. 2 capsules
12. 1 tablet
15. 1 tablet
18. 2 tablets

Practice Problems A

3. ciprofloxacin 1.5 gm by mouth once daily in the AM; two tablets; Take two tablets by mouth once daily in the morning
6. dilantin 0.5 g twice a day with breakfast and evening meal; five capsules; Take five capsules by mouth twice daily with breakfast and evening meal
9. pravastatin 20 mg by mouth daily at bedtime; two tablets; Take two tablets by mouth daily at bedtime
12. aspirin 10 grains by mouth every 4 to 6 hours as needed for aching—do not exceed 8 tablets every 24 hours; two tablets; Take two tablets by mouth every 4 to 6 hours as needed for aching. Do not take more than 8 tablets in any 24-hour period.
15. promethazine 0.0375 gm every 4 to 6 hours if needed for nausea and vomiting; 1 ½ tablets; Take 1 ½ tablets by mouth every 4 to 6 hours as needed for nausea and vomiting

18. Evista 0.12 gm by mouth daily; two tablets; Take two tablets by mouth daily

Practice Problems B

3. codeine sulfate 60 mg by mouth every 4 to 6 hours as needed for pain; four tablets; Take four tablets by mouth every 4 to 6 hours as needed for pain
6. ferrous sulfate 650 mg by mouth twice a day with breakfast and evening meal; two tablets; Take two tablets by mouth twice a day with breakfast and evening meal
9. Nitrostat 0.6 mg under tongue every 5 minutes × 3 doses as needed for angina—if no relief, call 9-1-1; one tablet; Place one tablet under tongue every 5 minutes for three doses as needed for angina; if no relief, call 9-1-1

Practice Problems C

3. Flagyl 250 mg by mouth twice daily for 7 days; 7 tablets; Take one-half tablet by mouth twice a day for 7 days
6. Valium 5 mg every morning for anxiety and 7 ½ mg at bedtime for sleep; 10 tablets; Take one tablet every morning for anxiety and 1 ½ tablets at bedtime for sleep
9. Septra DS twice daily for 7 days and then one tablet daily for 21 days; 35 tablets; Take one tablet twice daily for 7 days then one tablet daily for 21 days

Posttest

3. F; Tylenol 10 grains every 4 to 6 hours as needed for fever; two tablets; Take two tablets every 4 to 6 hours as needed for fever
6. D; diltiazem-SR 120 mg by mouth now then 60 mg by mouth daily; 31 capsules, two capsules; one capsule;

Take two capsules by mouth now then one capsule by mouth daily

9. tetracycline 500 mg four times daily for 5 days, then 500 mg twice daily for 5 days, then 500 mg daily for 5 days for acne; one capsule; 20 caps; 10 caps; 35 capsules; 2 g; 1 g; 500 mg; Take one capsule by mouth 4 times a day for 5 days, then one capsule by mouth twice a day for 5 days; then one capsule by mouth daily for 5 days
12. Urecholine 20 mg by mouth twice daily with meals for 10 days; A; two tablets twice daily; 40 tablets; Take two tablets by mouth twice daily with meals for 10 days
15. ampicillin 1 gm by mouth now, then 500 mg by mouth four times daily for 12 days; two capsules; one capsule; 50 capsules; Take two capsules by mouth now, then take one capsule by mouth four times a day for 12 days
18. Surfak one or two capsules by mouth at bedtime as needed; one or two capsules; 100 mg; Take one or two capsules by mouth at bedtime as needed

Chapter 8

Pretest

3. Tylenol 5 grains every 4 hours as needed for fever and aching; 10 mL
6. Zofran 2 mg intramuscularly 30 minutes before treatment; 1 mL
9. meperidine 75 mg intramuscularly at once; 1.5 mL
12. 1.9 mL; streptomycin 750 mg intramuscularly
15. 7.5 mL; erythromycin 0.3 g by mouth three times a day
18. 2 tsp; 10 mL; Benadryl 25 mg by mouth as needed

Practice Problems A

3. Diflucan suspension 35 mg by mouth daily; 3.5 mL

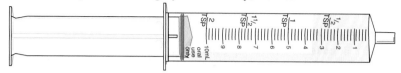

6. ranitidine syrup 150 mg twice a day every 12 hours; 10 mL

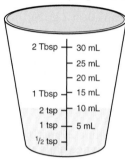

9. Lanoxin elixir 75 mcg twice daily if pulse is higher than 60; 1.5 mL; no
12. Vancocin HCl oral solution 250 mg twice a day for bacterial infection; 5 mL or 1 tsp
15. Duricef oral suspension 0.5 g every 6 hours with food; 10 mL
18. acetaminophen 60 mg every 4 hours as needed for fever and aching; 0.6 mL; two droppersful of 0.8 mL;

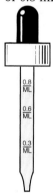

Practice Problems B

3. 1.8 mL
6.

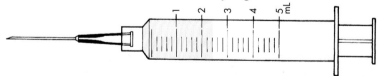

9. no; it is more accurate to use a 3-mL syringe marked in tenths of a milliliter;

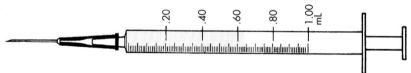

Practice Problems C

3. tobramycin 60 mg intramuscularly every 8 hours; 1.5 mL;

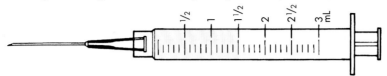

6. benztropine mesylate 1 mg intramuscularly daily; 1 mL

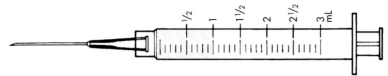

9. Amikin 250 mg intramuscularly every 8 hours; 1 mL;

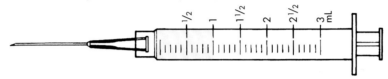

12. Cleocin phosphate 0.25 g intramuscularly at once and then every 8 hours; 1.7 mL;

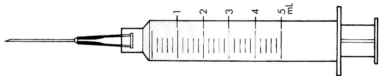

15. Depo-Provera 0.3 g intramuscularly every month; 0.75 mL
18. phenobarbital sodium 1 1/2 grains intramuscularly every 4 hours as needed for agitation; 0.75 mL; 90 mg;

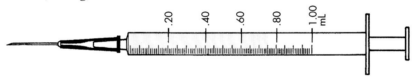

Posttest

3. penicillin V potassium oral solution 0.25 g by mouth four times daily; 10 mL; 2 tsp;

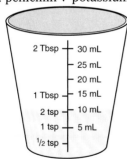

6. scopolamine 1/150 grain subcutaneously 30 minutes before surgery; 1 mL
9. diazepam 2 mg intramuscularly now and then every 6 hours as needed for anxiety; 0.4 mL
12. Cipro 0.4 g intravenously every 12 hours; 40 mL

15. Duricef 750 mg by mouth now, then 0.5 g every 12 hours; B; 7.5 mL; 1 1/2 tsp; 5 mL; 1 tsp;

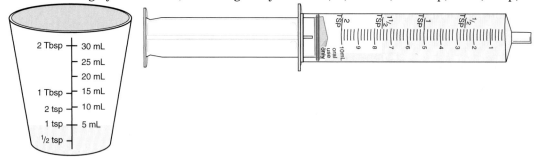

18. Garamycin 30 mg intramuscularly every 8 hours; 0.75 mL

Chapter 9

Pretest

3. 2 g; 4 mL; 3 mL; 1 mL; 0.5 mL

6. 61 mL; 39 mL; 125 mg/mL; 6 days and two doses into the seventh day

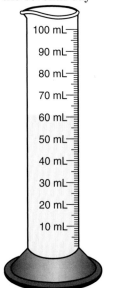

9. 1 g; sterile water for injection; 24 hours; 10 days; Ancef; cefazolin sodium; protect from light, store at controlled room temperature; 3 mL; 0.8 mL; 0.5 mL

Practice Problems A

3. 0.6 mL; 0.6 mL; 1.2 mL

Practice Problems B

3. 100 mL; water; 61 mL; add distilled water in two portions shake well after each addition; 125 mg/5 mL; 200,000 units/5 mL; 5 mL; 1/2 tsp; 5 days; 39 mL

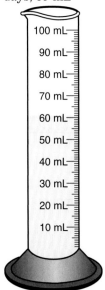

6. 3.5 mL; 1 gm; 375 mg; 1 hour; 1 hour; three vials; 1 mL; six vials; no only stable for 1 hour; 0.5 mL

9. 200 mg; sterile water for injection or bacteriostatic sterile water for injection; 10 mL; one dose

Posttest

3. 500 mg; 166.7 mg/mL; 2.7 mL; 250 mg; five vials; yes; yes if refrigerated for safety; 1.8 mL

6. 5 g; IM only; 9 mL; 1.3 mL (because 1.25 mL cannot be measured in a 3 mL syringe, the answer is rounded to 1.3 mL); one vial will last 10 days; 28 days at room temperature; 3.5 mL

9. 1.2 g; 1 mL; IM and IV; aqueous solution that contains some phenol; store between 15° and 30° C (59° and 86° F), do not refrigerate

Chapter 10

Pretest

 3. 24.6 mg tid
 6. 2.55 mL; 127.3 mcg; 2.6 mL
 9. 12.4 mL; 30.9 mg; 2 ½ tsp
12. 20 mg; 20 mL

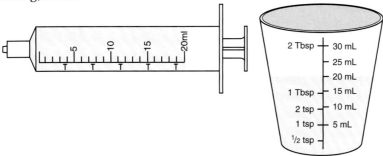

15. 6 mg; 0.24 mL; 0.24 mL

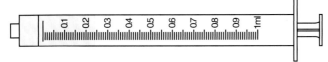

18. 153.4 mg; 3.8 mL; 306.8 mg/day

Practice Problems A

 3. 34.09 kg
 6. 15 kg
 9. 25.45 kg

Practice Problems B

 3. 2.5 mg; 2.5 mL; 1/2 tsp

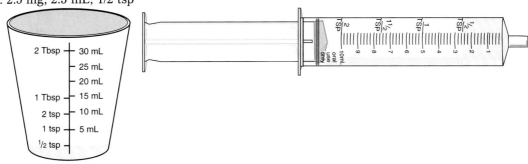

 6. 272.7 mg trimethoprim; 136.4 mg trimethoprim; 17.1 mL/dose; 3½ tsp
 9. 40 mg; 4 mL

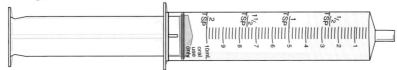

12. 400 mg; 5 mL; two tablets
15. 136.4 mg; 5.5 mL; 1 tsp; 1/2 tsp
18. 22.7 mg; 2.3 mL; 3-mL syringe

Practice Problems C

 3. 0.29 m²

Practice Problems D

3. 0.88 m²; 103.53 mg; 5.2 mL
6. 1.34 m²; 3.94 mg; 4 mL
9. 1.1 m²; 97.06 mg; 6.6 mL; 13.2 mL
12. 0.82 m²; 0.12 mg; 2.4 mL
15. 1.77 m²; 2.48 mg; 2.5 mL
18. 68.18 mg; 17.05 mg;
    6.8 mL

Practice Problems E

3. 7.5 mg; 1.88 mL; 1.9 mL
6. 26.67 mg; 1.07 mL; 1.1 mL; oral dose syringe

Posttest

3. 0.95 m²; 279.41 mg; 250 mg/5 mL; 5.6 mL
6. 136.35 mg; 6.5 mL
9. 13 mg; 0.4 mL

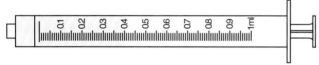

12. 1.75 mg; 17.5 mL; 0.44 mL

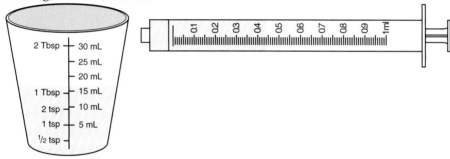

15. 1.75 m²; 113.75 mg; 5.7 mL; 150-mg vial

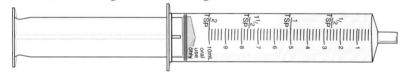

18. 409.09 mg; 136.36 mg; 3.6 mL

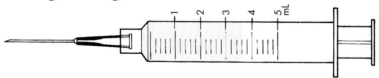

Chapter 11

Pretest

3. 1.5 mL; IM; 1.6 mL; 7 days

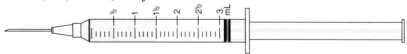

6. penicillin 500,000 units intramuscularly now and then every 6 hours; 2 mL; 2,500,000 U; five doses

9. 0.35 mL; 50-unit syringe

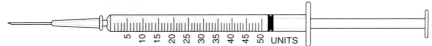

12. B; 0.85 mL; tuberculin (1 mL) syringe

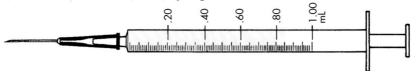

15. 1,000,000 units/mL; 7 days under refrigeration; 10 mL; Reconstituted to 1,000,000 units/mL @ Date/time and initials

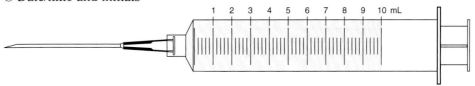

18. 15 mL; A; 3 tsp or 1 tbsp

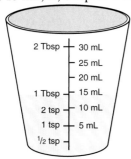

Practice Problems A

3. 3.13 mL; D; 3.2 mL; using a teaspoon, give 3/4 tsp for the closest dose

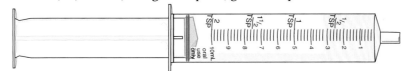

6. penicillin G 750,000 units intramuscularly every 12 hours; 2.5 mL

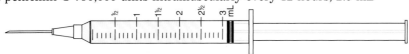

9. penicillin V oral suspension 200,000 units orally four times daily; 2.5 mL; 1/2 tsp

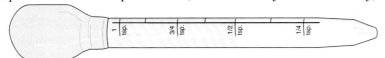

12. 500,000 units/mL; 1.8 mL; 0.9 mL; Refrigerate; Reconstituted to 500,000 units/mL @ Date/time and initials; 3-mL syringe should be used for doses of IM medications at or less than 3 mL

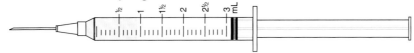

15. 5,000,000 units/day; 1.3 mL; 1.25 mL
18. two suppositories

Practice Problems B

3. D; A

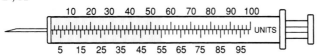

6. B; C

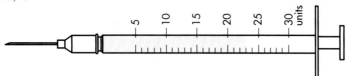

9. F; A

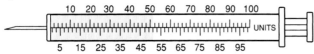

12. D and A; B

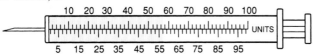

15. D and A; A

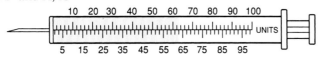

18. C; B

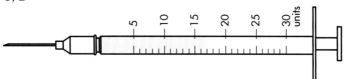

Practice Problems C

3. 0.4 mL

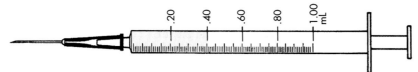

6. 0.75 mL

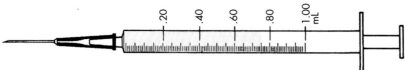

9. A; 0.75 mL

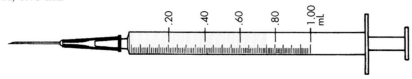

12. 0.6 mL; 9 minims

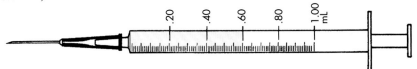

15. 0.12 mL; 9.5 mL

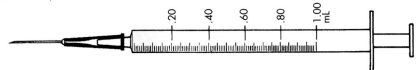

18. 0.8 mL; 1-mL tuberculin syringe

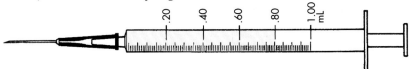

Practice Problems D

3. 7.5 mL

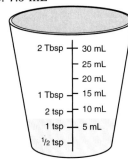

6. 18 mL

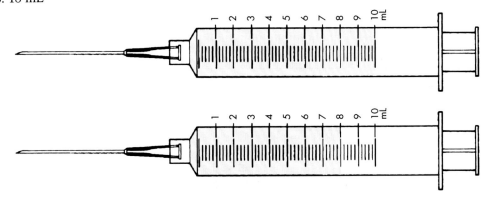

9. 15 mL

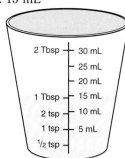

12. 7.46 mL; 7.5 mL

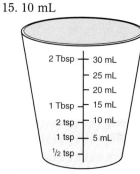

15. 10 mL

18. 5 mL

Practice Problems E

3. 5 g of sodium chloride in 100 mL of solution; 5 g/100 mL

6. 5 g formaldehyde in 100 mL of solution; 5 g/100 mL

9. 1 g of Zephiran chloride in 1000 mL of solution; 0.1 g/100 mL

12. 10 g povidone in 100 mL of solution; 378 g/3780 mL of solution

15. 500 mg magnesium sulfate in 1 mL of solution; 25 g/50 mL vial; 200 mEq/50 mL vial

Posttest

3. 0.38 mL

6. 0.5 mL

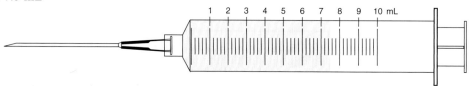

9. 7.5 mL

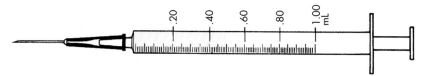

12. B and A; regular 22 units; NPH 18 units

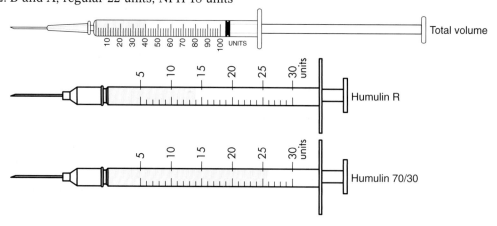

15. 0.25 mL

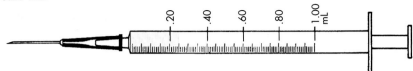

18. 1.7 mL

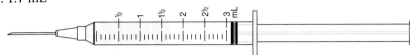

Chapter 12

Pretest

3. 125 mL; 2 mL/min; 42 gtts/min
6. 37 min; 30 gtts/min
9. 2.88 L; 2880 mL; three containers
12. 25 g; 25 min; 300 gtts/min
15. 92 gtts/min; 55 mL; 250 mg
18. 2 mL; 3.4 mL/min; 68 gtts/min

Practice Problems A

3. 1,050,000 units
6. 2.4 mL; 1,795,690 units
9. 5 mL; 19.8 g; 0.04 mg
12. 150 mg; 3 mL; 112.5 mg
15. 350 mg; 175 mg; 262.5 mg
18. 10 g/hr; 0.45 g

Practice Problems B

3. 16 gtts/min; 12.5 g; 2.3 g; 15.6 mL/hr
6. 63 gtts/min; 187.5 mg
9. 25 gtts/min; 1.4 g; 0.9 g; 313 mg
12. 80.9 mg; 10 gtts/min; 72.8 mg
15. 104 gtts/min; 9 g
18. four vials; no; 50 gtts/min; 20 mL; 600 mg

Practice Problems C

3. 240 min; 4 hr; yes; 41.7 mg
6. 13.3 hr
9. 13 hr and 54 min; 25 g; 2.25 g
12. 75 g; 6750 mg; 150 min; 2 hr and 30 min
15. 2.5 mL; 379 min; 6 hr and 19 min
18. 80 min; 30 gtts/min; two vials; 1 hr 20 min, 120 mL

Posttest

3. 4.2 mL/hr; 450 mg; 2500 mg; 24 hours; 0.6 mL
6. 1000 mL/8 hrs; three containers; 125 mL/hr; 2.1 mL/min; 630 mL; 31.3 g
9. 0.7 mL/min; 41.7 mL; 42 gtts/min
12. 15 mL; 1.1 mL/min; 66 mL/hr; 7.5 g; 22 gtts/min
15. 4.8 mL; 0.5 mL; four vials; 3.7 mL/min; stable for only 1 hour; 73 gtts/min
18. 10 mL; 4.3 mL/min; 172 gtts/min; 1.7 mg/min; 108 mL

Chapter 13

Pretest

3. sodium hypochlorite 10 g : 100 mL of solvent
6. 1 g of NaCl
9. 4.3 mL; 60.7 mL; 8.6 mL; 121.4 mL
12. five tablets; 325 mL
15. 450 g; 300 tablets
18. 100 mL; 150 mL

Practice Problems A

3. 576 mL
6. 1 g (1000 mg); 5%
9. 240 mL; 1760 mL
12. 0.3 mL; 0.6 mL; 0.75 mg
15. 0.4%; 25%; 120 mL
18. 150 g

Practice Problems B

3. 0.3 mg
6. 0.07 ounces; 2 mL
9. 750 mL; 750 mL
12. 1 : 4 (25 : 100 should be reduced)
15. 4.5 g
18. 285.7 mL; 214.3 mL

Practice Problems C

3. 103 mL; 137 mL
6. 150 mL; 100 mL
9. 1125 mL; 375 mL
12. 1500 mL; 1500 mL
15. 0.05 mL; 9.95 mL
18. 2.5 mL; 247.5 mL

Practice Problems D

3. 4.6 g of 25%; 15.4 g of 12%
6. 107.1 mL of 15%; 642.9 mL of 1%
9. 20 g of 15%; 30 g of 2.5%
12. 150 mL of D-10-W; 100 mL of D-5-W
15. 10.98 mL of 5% sodium chloride; 39.02 mL of 0.9% sodium chloride
18. 15 mL of dextrose 25%; 60 mL of D-5-W

Posttest

3. 50 mg
6. 375 mL; 1125 mL
9. 225 mL; 75 mL; 30 mL; 270 mL
12. 75 mL; 175 mL; eight ampules
15. 2880 mL
18. 833.3 mL of 8%; 1666.7 mL of 5%

Chapter 14

Pretest

3. 240 tablets; Topamax 25 mg 4 tablets twice daily for 1 month; Take four tablets twice a day for a month; Topamax 25 mg
6. 11 tablets; 200 mg; Take two tablets by mouth at once and repeat in 12 hours, then take one tablet daily for a week

9. 10 mL; 7.5 mL; five vials; 5 vials are necessary to obtain 5000 mg (5 gm) as each vial contains 1 g

12. 100-mL container; 2.5 mL; 25 mL; Take ½ tsp by mouth three times a day for 10 days

15. 60 mL/day; 15 mL; 16 doses; Take 3 teaspoons (or 1 tablespoon) by mouth four times a day as needed for pain.

Practice Problems A

3. 2.5 mL; no; N/A; 40 mL; ½ tsp; Take 2.5 mL by mouth every six hours for 10 days

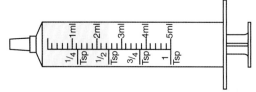

6. 140 mL; Keflex 250 mg/5 mL, 5 mL by mouth four times a day for 7 days; 150 mL; 10 mL; Take 1 teaspoonful by mouth four times a day for 7 days

9. 10 patches; Oxytrol 3.9 mg/dose, apply one patch every 3 days at 9 AM; Apply one patch every 3 days at 9 AM

12. two vials; 3 mL syringe for injection

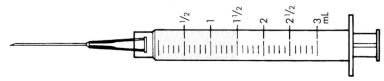

15. 30 tablets; 90 tablets; Glipizide 5 mg, one tablet by mouth every day; Take one tablet by mouth every day

18. 20 tablets; Take one tablet four times daily

Practice Problems B

3. 50 doses; Take two tablets by mouth daily

6. four doses; three vials

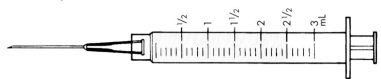

9. seven doses; four containers; Take four capsules each day 1 hour before a meal for tuberculosis

12. 40 days; Take one tablet each morning and ½ tablet each evening

15. 21 ampules; The medication is in ampules so each ampule can only be used once and the remainder must be properly discarded

18. 50 doses; Take two tablets three times a day after meals

Practice Problems C

3. 10 days; 120 tablets; Take four tablets by mouth daily

6. 31 days; Altace 5 mg # 62, one tablet twice a day for blood pressure; Take one tablet twice a day for blood pressure

9. 10 days; Pepcid 20 mg #20, one tablet by mouth twice daily; Take one tablet by mouth twice a day

12. 11 days; three vials

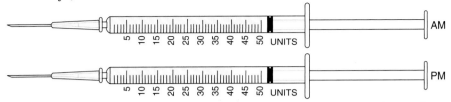

15. 25 days; 20 capsules; Take three capsules by mouth each morning and one capsule by mouth at bedtime for epilepsy
18. 15 days; Take two tablets by mouth twice a day

Posttest

3. nine patches; Apply a patch twice a week
6. 40 days; atenolol 50 mg # 60 tablets, 1 1/2 tablets daily; Take 1 ½ tablets every day
9. 7.5 mL; 900 mg; 225 mL; no; 1 ½ tsp; Take 1 ½ tsp by mouth three times a day

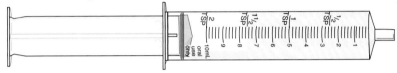

12. 90 capsules; 30 days; hydrochlorothiazide 12.5 mg, one capsule by mouth daily; Take one capsule by mouth every day
15. 15 days; amoxicillin 500 mg # 30, one capsule twice daily for infection; Take one capsule twice a day for infection
18. 56 capsules; Take two capsules by mouth twice a day for 14 days

Chapter 15

Note: Losses are shown in( ).

Pretest

3. $18.37; $13.50; $31.87
6. $3166.67
9. $16; ($1.50)

Practice Problems A

3. $14,901.67; $178,820

Practice Problems B

3. $3.60
6. $14.75
9. $0.55

Practice Problems C

3. 9%
6. 7.1%
9. 40.2%

Practice Problems D

3. $393.75
6. $4.93; $5.06; $5.39
9. $45.00

Practice Problems E

3. $79,205

Practice Problems F

3. $76,600; 20.3%; $29,200; $47,400

Practice Problems G

3. $13.85; $5.95
6. $21.80
9. $45.37

Practice Problems H

3. $960 annual profit; $613 annual profit

Practice Problems I

3. 150 tablets; 250 tablets; 9.5¢; 8.5¢; 5¢; one container
6. 215 tablets; 500 tablets/ container; one container; 16.5¢; 9.2¢; 8.1¢

Practice Problems J

3. 18 turnovers/6 months
6. no; 1.16 turnovers/2 month; 6.9 turnovers/year

Practice Problems K

3. no; $1.74 overage
6. $1358.70; no–everything balances; N/A

Posttest

3. $252;$126; 81¢; $60.75
6. $94.79; $29.98; $1.53/tablet;
9. $51.56; $22.06; $26.64; $11.19; $18.77; $13.08; prescription for $34.50

Ansel HC: Pharmaceutical Calculations, ed 13, Baltimore, 2009, Lippincott Williams & Wilkins.

Brown M, Mulholland JM: Drug Calculations: Ratio and Proportion Problems for Clinical Practice, ed 9, St. Louis, 2012, Mosby.

Chernecky C, Infortuna MH, Macklin D: Sunders Nursing Survival Guide: Drug Calculations and Drug Administration, ed 2, Philadelphia, 2006, Saunders.

Dison N: Simplified Drugs and Solutions for Health Care Professionals, ed 11, St. Louis, 1997, Mosby.

Fulcher EM, Soto CD, Fulcher RM: Pharmacology: Principles & Applications, ed 3, St. Louis, 2012, Saunders.

Kee J, Hayes E, McCuistion LE: Pharmacology: A Nursing Process Approach, ed 7, St. Louis, 2012, Saunders.

Kee JL, Marshall SM: Clinical Calculations: With Applications to General and Specialty Areas, ed 6, St. Louis, 2009, Saunders.

Morris DG: Calculate with Confidence, ed 5, St. Louis, 2010, Mosby.

Nasrawi CW, Allender, JA: Quick and Easy Dosage Calculations: Using Dimensional Analysis, ed 1, Philadelphia, 1999, Saunders.

Ogden SJ, Fluharty LK: Calculation of Drug Dosages, ed 9, St. Louis, 2012, Mosby.

CREDITS

Chapter 3

Figure 3-1. From Brown M, Mulholland JM: *Drug Calculations: Process and Problems for Clinical Practice*, ed 8, St. Louis, Mosby, 2008.

Chapter 4

Figure 4-3. Modified from Fulcher EM, Soto CD, Fulcher RM: *Pharmacology: Principles & Applications*, ed 3, St. Louis, Saunders, 2012.

Chapter 6

Figure 6-1. From Fulcher EM, Soto CD, Fulcher RM: *Pharmacology: Principles & Applications*, ed 3, St. Louis, Saunders, 2012.
Figure 6-2. Forms courtesy Clarian Health, Indianapolis, IN.

Chapter 8

Figure 8-1. From Fulcher EM, Soto CD, Fulcher RM: *Pharmacology: Principles & Applications*, ed 3, St. Louis, Saunders, 2012.
Figure 8-2. Kee J, Hayes E, McCuistion LE: *Pharmacology: A Nursing Process Approach*, ed 7, St. Louis, Saunders, 2012.
Figure 8-3. A, From Brown M, Mulholland JM: *Drug Calculations: Process and Problems for Clinical Practice*, ed 8, St. Louis, Mosby, 2008. **B,** From Fulcher EM, Soto CD, Fulcher RM: *Pharmacology: Principles & Applications*, ed 3, St. Louis, Saunders, 2012.
Figure 8-4. From Fulcher EM, Soto CD, Fulcher RM: *Pharmacology: Principles & Applications*, ed 3, St. Louis, Saunders, 2012.
Figure 8-5. Modified from Kee J, Hayes E, McCuistion LE: *Pharmacology: A Nursing Process Approach*, ed 7, St. Louis, Saunders, 2012.
Figure 8-6. From Clayton BD, Stock, YN, Cooper S: *Basic Pharmacology for Nurses*, ed 15, St. Louis, Mosby, 2010.
Figure 8-7. From Potter P, Perry A: *Fundamentals of Nursing*, ed 8, St. Louis, Mosby, 2013.
Figure 8-8. From Fulcher EM, Soto CD, Fulcher RM: *Pharmacology: Principles & Applications*, ed 3, St. Louis, Saunders, 2012.
Figure 8-9. Courtesy and copyright Becton, Dickinson and Company.
Figure 8-10. From Brown M, Mulholland JM: *Drug Calculations: Process and Problems for Clinical Practice*, ed 8, St. Louis, Mosby, 2008.

Figure 8-11. From Fulcher EM, Soto CD, Fulcher RM: *Pharmacology: Principles & Applications*, ed 3, St. Louis, Saunders, 2012.
Figure 8-12. From Fulcher EM, Soto CD, Fulcher RM: *Pharmacology: Principles & Applications*, ed 3, St. Louis, Saunders, 2012.
Figure 8-13. From Hopper T: *Mosby's Pharmacy Technician: Principles & Practice*, ed 3, St. Louis, Saunders, 2011.

Practice Problems and Posttest

Syringes from Fulcher EM, Soto CD, Fulcher RM: *Pharmacology: Principles & Applications*, ed 3, St. Louis, Saunders, 2012; Brown M, Mulholland JM: *Drug Calculations: Process and Problems for Clinical Practice*, ed 8, St. Louis, Mosby, 2008.
Medication cups from Fulcher EM, Soto CD, Fulcher RM: *Pharmacology: Principles & Applications*, ed 3, St. Louis, Saunders, 2012; From Ogden SJ, Fluharty LK: *Calculation of Drug Dosages*, ed 9, St. Louis, Mosby, 2012.
Medication spoon, dropper, and oral syringe from Fulcher EM, Soto CD, Fulcher RM: *Pharmacology: Principles & Applications*, ed 3, St. Louis, Saunders, 2012.

Chapter 9

Figure 9-6. From Brown M, Mulholland JM: *Drug Calculations: Process and Problems for Clinical Practice*, ed 8, St. Louis, Mosby, 2008.

Chapter 10

Figure 10-1. Modified from data by E Boyd and CD West. In Behrman RE, Vaughan VC: *Nelson Textbook of Pediatrics*, ed 14, Philadelphia, Saunders, 1992.
Figure 10-2. From Lentner C: Geigy Scientific Tables, ed 8, vol 1, Basel, Switzerland, Ciba-Geigy, 1981.
Figure 10-3. Modified from data by E Boyd and CD West. In Behrman RE, Kliegman RM, Jenson HB: *Nelson Textbook of Pediatrics*, ed 16, Philadelphia, Saunders, 2000.

Practice Problems and Posttest

Syringes from Fulcher EM, Soto CD, Fulcher RM: *Pharmacology: Principles & Applications*, ed 3, St. Louis, Saunders, 2012; Kee JL, Marshall SM: *Clinical Calculations: With Applications to General and Specialty Areas*, ed 7, St. Louis, Saunders, 2013; From Brown M, Mulholland JM: *Drug Calculations: Process and Problems for*

654

Clinical Practice, ed 8, St. Louis, Mosby, 2008.

Medication cup from Ogden SJ, Fluharty LK: *Calculation of Drug Dosages*, ed 9, St. Louis, Mosby, 2012.

Medication spoon, dropper, and oral syringe from Fulcher EM, Soto CD, Fulcher RM: *Pharmacology: Principles & Applications*, ed 3, St. Louis, Saunders, 2012.

Chapter 11

Figure 11-3. A-C, From Brown M, Mulholland JM: *Drug Calculations: Process and Problems for Clinical Practice*, ed 8, St. Louis, Mosby, 2008. **D,** From Kee JL, Marshall SM: *Clinical Calculations: With Applications to General and Specialty Areas*, ed 7, St. Louis, Saunders, 2013.

Practice Problems and Posttest

Syringes from Fulcher EM, Soto CD, Fulcher RM: *Pharmacology: Principles & Applications*, ed 3, St. Louis, Saunders, 2012; Kee JL, Marshall SM: *Clinical Calculations: With Applications to General and Specialty Areas*, ed 7, St. Louis, Saunders, 2013; From Brown M, Mulholland JM: *Drug Calculations: Process and Problems for Clinical Practice*, ed 8, St. Louis, Mosby, 2008.

Medication cup from Ogden SJ, Fluharty LK: *Calculation of Drug Dosages*, ed 9, St. Louis, Mosby, 2012.

Medication spoon, dropper, and oral syringe from Fulcher EM, Soto CD, Fulcher RM:

Pharmacology: Principles & Applications, ed 3, St. Louis, Saunders, 2012.

Chapter 12

Figure 12-1. A and **B**, From Brown M, Mulholland JM: *Drug Calculations: Process and Problems for Clinical Practice*, ed 8, St. Louis, Mosby, 2008. **C,** From Potter P, Perry A: *Fundamentals of Nursing*, ed 8, St. Louis, Mosby, 2013.

Figure 12-2. From Morris DG: *Calculate with Confidence*, ed 5, St. Louis, Mosby, 2010.

Table 12-1. Modified from Brown M, Mulholland JM: *Drug Calculations: Process and Problems for Clinical Practice*, ed 8, St. Louis, Mosby, 2008.

Posttest

Syringes from Fulcher EM, Soto CD, Fulcher RM: *Pharmacology: Principles & Applications*, ed 3, St. Louis, Saunders, 2012; Kee JL, Marshall SM: *Clinical Calculations: With Applications to General and Specialty Areas*, ed 7, St. Louis, Saunders, 2013; From Brown M, Mulholland JM: *Drug Calculations: Process and Problems for Clinical Practice*, ed 8, St. Louis, Mosby, 2008.

Medication cup from Ogden SJ, Fluharty LK: *Calculation of Drug Dosages*, ed 9, St. Louis, Mosby, 2012.

Medication spoon, dropper, and oral syringe from Fulcher EM, Soto CD, Fulcher RM: *Pharmacology: Principles & Applications*, ed 3, St. Louis, Saunders, 2012.

Active ingredients Chemicals in pure, undiluted forms that affect body function

Act-O-Vial System Two-section vial divided by a seal holding a premeasured active ingredient in the lower section and a premeasured diluent in the upper section; mixing occurs when the two sections of the vial are combined either through puncturing the seal or moving the seal through pressure; similar to Mix-O-Vial

Adolescence From 13 through 17 years of age

Alligation Mathematical method for determining the necessary amount of two solutes of different percentage strengths to prepare a compound to a given percentage strength

Alligation medial Calculation method by which the weighted average percentage strength of a mixture of two or more substances of known quantity and concentration may be determined

Ambulatory care Patient care in an outpatient setting; health care provided on an outpatient basis so that those who are treated in a health care facility depart after treatment on the same day

Ampule Small glass container that is sealed and holds a single dose of medication, usually for injection

Anatomy Study of the structure of the body

Anticoagulant Substance that stops or delays the clotting of blood

Apothecary system One of the oldest measurement systems used to calculate drug orders using measurements such as grains and minims

Arabic numerals The numbers 1, 2, 3, and the like

Assets Any property owned by the business

Auxiliary label Label added to prescriptions to provide supplementary instructions

Average wholesale price (AWP) Price that a pharmacy theoretically pays for its medications; this price is theoretical because discounts, sales, special deals, and the like may influence the actual wholesale price

Avoirdupois system English system of weights in which 1 pound equals 16 oz to 7000 grains equals 1 pound

Body surface area (BSA) Means of calculating doses of medication on the basis of weight and height using a nomogram

Buccal Between the gum and cheek; medications dissolved between the gum and cheek

Capitation fee Set amount of third-party money paid monthly to the pharmacy for a specific patient without regard to number of prescriptions filled

Cash flow Rate of receipts and expenses for the business

Celsius (Centigrade) System of measuring temperature with 0° being the freezing point and 100° being the boiling point of water

Chemistry Study of elements, their compounds, and the molecular structure and interactions of matter

Clark's rule Means of calculating a child dose of medication from an adult dose on the basis of the child's weight in pounds

Complex fraction Fractions in which the numerator, denominator, or both are fractional units

Continuous infusion Introduction of a substance such as IV fluids or interstitial fluids over a period of time without interruption

Conversion factor, time Factor needed to change from one unit of time to another such as hours to minutes

Conversion factor, volume Factor needed to change from one unit of volume to another between measuring systems or within a measuring system, such as liters to milliliters

Daily cash or sales report Report made at the end of each day that summarizes the sales, discounts, amount of cash, checks, refunds, and credit card charges that have occurred in the day's operations

Decimal Number system based on the number 10, and progressions of 10s

Decimal place Place values found to the right of the decimal point

Denominator Bottom number of a fraction

Depot Long-acting oil based medications that are gradually released for prolonged drug administration

Depreciation Decrease in value of an asset based on total value of an asset, the estimated length of use of the asset, and its value at disposal

Diluent Agent that dilutes a substance; in pharmacology, the liquid added to a powder to change the solid to a liquid or to dilute another liquid

Dilution Process of making a more concentrated solution less concentrated

Dimensional analysis Mathematical means of manipulating units or the dimension given to numbers to cancel unwanted units when converting unit equivalency; an advanced form of ratio and proportion

Discounts or markdowns Subtraction of a percentage amount from the markup price of an item which lowers the actual price by the given percentage; also called markdown or sales discount

Dividend Number that is being divided in division

Divisor Number by which another number is divided

Dosage Size, amount, and number of doses of a medication for therapeutic care

Dosage available (DA) Amount of medication available for doses

Dosage form (DF) Physical/structural character of a dose

Dosage (Dose) strength Weight of active ingredient(s) in a dose

Dosage strength available Strength or weight of medication available for doses

Dose Amount of a medication to be administered at one time

Dose ordered (DO) Amount of medication ordered for a single dose

Dose time Amount of time needed to administer medication

Dose to be given (DG) Amount of medication such as, number of tablets or amount of liquid volume, to be administered as a dose

657

Dose volume Volume of medication administered at a given time

Drop factor Size of drop from the drip chamber found on IV tubing (drops/mL)

Early childhood From 1 through 5 years of age

Elixir Clear, sweetened, flavored medication containing alcohol and water

Enteric-coated Coating on tablets that allows medication to pass through the stomach unchanged and prevents absorption before reaching the intestines

Extremes First and last number found in a proportion

Fahrenheit System of measuring temperature with 32° being the freezing point and 212° being the boiling point of water

Flow rate Speed at which IV medications are infused depending on physician's order; usually drops/minute

Fraction Part of a whole number expressed as a decimal or with a numerator and denominator

Fried's rule Means of calculating an infant dose of medication from an adult dose on the basis of the infant's age in months

Generic name Official nonproprietary name given to a drug by the U.S. Food and Drug Administration

Graduates Containers marked with progressive series of lines or markers usually in the metric system, for measuring specified amounts of liquids or solids

Gross margin Difference between the selling price and the purchase price; can be affected by the total inventory available

Gross profit Difference in purchase price of merchandise and the income or markup of the inventory

Improper fraction Fraction in which the numerator is equal to or greater than the denominator; a fraction that is greater than 1

Indication Reason to prescribe a medication

Infant From age 1 month to 1 year

Inpatient Patient who has been admitted to a health care facility such as a hospital for at least a 24-hour or overnight stay

Inscription Part of prescription that indicates the name of the drug and dosage prescribed

International units System of measure for international technical and scientific work based on metric system

International System of Units (SI) (or metric system) Internationally accepted system of measurement of mass, length, and time based on international units

Intradermal Into or within the dermis of skin

Intramuscular Into or within muscle

Intravenous Into or within vein

Inventory Listing of merchandise on hand summarizing the quantity of each item and its respective cost

Inversion To turn upside down, as with a fraction, or to interchange the terms of a ratio

Late childhood From age 6 years through 12 years

Lowest term Form of a fraction in which no common number will divide into both the numerator and denominator evenly

Lyophilized Freeze dried

Macrodrip infusion sets Infusion sets used for measuring the rate of IV fluids; macrodrip sets supply large drops (10 to 20 drops/mL) of fluid called macrodrops

Maintenance therapy Using IV fluids to provide necessary nutrients to meet daily needs for water, electrolytes, and glucose

Markup Difference found when the wholesale price is subtracted from the retail price

Markup percentage Calculation done by dividing the cost of the item into the difference between the selling price and the cost

Means Second and third numbers found in a proportion

Measurable amount The quantity of medication that can be most accurately measured on the utinsel available

Medication order Written or verbal direction for administration of medication in a health care setting

Medication strength Concentration of active ingredient in a medication

Meniscus Curved line that develops on the upper surface of a liquid when the liquid is poured into a container

Metric system Decimal measurement system considered to be the international standard for scientific and industrial measurements, using grams, liters, and meters

Microbiology Study of microscopic organisms

Microdrip infusion sets Infusion sets used for measuring the rate of IV fluids; microdrip sets supply small drops (e.g., 60 drops/per mL) called microdrops; other microdrip sets provide 50, 100, or 150 drops/mL

Military time (International Standard Time) System of time that recognizes a 24-hour notation of hours and minutes

Milliequivalent Weight of drug in volume of solution; number of grams of solute dissolved in 1 mL of normal solution

Mixed number Number that contains a whole number and a fraction

Multiplicand Number that is to be multiplied or is multiplied by another

Multiplier Number that is used to multiply another number

National Drug Code (NDC) Unique number on drug label that identifies manufacturer, product, and size of container

Neonate From birth to 1 month

Net income (bottom line) Selling price less the purchase price and expenses

Nomogram A graph, diagram, or chart that shows a relationship between numerical variables, such as height and weight

Numerator Top number found in a fraction

Oral medications Medications taken by mouth

Overhead Expenses of a business not including cost of inventory, such as rent, wages, utilities, insurance, and other costs of doing business

Par level Predetermined point for reordering inventory; inventory to be kept on hand

Parenteral Medications given through skin by injection

Patent, Patency State in which an object is open or evident

Percentage Means of expressing a portion of 100 parts

Pharmacokinetics Processing of drugs in body or movement of drugs through body

Pharmacology Study of drugs, their uses, and their interactions with living systems

Pharmacotherapeutics Effects of drugs on body in treatment of conditions and diseases

Physiology Study of processes and function of the human body

Piggyback Special coupling into primary IV lines allowing supplementary solutions to be added for administration into current IV administration set

Powder displacement Amount of solute that causes displacement in total volume of medication

Powder volume Space occupied by dry powder or freeze-dried (lyophilized or crystalline) active ingredient related to total volume of medication following reconstitution with indicated diluent

Prescription Written order by licensed health care professional for dispensing or administering medications

Product Number obtained by multiplying two numbers together

Profit Difference found when expenses are subtracted from income obtained from sales

Profit margin Percentage found when net profit is divided by sales

Proper fraction Fraction in which the numerator is less than the denominator

Prophylaxis Using a biological, chemical, or mechanical agent to prevent disease by preventing the cause of disease, such as infectious agents, from entrance to the body

Proportion Comparative relationship between the parts; one or more ratios that are compared

Psychology Study of behavior and the functions and processes of the mind, as related to the social and physical environment

Pulvule Capsule filled with medication in powdered form

Quotient Number obtained when one number is divided by another

Ratio Means of describing the relationship between two numbers

Ratio strength Strength of weak solutions or liquid preparations expressed in ratio terms; because all ratios may be stated as parts of 100, same as expressing percentage strength

Reconstitution Process of adding fluid, such as water or saline, to powdered or cystalling form of medication, making a specific liquid dosage strength

Remainder Number that is left after completing subtraction; in division the number left after division

Replacement therapy When a deficit of fluids or electrolytes is present in the body, providing needed fluids or electrolytes to meet these needs

Restorative therapy Day-by-day restoration of vital fluids and electrolytes using IV therapy to replace body's deficit

Roman numerals Numbers that use Roman letters such as I for 1, V for 5, and the like

Round/Rounding To calculate a number to a desired place value when exact number is unknown; adjustment made to the desired place by changing numbers to the right

Scheduled medications Classification of medications with the potential for abuse and misuse

Scored tablet Tablet containing an indention for ease of breaking into equal parts

Signa (Sig) Part of prescription that indicates dosage of medication to be taken

Solute Substance dissolved in a solution or semisolid

Solvent Substance in which a solute is dissolved, either liquid or semisolid

Stock medication Medication kept on hand for use in preparing prescriptions; medication of a higher percentage of active ingredient that is used to prepare a medication of a lower percentage

Subcutaneous Beneath skin; medications injected into subcutaneous tissue

Sublingual Under tongue; medications dissolved under the tongue

Superscription Part of prescription designated with symbol ℞

Suspension Medication consisting of small particles that are not dissolved but are dispersed throughout liquid

Syrup Aqueous solution sweetened with sugar or a sugar substitute to disguise taste

Tincture Alcohol-based liquid used as a skin preparation

Toxicology Study of adverse toxic reactions or toxic levels of chemicals and drugs

Trade/Brand name Name given to a medication by manufacturer

Turnover rate Rate at which inventory is sold over a specified period of time

U.S. customary system (household system) System of measurement based on common kitchen measuring devices

Unit Basic measurement used to indicate strength of some medications; strength of units is particular to that medication and is not comprehensive

Vehicle Inert substance in which medication is mixed for administration

Vial Glass or plastic container with metal-enclosed rubber seal for injectable medications; may hold single or multiple doses

Viscosity Thickness of liquid substance

Whole number Numeral consisting of one or more digits; number that is not followed by fraction or decimal

Young's rule Means of calculating a child dose of medication based on child's age

Index

Page numbers followed by "f" indicate figures, "t" indicate tables, and "b" indicate boxes.